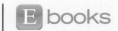
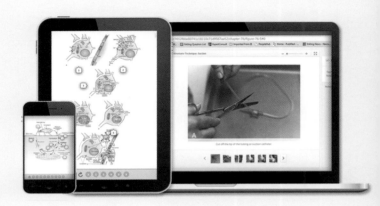
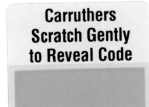

# Soft Tissue Augmentation

**Procedures in Cosmetic Dermatology**
**Series Editor: Jeffrey S. Dover MD, FRCPC, FRCP**
**Associate Editor: Murad Alam MD, MSCI**

Chemical Peels
Second edition
Rebecca C. Tung MD and Mark G. Rubin MD
ISBN 978-1-4377-1924-6

Treatment of Leg Veins
Second edition
Murad Alam MD, MSCI and Sirunya Silapunt MD
ISBN 978-1-4377-0739-7

Body Contouring
Bruce E. Katz MD and Neil S. Sadick MD, FAAD, FAACS,
FACP, FACPh
ISBN 978-1-4377-0739-7

Non-Surgical Skin Tightening and Lifting
Murad Alam MD, MSCI and Jeffrey S. Dover MD, FRCPC,
FRCP
ISBN 978-1-4160-5960-8

Botulinum Toxin
Fourth edition
Alastair Carruthers MA, BM, BCh, FRCPC, FRCP(Lon) and
Jean Carruthers MD, FRCSC, FRC(Ophth), FASOPRS
ISBN 978-0-323-47659-1

Soft Tissue Augmentation
Fourth edition
Jean Carruthers MD, FRCSC, FRC(Ophth), FASOPRS and
Alastair Carruthers MA, BM, BCh, FRCPC, FRCP(Lon)
ISBN 978-0-323-47658-4

Body Shaping: Skin Fat Cellulite
Jeffrey Orringer MD, Jeffrey S. Dover MD, FRCPC, FRCP
and Murad Alam MD, MSCI
ISBN 978-0323321976

Cosmeceuticals
Third edition
Zoe Diana Draelos MD, Murad Alam MD, MSCI and Jeffrey
S. Dover MD, FRCPC, FRCP
ISBN 978-0-323-29869-8

Lasers and Lights
Fourth edition
George Hruza MD and Elizabeth Tanzi MD
ISBN 978-0-323-48006-2

Photodynamic Therapy
Second edition
Mitchel P. Goldman MD
ISBN 978-1-4160-4211-2

Liposuction
C. William Hanke MD, MPH, FACP and Gerhard Sattler MD
ISBN 978-1-4160-2208-4

Scar Revision
Kenneth A. Arndt MD
ISBN 978-1-4160-3131-4

Hair Transplantation
Robert S. Haber MD and Dowling B. Stough MD
ISBN 978-1-4160-3104-8

Blepharoplasty
Ronald L. Moy MD and Edgar F. Fincher MD
ISBN 978-1-4160-2996-0

**For Elsevier**
Content Strategist: Belinda Kuhn
Content Development Specialist: Humayra Rahman Khan
Project Manager: Srividhya Vidhyashankar
Design: Miles Hitchen
Illustration Manager: Nichole Beard

**PROCEDURES IN COSMETIC DERMATOLOGY**

# Soft Tissue Augmentation

## Fourth Edition

Edited by

**Jean Carruthers** MD, FRCSC, FRC (OPHTH), FASOPRS
Clinical Professor, Department of Ophthalmology and Visual Science,
University of British Columbia, Vancouver, BC, Canada

**Alastair Carruthers** MA, BM, BCh, FRCPC, FRCP(Lon)
Clinical Professor, Department of Dermatology and Skin Science,
University of British Columbia, Vancouver, BC, Canada

Series Editor
**Jeffrey S. Dover** MD, FRCPC, FRCP
Director, SkinCare Physicians, Chestnut Hill, MA; Associate Clinical Professor of Dermatology,
Yale University School of Medicine; Adjunct Associate Professor of Dermatology,
Brown Medical School, Providence, RI, USA

Associate Editor
**Murad Alam** MD, MSCI
Professor of Dermatology, Otolaryngology, and Surgery; Chief, Section of Cutaneous and Aesthetic
Surgery; Vice-Chair, Department of Dermatology, Northwestern University, Chicago, IL, USA

ELSEVIER
Edinburgh  London  New York  Oxford  Philadelphia  St Louis  Sydney  Toronto  2018

# ELSEVIER

First edition 2005
Second edition 2008
Third edition 2013

**Notices**

Knowledge and best practice in this field are constantly changing. As new research and experience broaden our understanding, changes in research methods, professional practices, or medical treatment may become necessary.

Practitioners and researchers must always rely on their own experience and knowledge in evaluating and using any information, methods, compounds, or experiments described herein. In using such information or methods they should be mindful of their own safety and the safety of others, including parties for whom they have a professional responsibility.

With respect to any drug or pharmaceutical products identified, readers are advised to check the most current information provided (i) on procedures featured or (ii) by the manufacturer of each product to be administered, to verify the recommended dose or formula, the method and duration of administration, and contraindications. It is the responsibility of practitioners, relying on their own experience and knowledge of their patients, to make diagnoses, to determine dosages and the best treatment for each individual patient, and to take all appropriate safety precautions.

To the fullest extent of the law, neither the Publisher nor the authors, contributors, or editors, assume any liability for any injury and/or damage to persons or property as a matter of products liability, negligence or otherwise, or from any use or operation of any methods, products, instructions, or ideas contained in the material herein.

ISBN: 978-0-323-47658-4
E-ISBN: 978-0-323-48008-6

**ELSEVIER** your source for books, journals and multimedia in the health sciences

**www.elsevierhealth.com**

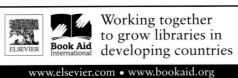

Working together to grow libraries in developing countries

www.elsevier.com • www.bookaid.org

The publisher's policy is to use paper manufactured from sustainable forests

Printed in China
Last digit is the print number: 9 8 7 6 5 4 3 2 1

# Contents

# Video contents

# Series preface

Much has changed since the first edition of this series. Non-invasive and minimally invasive cosmetic procedures, as pioneered by dermatologists, have become increasingly adopted by physicians and well-accepted by patients. Cosmetic dermatologic surgery procedures have been refined and improved. Interventions have become more effective, and also safer and more tolerable with increasing benefit:risk ratios. Combination cosmetic regimens that include multiple procedure types have been shown to achieve results comparable to those with more invasive procedures. And new devices and technologies continue to be introduced.

And how best to keep up with these advances and to ensure your offerings are state of the art and at the cutting edge? The newest edition of the Procedures in Cosmetic Dermatology series keeps you there, and for those starting out in the field these texts quickly introduce you and bring you to the state of the art. Each book in this series is designed to quickly impart basic skills as well as advanced concepts in an easy-to-understand manner. We focus not on theory but on how-to. Our expert book editors and chapter authors will guide you through the learning process efficiently, so you can soon get back to treating patients.

The authors are leading dermatologists in the field. Dermatologists' role in cosmetic medicine has continued to expand. Research has revealed that primary care physicians and the general public view dermatologists as the experts in less invasive cosmetic procedures. A nationwide advanced fellowship program in cosmetic dermatologic surgery has been initiated to train the next generation of dermatologists to the highest standards.

What has not changed is physicians' need for clear, concise, and current direction on procedure techniques. Physicians need to be proficient in the latest methods for enhancing appearance and concealing the visible signs of aging.

To that end, we hope that you, our reader, find the books enjoyable and educational.

We thank our many contributors and wish you well on your journey of discovery.

Jeffrey S. Dover MD, FRCPC, FRCP and
Murad Alam MD, MSCI

v

# Series preface first edition

Although dermatologists have been procedurally inclined since the beginning of the specialty, particularly rapid change has occurred in the past quarter century. The advent of frozen section technique and the golden age of Mohs skin cancer surgery has led to the formal incorporation of surgery within the dermatology curriculum. More recently technological breakthroughs in minimally invasive procedural dermatology have offered an aging population new options for improving the appearance of damaged skin.

Procedures for rejuvenating the skin and adjacent regions are actively sought by our patients. Significantly, dermatologists have pioneered devices, technologies, and medications, which have continued to evolve at a startling pace. Numerous major advances including virtually all cutaneous lasers and light-source-based procedures, botulinum exotoxin, soft tissue augmentation, dilute anesthesia liposuction, leg vein treatments, chemical peels, and hair transplants have been invented or developed and enhanced by dermatologists. Dermatologists understand procedures, and we have special insight into the structure, function, and working of skin. Cosmetic dermatologists have made rejuvenation accessible to risk-averse patients by emphasizing safety and reducing operative trauma. No specialty is better positioned than dermatology to lead the field of cutaneous surgery while meeting patient needs.

As dermatology grows as a specialty, an ever-increasing proportion of dermatologists will become proficient in the delivery of different procedures. Not all dermatologists will perform all procedures, and some will perform very few, but even the less procedurally directed among us must be well versed in the details to be able to guide and educate our patients. Whether you are a skilled dermatologic surgeon interested in further expanding your surgical repertoire, a complete surgical novice wishing to learn a few simple procedures, or somewhere in between, this book and this series are for you.

The volume you are holding is one of a series entitled "Procedures in Cosmetic Dermatology." The purpose of each book is to serve as a practical primer on a major topic area in procedural dermatology.

If you want to make sure you find the right book for your needs, you may wish to know what this book is and what it is not. It is not a comprehensive text grounded in theoretical underpinnings. It is not exhaustively referenced. It is not designed to be a completely unbiased review of the world's literature on the subject. At the same time, it is not an overview of cosmetic procedures that describes these in generalities without providing enough specific information to actually permit someone to perform the procedures. And importantly, it is not so heavy that it can serve as a doorstop or a shelf filler.

What this book and this series offer is a step-by-step, practical guide to performing cutaneous surgical procedures. Each volume in the series has been edited by a known authority in that subfield. Each editor has recruited other equally practical-minded, technically skilled, hands-on clinicians to write the constituent chapters. Most chapters have two authors to ensure that different approaches and a broad range of opinions are incorporated. On the other hand, the two authors and the editors also collectively provide a consistency of tone. A uniform template has been used within each chapter so that the reader will be easily able to navigate all the books in the series. Within every chapter, the authors succinctly tell it like they do it. The emphasis is on therapeutic technique; treatment methods are discussed with an eye to appropriate indications, adverse events, and unusual cases. Finally, this book is short and can be read in its entirety on a long plane ride. We believe that brevity paradoxically results in greater information transfer because cover-to-cover mastery is practicable.

We hope you enjoy this book and the rest of the books in the series and that you benefit from the many hours of clinical wisdom that have been distilled to produce it. Please keep it nearby, where you can reach for it when you need it.

Jeffrey S. Dover MD, FRCPC, FRCP and
Murad Alam MD, MSCI

# Preface

*"To improve is to change; to be perfect is to change often".*
Winston Churchill

Since our third edition in the *Procedures in Cosmetic Dermatology* Series there has been an unprecedented amount of change in the field of soft tissue augmentation!

The concept of the three-dimensional filler approach has rapidly expanded with the development of new fillers, new methods of administering fillers, new anatomical concepts, new appreciation of the three-dimensional subcutaneous anatomy and consequent safety. A fresh appreciation of the best modalities to use in combination including fillers, neuromodulators and energy-based devices has been thoroughly explored as has the relationship of these approaches to traditional surgery.

The use of CT and MRI scans has given a pictorial improvement in our understanding of the various causes of facial deflation. We always saw the loss of facial fat associated with aging, but improved understanding of specific facial fat compartmentalization with age-related atrophy and descent has enabled us to more accurately reflate these collapsed compartments for a more natural result.

Loss and inward rotation of facial bone in the upper, mid and lower face begins earlier in women than in men, but appreciating the trends in age-related bony atrophy are as important as perceiving the changes in facial fat.

The improvement in our understanding of facial skin descent and expansion (dermatochalasis) due to collagen and elastin loss, its treatment and prevention have iced the facial cake. An appreciation of the similarities and differences in treating facial skin in all Fitzpatrick and Glogau skin types is so important.

After all, it is important to put the replacement volume where it will be seen to improve the facial aesthetic in our patient's specific cultural milieu.

The concept of filler erasability has further elevated the popularity of the HA fillers and hyaluronidase is in every office. Moreover, when other fillers come to market we can hope that an "eraser" will be available at the same time.

Longer-lasting semi-permanent and permanent fillers also have their place in our therapeutic armamentarium. The calcium hydroxylapatite fillers, poly-L-lactic acid, liquid injectable silicone and PMMA in bovine collagen suspension are all approved for facial augmentation, and we expect more classes of fillers to become available.

Finally, we turn to the most important feature of all: our patients! No-one likes pain, and the introduction of the admixture of local anesthetic with fillers spearheaded by Marianno Busso, MD, has indeed allowed many more patients to avail themselves of this successful treatment. His work has stimulated us all to blend fillers so as to enhance patient comfort.

Finally, we feel the world of fillers will change yet again with their perception as drugs not devices. In other words, using the presence of a filler to cause collagen deposition and long-term natural correction is a very important concept.

The filler world has changed dramatically in the past few years. We hope that you enjoy this changed world as much as we do.

Jean Carruthers MD, FRCSC, FRC (OPHTH), FASOPRS
Vancouver, BC, Canada

# List of contributors

The editor(s) would like to acknowledge and offer grateful thanks for the input of all previous editions' contributors, without whom this new edition would not have been possible.

**Mathew M. Avram MD, JD**
Director, MGH Dermatology Laser & Cosmetic Center, Massachusetts General Hospital, Harvard Medical School, Boston, MA, USA

**Raul Alberto Banegas MD**
Plastic Surgeon, Centro Arenales, Buenos Aires, Argentina

**Katie Beleznay MD, FRCPC, FAAD**
Clinical Instructor, Department of Dermatology, University of British Columbia, Vancouver, BC, Canada

**Jeanette M. Black MD**
Dermatologist, Skin Care and Laser Physicians of Beverly Hills, Los Angeles, CA, USA

**Joanna G. Bolton MD, FAAD**
ASDS Cosmetic Dermatologic Surgery Fellow, Cosmetic Laser Dermatology, San Diego, CA, USA

**André Vieira Braz MD**
Dermatologist, Clinical, Surgical and Cosmetic, Dermatology Clinic, Rio de Janeiro, RJ, Brazil

**Harold J. Brody MD**
Clinical Professor of Dermatology, Emory University School of Medicine, Atlanta, GA, USA

**Alastair Carruthers MA, BM, BCh, FRCPC, FRCP(Lon)**
Clinical Professor, Department of Dermatology and Skin Science, University of British Columbia, Vancouver, BC, Canada

**Jean Carruthers MD, FRCSC, FRC (OPHTH), FASOPRS**
Clinical Professor, Department of Ophthalmology and Visual Science, University of British Columbia, Vancouver, BC, Canada

**Gabriela Casabona MD**
Director at Clinica Vida Cosmetic, Laser and Mohs Surgery Center, New York, NY, USA

**Kyle M. Coleman MD**
Co-Owner, Etre, Cosmetic Dermatology and Laser Center, New Orleans, LA, USA

**William P. Coleman III MD**
Clinical Professor of Dermatology; Adjunct Professor of Surgery (Plastic Surgery), Tulane University Health Sciences Center, New Orleans, LA, USA

**Steven Dayan MD**
Clinical Assistant Professor, University of Illinois, Chicago, IL, USA

**Jeffrey S. Dover MD, FRCPC, FRCP**
Director, SkinCare Physicians, Chestnut Hill, MA; Associate Clinical Professor of Dermatology, Yale University School of Medicine; Adjunct Associate Professor of Dermatology, Brown Medical School, Providence, RI, USA

**Jason J. Emer MD**
Private Practice, The Roxbury Institute, Beverly Hills, CA, USA

**Sabrina Guillen Fabi MD, FAAD, FAACS**
Dermatologist, Cosmetic Laser Dermatology, Volunteer Assistant Clinical Professor, Department of Medicine/Dermatology, University of California, San Diego, CA, USA

**Steven Fagien MD**
Oculoplastic Surgeon, Private Practice, Aesthetic Eyelid Plastic Surgery, Boca Raton, FL, USA

**Rebecca Fitzgerald MD**
Dermatologist, Private Practice, Los Angeles, CA, USA

**Laurel Naversen Geraghty MD**
Dermatologist, Dermatology and Laser Associates of Medford, Medford, OR, USA

**Marguerite Germain MD**
Dermatologist, Private Practice, Mt Pleasant, SC, USA

**Richard G. Glogau MD**
Clinical Professor of Dermatology, University of California, San Francisco, CA, USA

**Greg J. Goodman MD, FACD, GradDipClinEpi**
Associate Professor, Monash University, Clayton, Victoria, and Chief of Surgery, Skin and Cancer Foundation Inc., Carlton, Victoria, Australia

**Adele Haimovic MD**
Dermatologist, SkinCare Physicians, Chestnut Hill, MA, USA

**Bhushan Hardas MD, MBA**
Chief Scientific Officer (Devices), Therapeutic area head of Dermatology and Aesthetics, Allergan, Irvine, CA, USA

**Shannon Humphrey MD, FRCPC, FAAD**
Clinical Assistant Professor, Director of CME, Department of Dermatology and Skin Science, University of British Columbia, Vancouver, BC, Canada

**Omer Ibrahim MD**
Dermatologist, SkinCare Physicians, Chestnut Hill, MA, USA

**Derek H. Jones, MD**
Founder and Director, Skin Care and Laser Physicians of Beverly Hills; Clinical Associate Professor, Dermatology, University of California, Los Angeles, CA, USA

**Isabela Tollini Jones MD**
ASDS Cosmetic Dermatologic Surgery Fellow, Cosmetic Laser
Dermatology, San Diego, CA, USA

**Shilpi Khetarpal MD**
Dermatologist, Cleveland Clinic Foundation, Cleveland, OH,
USA

**Val Lambros MD, FACS**
Assistant Clinical Professor, Plastic Surgery, University of
California at Irvine, Irvine, CA, USA

**Bassel H. Mahmoud MD, PhD**
Dermatologist, Lahey Hospital and Medical Centre, Burlington,
MA, USA

**Paula Marchese MD**
Assistant at Clinica Vida Cosmetic, Laser and Mohs Surgery
Center, New York, NY, USA

**Kavita Mariwalla MD**
Dermatologist, Mariwalla Dermatology, West Islip, NY, USA

**Gary D. Monheit MD**
Dermatologist, Total Skin and Beauty, Birmingham, AL, USA

**Jose R. Montes MD**
Associate Professor and Director, José Raúl Montes Eyes &
Facial Rejuvenation, San Juan, Puerto Rico

**Diane K. Murphy MBA**
Consultant, Allergan, Irvine, CA, USA

**Rhoda S. Narins MD, FAAD**
Medical Director, Dermatology Surgery and Laser Center, New
York, NY, USA

**David M. Ozog MD, FAAD**
Director of Cosmetic Dermatology, Division of Mohs
and Dermatological Surgery, Vice-Chair Department of
Dermatology, Henry Ford Hospital, Detroit, MI, USA

**Berthold J. Rzany MD, ScM**
Professor, Rzany & Hund, Private Practice for Dermatology and
Aesthetic Medicine, Berlin, Germany

**Neil S. Sadick MD, FAAD, FAACS, FACP, FACPh**
Clinical Professor, Weill Cornell Medical College, Cornell
University, New York, NY, USA

**Gerhard Sattler, MD**
Founder, Medical Director, Rosenparkklinik, Darmstadt,
Germany

**Sonja Sattler MD**
Founder, Financial Director, Rosenparkklinik, Darmstadt,
Germany

**Kyle Koo-II Seo MD, PhD**
Clinical Associate Professor, Department of Dermatology, Seoul
National University College of Medicine, Seoul, South Korea

**Renee Sheinin MD**
Dermatology Resident, Henry Ford Health System, Detroit,
MI, USA

**Kevin C. Smith MD, FRCPC**
Private Practice, Niagara Falls Dermatology and Skin Care
Centre Ltd, Niagara Falls, ON, Canada

**Ada R. Trindade de Almeida MD**
Dermatologist, Dermatologic Clinic, Hospital do Servidor
Público Municipal de São Paulo; Private Practice, São Paulo,
Brazil

**Heidi A. Waldorf MD**
Waldorf Dermatology Aesthetics; Director, Laser & Cosmetic
Dermatology; Mount Sinai Hospital; Associate Clinical
Professor, Department of Dermatology, Icahn School of
Medicine of Mount Sinai, New York, NY, USA

**Monique Vanaman Wilson MD**
ASDS Cosmetic Dermatologic Surgery Fellow, Cosmetic Laser
Dermatology, San Diego, CA, USA

**Birgit Wörle MD**
Dermatologist, Phlebologist, Hirslanden Klinik, Meggen,
Switzerland

# Acknowledgments

Dr Stuart Maddin is the godfather of Canadian dermatology. When we first returned to Vancouver from our postgraduate training in 1977, Alastair was enticed to write part of Stuart's latest textbook. This led to San Francisco fellowships in 1982: in dermatologic surgery for Alastair and in the ophthalmological use of botulinum toxin A for Jean. Stuart's vision of the future of procedural dermatology has since been proven indelibly and we are both so grateful to him for his charm, intellect, continuous energy and belief in our work. Fortunately for this new world of fillers, the demographics were perfect. The baby boom generation was just starting to deflate as bovine collagen was FDA-approved in the early 1980s! In these very early days we were also surrounded by dermatologists who were equally fascinated by the revolutionary new ability to treat the aging process: Hal Brody, Bill Coleman, Rick Glogau, Arnie Klein, Nick Lowe, Steve Mandy, Gary Monheit, Rhoda Narins, Sam Stegman, Ted Tromovitch, and Luitgard Wiest, amongst others. We have learned so much from you all: you have made this path the best!

A look at the authors of this book will show that the magic continues: new ideas, superb chapter contributions and videos have come from the Coleman family, from Steve Fagien, Shannon Humphrey, Derek Jones, Bert Rzany, Kyle Seo, Ada Trindade de Almeida, and Susan Weinkle, amongst others. We thank you.

Our office clinical and research teams are responsible for huge amounts of data collection, photography and patient followup. Without their dedication and their joy in this work we would never have the data to write about and teach with. We humbly thank you all.

Our three sons, their partners and our grandsons have given us so much love and encouragement over the years.

We love you all and we cherish all the times we have shared together. Now that this book is finished, there will be even more time!

Jean Carruthers MD, FRCSC, FRC (OPHTH), FASOPRS and Alastair Carruthers MA, BM, BCh, FRCPC, FRCP(Lon)

# Dedication

We dedicate this volume to our children and their families. Our sons were young when the botulinum toxin story began and they have regarded the efforts of their parents to cope with this accidental discovery with tolerance and increasing pride over the years. We have appreciated the support and encouragement they have given us (rather than the other way round). The love they have given us means we are indeed fortunate!

Alastair Carruthers MA, BM, BCh, FRCPC, FRCP(Lon)
and Jean Carruthers MD, FRCSC, FRC (OPHTH),
FASOPRS

To the women in my life: my grandmothers, Bertha and Lillian, my mother, Nina, my daughters, Sophie and Isabel, and especially to my wife, Tania. For their never-ending encouragement, patience, support, love, and friendship. To my father, Mark – a great teacher and role model; to my mentor, Kenneth A. Arndt for his generosity, kindness, sense of humor, joie de vivre, and above all else curiosity and enthusiasm.

Jeffrey S. Dover MD, FRCPC, FRCP

Elsevier's dedicated editorial staff has made possible the continuing success of this ambitious project. The team led by Belinda Kuhn, Humayra Khan and the production staff have refined the concept for this new edition while maintaining the series' reputation for quality and cutting-edge relevance. In this, they have been ably supported by the graphics shop, which has created the signature high-quality illustrations and layouts that are the backbone of each book. We are also deeply grateful to the volume editors, who have generously found time in their schedules, cheerfully accepted our guidelines, and recruited the most knowledgeable chapter authors. And we especially thank the chapter contributors, without whose work there would be no books at all. Finally, I would also like to convey my debt to my teachers, Kenneth Arndt, Jeffrey Dover, Michael Kaminer, Leonard Goldberg, and David Bickers, and my parents, Rahat and Rehana Alam.

Murad Alam MD, MSCI

# Introduction

Jean Carruthers, Alastair Carruthers

## Summary and Key Features

- Knowledge of the subcutaneous neurovascular, bony, and muscular anatomy of each region of the face is increasingly important. Understanding of the aesthetic desires of each subject and careful targeted volumization is the key to aesthetic success with facial fillers.

- Understanding different regional concepts of beauty and the use of validated assessment scales have aided in achieving optimal outcomes.

- Reversers and better pain management have enhanced augmentation procedures. Better understanding of anatomy and improved injection techniques have reduced vascular occlusion complications.

- Three-dimensional fillers are now seen as stimulators of neocollagenesis, thus improving the texture of facial skin from the "inside."

In 1885 two extremely powerful European figures, Kaiser Wilhelm and Chancellor Bismarck, decided to announce the new age of retirement, age 65. At that time the median age in the population was 16. Nowadays it is 41.7.[1]

In addition, adults are currently working longer and living better and are much more educated about the ways to live a healthy lifestyle. They are also very pressed for time because they are not only looking after their children and grandchildren but also are taking care of their aging parents.

There are also significant stresses from the workplace, in that older workers are competing for work and promotions with younger colleagues.

The new world of noninvasive rejuvenation is perfectly timed to assist them to recover and maintain their youthful and empowered appearance.

In the ASDS Consumer Survey on Cosmetic Dermatologic Procedures[2] of 7315 individuals surveyed, 5 in 10 were considering a cosmetic procedure for aesthetic indications not only in the face but also over the entire body. They wished to look as young as they felt, to appear more attractive, and to feel more confident.[1]

In 2014 nearly half of all cosmetic patients in the United States requesting noninvasive or minimally invasive interventions received multiple cosmetic procedures at the same time.[2] They are also most interested in procedures that give little or no downtime.

Synthetic fillers, such as hyaluronans, calcium hydroxylapatite, poly-L-lactic acid, and silicone, allow three-dimensional volumization without a prior harvesting procedure. Local tumescent anesthesia liposuction allows autologous product to be used for volumization.

The anatomic structures of facial aging of bone, fat, and skin have been further studied by computed tomography (CT), magnetic resonance imaging (MRI) scans, and detailed anatomic cadaver dissection which have allowed us to visualize accurately the underlying age-related changes. A new descriptive language of age-related facial changes using facial scales has been published, demonstrating their value in improving communication not only with our patients in our clinics, but also with each other as we work together toward better treatments.[3]

Patient-reported outcomes (PROs) have become the standard for assessing treatment outcomes from the patient's point of view. Published validated questionnaires, such as the Facial Line Outcomes (FLO) and Self-Perception of Age (SPA), can be used as easily in the clinic as in the research setting. Several validated PROs are used both by patients and by the treating and evaluating physician—such as the Lip Fullness Scale (LFS) and Look and Feel of the Lips (LAF) scale, as well as the severity scales for Perioral Lines at Rest (POL), Perioral Lines at Maximum Contraction (POLM), and Oral Commissure Severity (OCS), and the Face-Q scales.[4–9] The recognition that the patient's opinion is all important and must thus be recorded, studied, and understood is a gift of the field of aesthetic medicine.

Patients prefer their treatments to be as pain-free as possible. In the past decade, we have learned that educating our subjects dramatically reduces their anxiety, as does topical chilling with ice and topical anesthesia and "talkesthesia." Pain control for facial injections has largely evolved away from trigeminal nerve blocks, with the common addition of lidocaine to injected fillers. The addition of saline to dilute the filler decreases cohesiveness, allowing for smooth delivery and the ability to distribute the product evenly by gentle massage.

Reversibility has also become a cornerstone of facial filler injections. Hyaluronidase is an enzyme that will catabolize any hyaluronic acid (HA) filler, sometimes within 24 hours. New classes of fillers may be produced with custom-made "erasers" in the future. Post-treatment bruising can now be treated immediately using intense pulsed light at moderate settings, which allows the bruise to be absorbed within 24 to 48 hours instead of 7 to 10 days.

All subjects are aware that they will see an immediate filler effect with the desired new contour. They may not be aware of the neocollagenesis that occurs with the filler apparently stimulating the development of new collagen in the dermis,[3] which will give a more reflectant glowing facial skin.

The past century has seen an explosion of development of new fillers and their global acceptance by a patient population that would rather look restored and younger without the trauma and downtime of surgery. Indeed, the introduction of noninvasive or minimally invasive injectable procedures represents a significant shift in the approach to facial rejuvenation. According to the website of the American Society of Aesthetic Plastic Surgeons 2016, injectables overall saw a 21% increase in 2015.[10]

## References

1. *Median Age of the world's population*. Wikipedia.org. Accessed Oct 22, 2016.
2. *ASDS Consumer survey on cosmetic Dermatologic Procedures*. 2016.
3. Carruthers J, Burgess C, Day D, Fabi SG, Goldie K, Kerscher M, Nikolis A, Pavicic T, Rho NK, Rzany B, Sattler G, Sattler S, Seo K, Werschler WP, Carruthers A. Consensus Recommendations for Combined Aesthetic Interventions in the Face Using Botulinum Toxin, Fillers, and Energy-Based Devices. *Dermatol Surg*. 2016;0:1–12.
4. Carruthers A, Carruthers J, Hardas B, et al. A validated lip fullness rating scale. *Dermatol Surg*. 2008a;34(suppl 2):S161–S166.
5. Carruthers A, Carruthers J, Hardas B, et al. A validated marionette lines rating scale. *Dermatol Surg*. 2008b; 34(suppl 2):S167–S172.
6. Carruthers A, Carruthers J, Hardas B, et al. A validated crow's feet rating scale. *Dermatol Surg*. 2008c;34(suppl 2):S173–S178.
7. Carruthers A, Carruthers J, Hardas B, et al. A validated hand grading rating scale. *Dermatol Surg*. 2008d;34(suppl 2):S179–S183.
8. Carruthers J, Carruthers A, Monheit GD, Davis PG, Tardie G. Multicenter, randomized, parallel-group study of onabotulinumtoxinA and hyaluronic acid dermal fillers (24-mg/mL smooth, cohesive gel) alone and in combination for lower facial rejuvenation: satisfaction and patient-reported outcomes. *Dermatol Surg*. 2011;36(suppl 4):2135–2145.
9. Carruthers J, Flynn TC, Geister TL, et al. Validated assessment scales for the mid face. *Dermatol Surg*. 2012;38:320–332.
10. *American Society for Aesthetic Plastic Surgery website*. Accessed 22 Oct 2016.

## Further reading

Carruthers A, Carruthers J, Hardas B, et al. A validated lip fullness rating scale. *Dermatol Surg*. 2008;34(suppl 2): S161–S166.

Carruthers A, Carruthers J, Hardas B, et al. A validated marionette lines rating scale. *Dermatol Surg*. 2008; 34(suppl 2):S167–S172.

Carruthers A, Carruthers J, Hardas B, et al. A validated crow's feet rating scale. *Dermatol Surg*. 2008c;34(suppl 2):S173–S178.

Carruthers A, Carruthers J, Hardas B, et al. A validated hand grading rating scale. *Dermatol Surg*. 2008d;34(suppl 2): S179–S183.

Carruthers J, Carruthers A, Monheit GD, Davis PG, Tardie G. Multicenter, randomized, parallel-group study of onabotulinumtoxinA and hyaluronic acid dermal fillers (24-mg/mL smooth, cohesive gel) alone and in combination for lower facial rejuvenation: satisfaction and patient-reported outcomes. *Dermatol Surg*. 2011;36(suppl 4):2135–2145.

Carruthers J, Flynn TC, Geister TL, et al. Validated assessment scales for the mid face. *Dermatol Surg*. 2012;38:320–332.

Carruthers JDA, Glogau R, Blitzer A, Facial Consensus Group Faculty. Advances in facial rejuvenation: botulinum toxin type A, hyaluronic acid dermal fillers, and combination therapies: consensus recommendations. *Plast Reconstr Surg*. 2008;121(suppl 5):S5–S30.

Fagien S, Carruthers J. A comprehensive review of patient reported satisfaction with botulinum toxin type A for aesthetic procedures. *Plast Reconstr Surg*. 2008;122:1915–1925.

# Fillers: paradigm shifts produce new challenges

### Richard G. Glogau

## Summary and Key Features

- A shift in treatment concept from two-dimensional to three-dimensional.
- Volume replacement rather than static wrinkle correction.
- Twenty years of collagen injectables replaced with hyaluronic acid (HA) gels.
- More robust—denser, harder, greater lift—HA gels introduced.
- Newer products are niche variations of existing HA technology.
- More robust fillers require deeper application.
- Deeper placement involves exposure to vascular communications with retinal artery and branches of carotid artery.
- Treatment of the temple area involves potential middle temporal vein injection, which can cause pulmonary or cerebral embolism.
- Intravascular injection or vascular compression from robust agents can cause catastrophic consequences.
- Risk factors include filler particle size, pressure generated, and speed of injection.
- Volume replacement gives satisfying aesthetic improvement unachievable by other means.
- Location of injection is key to avoiding risk and providing cosmetic benefit.

*1926 real estate classified ad in the Chicago Tribune:*
*"Attention salesmen, sales managers: location, location, location, close to Rogers Park."*
William Safire, June 26, 2009, *New York Times Magazine*

When this topic was reviewed in the 2012 edition of *"Soft Tissue Augmentation,"* we pointed out the shift in aesthetics that was occurring. Fillers were moving from treatment of static wrinkles in the two-dimensional plane to correcting the three-dimensional volume changes in the aging face. What started out as very small and arbitrary amounts of material (0.5 and 1.0 mL syringes of bovine collagen or occasional microdroplets of silicone) in the 1970s and an unblinking focus on the single line or small dermal acne scar, suddenly blossomed into greater volumes of filler, especially with the introduction of hyaluronic acid (HA) gels. With the blockbuster aesthetic impact of botulinum toxin on the muscles of facial expression, the tools were at hand to address a second significant component of facial aging: the dramatic loss of subcutaneous and deep tissue volume associated with the aging face.

The single syringe of collagen commercially available for 25 years was completely inadequate to address the tasks at hand. The markets began to respond with a virtual flood of new filler products—HA gels, polylactic acid (PLA), calcium hydroxylapatite (CaHA), polymethylmethacrylate (PMMA)—and a renewed interest in two filler agents that had been in use before: silicone and fat. After 20 years of three fillers—collagen, silicone, and fat—the aesthetic market expanded in 5 years to more than 300 commercially available forms of injectable filler worldwide, with more coming every year.

The HA gels are now available in a variety of densities, with added lidocaine, and they constitute the lion's share of the filler market in North America at the present time. Although Restylane was the first HA filler product US Food and Drug Administration (FDA)-approved to enter the US market, it was quickly followed by the Juvéderm family of fillers and has been joined by other injectable products of different compositions: Sculptra (Dermik Laboratories, Sanofi-Aventis, Bridgewater, New Jersey), a PLA filler, Radiesse (BioForm Medical, San Mateo, California), a CaHA filler, Bellafill (Suneva, San Diego, California), a PMMA filler, and Belotero (Merz, Frankfurt a.M., Germany), an HA gel filler for fine lines.

In 2012 we pointed out that many of the products were coming from European manufacturers and described two interesting agents, Aquamid (Contura, Soeborg, Denmark), a polyacrylamide gel, and Ellansé (AQTIS, Utrecht, Netherlands), polycaprolactone microspheres in carboxymethyl cellulose gel. Neither product currently has made it through the FDA approval process. Other HA gel fillers, such as the Emervel family of fillers (Galderma, S.A., Lausanne, Switzerland), are in trial or are awaiting FDA approval. What changes in professional market demand and perception are now driving the process forward? What have we learned since 2012?

As a result of the influx of new fillers, together with a heightened appreciation of the three-dimensional nature of volume loss in the aging face, there was a rapid increase in volume of material being injected into the deeper compartments of the face, frequently giving more significant and natural improvements to the aging face. Convex contours of the cheek in particular, but also the temples, lips, chin, eyes, were subtly restored to younger volumes in ways that traditional incisional surgery could not address. Whole new areas of application were suddenly available to the injector.

Homologous fat, which was a readily available by-product of liposuction techniques introduced in the early 1980s, was the only true volume injectable. Many liposuction surgeons tried various harvesting and processing techniques as they recycled the unwanted fat from abdomens and hips to various places on the face and body. However, for the most part the results were inconsistently dependable, not long-lasting for the majority of patients, and occasionally producing unwanted asymmetric outcomes. But the use of fat did increase further understanding of the nature and distribution of the subcutaneous fat compartments in the aging face. For example, noninvasive magnetic resonance imaging (MRI) and imaging techniques estimate the volume of the midface subcutaneous fat at somewhere between 13 and 17 mL per side[1]—not a deficit likely to be repaired with a single syringe of any material!

HA fillers have become the dominant filler in the United States and global markets. They are stable at room temperature, available "off the shelf," and were manufactured in single preloaded syringes, very reminiscent of the old collagen injections. They provide good reversibility with hyaluronidase, an important safety consideration. They provide more immediate "lift" than the collagen fillers that preceded them, have longer duration of action, and require no allergy skin testing prior to treatment. They are easily injected through small-gauge needles, 30 gauge and smaller. Because they are derived from bacteria, they do not share the problems of animal-derived proteins like the collagen products.

The evolution of the HA gel products has made some technologic improvements in the products. One approach has been to vary the concentration of the HA gel. Another is to vary the degree of cross-linking between the polymer chains, and another significant improvement was the addition of lidocaine for increased comfort of injection. Changes in density and cross-linking variously affect the rheology of the materials and can improve duration, lift, and ease of injection through small-gauge needles.

Some of these changes have produced "niche" products for specific anatomic areas or applications: Restylane Silk (Galderma), and Volbella (Allergan) for lip augmentation, Volift (Allergan) for nasolabial folds, and Voluma (Allergan) and Restylane Lift (Galderma, formerly Perlane-L) for midface augmentation. However, the shared characteristic of all these "niche" fillers is that they are not "dermal" fillers but are placed in the deep subcutaneous, submucosal, or submuscular space, often just above the periosteum. Each of these products offers a nuanced variation of the earlier HA gel fillers to appeal to physicians and patients alike.

However, the hallmark of the popular HA fillers is their adaptability, tolerability, and reversibility. Injectors can easily pick two or three of the available HA fillers and by diluting them slightly, they can often make one of the standard HA fillers perform satisfactorily in different anatomic depths. Although such activity must be recognized as "off-label" use of approved medical devices, the practice appears widespread as physicians and patients seek treatment of a variety of anatomic locations and aesthetic indications in a single office visit.

The challenge for the treating physician is to select the suitable agent and place it appropriately in the given anatomic location to produce the desired aesthetic result. In the 1970s and early 1980s when bovine collagen injections were in use, wrinkles were the aesthetic target, the placement was in the dermis, and the postinjection side effects were predictably local bruising at the site of injection. As the aesthetic range gradually included defects with some depth, like expression lines, vascular occlusions began to appear, particularly ischemic accidents in the supratrochlear vessels (from treatment of the glabellar lines), the angular branch of the facial artery (treatment of nasolabial folds), or the occlusion of the labial artery (lip augmentation).

These vascular accidents appeared to increase in number when the shift occurred from the original Zyderm collagen to Zyplast, a collagen product in which the collagen polymers were cross-linked to produce longer duration of effect. Zyplast was much more slippery than Zyderm, and injectors could inadvertently inject the entire syringe with one push on the plunger, potentially contributing to vascular accidents. Although debate swirled about the underlying cause of these occlusions (intravascular vs. extravascular compression,[2] hemostatic effect of the collagen vs. mass effect of the bolus in the vessel), the nature of the phenomenon was that (1) it was irreversible—nothing existed to dissolve the collagen, and (2) it required the injection to occur below the dermis in the subcutaneous space, where the smaller arteries came close to the surface anatomy.

The evolution of use of the HA gel fillers followed the same process, although the dermal placement of these materials was certainly less common. Restylane, because of the particulate nature of the HA, produced a color shift known as the Tyndall effect when it was injected too superficially. However, it certainly did not take much time for the occlusive accidents to be seen with HA treatment of the glabellar creases, nasolabial folds at the base of the nose, and labial arteries, among others. The next evolutionary step was to use the HA fillers to go even deeper in the soft tissue to address true volume deficits: loss of premalar and malar fat, perioral volume loss, atrophy along the mandibular ridge, and loss of fat in the temples, forehead, and nose.

The filler materials themselves became robust, providing greater lift, duration, and volume. They required larger-caliber needles to inject the material that can allow greater aliquots of material to be injected with greater speed and higher pressures than possible with smaller needles. But the catastrophic vascular complications of retinal artery embolization in the literature reflect the deeper anatomy being targeted, along with many of the facial arteries sharing circulation with the retinal artery.

Several superficial arteries of the facial vasculature are distal branches of the ophthalmic artery (supraorbital, supratrochlear, dorsal nasal, and angular artery of the nose) (Fig. 2.1). The danger is not limited to the arterial side of the circulation. In the temple area, a frequent site of unwanted atrophy and an aesthetic target for deep filler injections, the middle temporal vein (MTV) communicates with the cavernous sinus through the periorbital veins and the pulmonary artery via the internal jugular vein,[3] requiring judicious placement of filler in the immediate periosteal space to avoid intravascular injection of the MTV and potential vision loss or pulmonary and cerebral embolism.

Unfortunately, only small amounts of filler are required to produce retrograde injection from the distal branches to the retinal artery, reportedly as little as 0.5 mL of material. Although fortunately these deep vascular complications with retrograde embolism are quite rare, they warrant a careful understanding of both the potentially problematic vasculature and available techniques to lessen the risk of the injections.[4] The inextricable link between speed of injection and risk of side effect has been demonstrated in clinical trials.[5] In addition, suggestions have been made to use smaller syringes (reducing pressure), blunt cannulae (less chance of direct vessel cannulation), multiple small aliquots rather than large single amounts, aspiration before injection to confirm location of the needle tip, use of vasoconstrictors in the area before injecting filler to reduce vessel caliber, and moving the needle or cannula slightly while injecting to avoid intravascular puncture. Consider injecting across the vessel's path rather than parallel to it to minimize intravascular injection.

Although vascular accidents have been reported with all manner of filler, fat clearly seems to run a higher risk, probably secondary to the higher pressures and larger particle sizes injected. Along with other permanent or semipermanent fillers, such as CaHA, PMMA, PLA, and silicone, there is no chance of removing or dissolving the offending filler in case of vascular accident. HA gel fillers offer a chance to ameliorate some cases of vascular occlusion if the occlusion is in the superficial vasculature (e.g., glabellar ischemia, angular artery ischemia, or labial artery

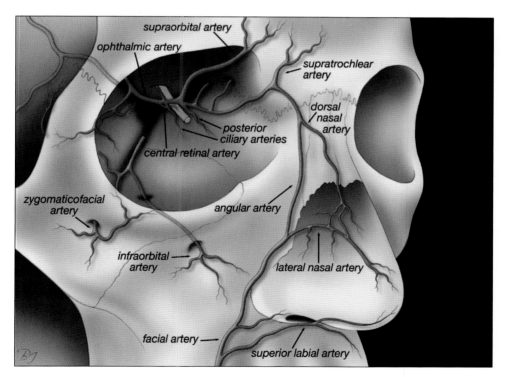

**Figure 2.1** The potential for retrograde communication and embolism to the central retinal artery can be traced to the facial artery, lateral nasal artery, dorsal nasal artery, infraorbital artery, zygomaticofacial artery, supratrochlear artery, supraorbital artery, and even the superior labial artery. *Reprinted from Lazzeri D, Agostini T, Figus M, Nardi M, Pantaloni M, Lazzeri S. Blindness following cosmetic injections of the face, Plast Reconstr Surg. 2012;129(4):995–1012. p 1006.*

occlusion).[6] In these cases flooding the area with hyaluronidase (Vitrase, Bausch + Lomb, Bridgewater, New Jersey), using topical nitropaste 2% (Nitro-Bid, Fougera, Melville, New York),[7] and supportive care with aspirin, emollient, and dressings may help minimize the damage.[8]

However, if deeper vascular occlusion has occurred (vision changes, symptoms of stroke, etc.), the time pressure is acute. Permanent retinal blindness occurs after 60 to 90 minutes. Emergency consultation with ophthalmology and neurology is required. Recovery of function is usually marginal at best. Use of hyaluronidase in the retroorbital space may have theoretical benefit but the use is not established.[9–11]

In addition to the vascular complications that occur at the time of treatment, the robust HA fillers for deeper placement have been reported to cause a late-onset inflammatory nodular reaction, which can be persistent and requires corticosteroids, hyaluronidase, and repeat treatments to manage.[12] While they appear relatively infrequently, they are another potential problem to be managed as fillers moved from superficial to deep placement.

The upside to the transition to deeper placement of more robust fillers has been achievement of greater duration of effect and in most cases a more natural-appearing reversal of the loss of facial volumes that are lost in an aging face. In particular, the replacement of midface volumes has an effect on appearance that cannot be readily achieved by other means, including cold steel surgery. Following the adoption curve of many new, innovative therapies, there can be a tendency to overtreat in the initial transition to the newer materials and techniques. We see far too many patients with overfilled mid-faces and malar eminences, usually with overfilled lips to go along with it. However, the aesthetically intelligent injector can address superficial, medium, and deep defects using either a variety of niche filler products or various dilutions of a single product to produce natural results.

Although the manufacturers obviously prefer the targeted niche approach to differentiate their products from the competition, many patients and physicians are sensitive to the costs incurred by using multiple syringes of different products. The use of more than one syringe of a single product can address multiple anatomic sites and various depths and seems to be a trend. In addition, the use of combination therapy to address skin texture, repetitive movement of muscles of expression, and smaller volume changes (above the brow, above the upper lip, along the jaw line, earlobes, etc.) separate the experienced injectors from the ordinary, but there can be no doubts that the progression to deeper fillers can make all of us look better. Remember: location, location, location.

## References

1. Barrera JE, Most SP. Volumetric imaging of the malar fat pad and implications for facial plastic surgery. *Arch Facial Plast Surg.* 2008;10(2):140–142.
2. Chang SH, Yousefi S, Qin J, et al. External compression versus intravascular injection: a mechanistic animal model of filler-induced tissue ischemia. *Ophthal Plast Reconstr Surg.* 2016;32:261–266.
3. Tansatit T, Apinuntrum P, Phetudom T. An anatomical study of the middle temporal vein and the drainage vascular networks to assess the potential complications and the preventive maneuver during temporal augmentation using both anterograde and retrograde injections. *Aesthetic Plast Surg.* 2015;39(5):791–799.
4. Beleznay K, Carruthers JD, Humphrey S, Jones D. Avoiding and treating blindness from fillers: a review of the world literature. *Dermatol Surg.* 2015;41(10):1097–1117.
5. Glogau RG, Kane MA. Effect of injection techniques on the rate of local adverse events in patients implanted with nonanimal hyaluronic acid gel dermal fillers. *Dermatol Surg.* 2008;34(suppl 1):S105–S109.
6. DeLorenzi C. Complications of injectable fillers, part 2: vascular complications. *Aesthet Surg J.* 2014;34(4):584–600.
7. Kleydman K, Cohen JL, Marmur E. Nitroglycerin: a review of its use in the treatment of vascular occlusion after soft tissue augmentation. *Dermatol Surg.* 2012;38(12):1889–1897.
8. Cohen JL, Biesman BS, Dayan SH, et al. Treatment of hyaluronic acid filler-induced impending necrosis with hyaluronidase: consensus recommendations. *Aesthet Surg J.* 2015;35(7):844–849.
9. Goodman GJ, Clague MD. A rethink on hyaluronidase injection, intraarterial injection, and blindness: is there another option for treatment of retinal artery embolism caused by intraarterial injection of hyaluronic acid? *Dermatol Surg.* 2016;42(4):547–549.
10. Fagien S. Commentary on a rethink on hyaluronidase injection, intra-arterial injection and blindness. *Dermatol Surg.* 2016;42(4):549–552.
11. Steinsapir KD. Treating filler related visual loss. *Dermatol Surg.* 2016;42(4):552–554.
12. Beleznay K, Carruthers JD, Carruthers A, Mummert ME, Humphrey S. Delayed-onset nodules secondary to a smooth cohesive 20 mg/mL hyaluronic acid filler: cause and management. *Dermatol Surg.* 2015;41(8):929–939.

## Further reading

Lazzeri D, Agostini T, Figus M, Nardi M, Pantaloni M, Lazzeri S. Blindness following cosmetic injections of the face. *Plast Reconstr Surg.* 2012;129(4):995–1012.

# 3

# Facial attractiveness and the central role of volume

## Greg J. Goodman

## Introduction

The issue practitioners are facing is that we are now able to positively impact on most of our patient's appearance in ways we never could before. To take on that responsibility we need to understand what is our desired result. Central to this is an understanding of what is beauty, as there is little doubt that it is beauty that we are ultimately trying to achieve. To successfully manage patients we start by understanding why beauty exists, why it is important to our patients, and how to enhance this. In addition, we need to tackle the concept of universality of beauty across ethnicities.

## The very existence of beauty

Arguably, beauty is innate and is about survival itself.[1] By recognizing what is good and bad around us in terms of beauty or ugliness we are likely to choose good (or beautiful) and avoid bad or harmful (ugly).[2,3]

Many different professions have studied attractiveness and beauty—psychologists,[4–9] neuroscientists,[10] biologists, human behaviorists,[11] anthropologists, dentists and orthodontists,[12] dermatologists and surgeons,[13–15] as well as other specialties[16]—all approaching this topic from their own unique perspectives.

Attractiveness may seem a frivolous topic but with the prospect for a more fulfilling life enhanced purely by its presence or absence,[17,18] it clearly has an important function.

### Pearl 1

Attractiveness appreciation is an innate human skill, with all senses participating but the visual sense dominating.

Given that our visual sense is the strongest, it is no surprise that our appreciation of facial appearance is rapid, efficient, and even in a subliminal way a very important part of mate selection. Therefore maximizing facial attractiveness is uppermost in all our patients' hearts and minds. Although movement and surface-related issues are undoubtedly important aspects in a beautiful face, arguably volume is the most important (Fig. 3.1).

Volume is central to rejuvenation of the aging face or facial improvement at any age and plays a pivotal role in our visual clues when assessing facial beauty and handsomeness.

The appraisal of beauty and recognition of another's face take only a fraction of a second.[19,20] Brain responses to facial beauty have been widely studied.[21–23] Magnetic resonance imaging (MRI) has shown that beauty results in widespread brainwave activity that directly correlates to the degree of facial attractiveness.[24] In another study, performing a task was found to take longer if one was distracted by an attractive facial image, even if it was outside direct vision. In other words, facial beauty automatically competes with any other task we are doing.[25]

### Pearl 2

Although we very quickly assess beauty, the exact mechanism of how remains elusive.

Question: What are the principles that underpin our understanding of beauty?

The total attractiveness of an individual is not quite the same as facial beauty. Attractiveness is a total package and may relate to how a person moves,[26] appearance of fitness,[27] and how one expresses himself or herself,[28] sounds,[29] or thinks.[30] It may relate to their power or success, to the reputation they have, how they relate to others, and many other facets that go in to making an individual who they are.

Attractiveness in humans is certainly not limited to the face. A determinant of female attractiveness and beauty is termed the ogee curve. This curve is simply a convexity followed by a concavity, which is best appreciated by the example of the classic 1950s pinup, in which we see a convexity on either side of a concavity at the waistline. The waist–hip ratio (WHR) is one of the most alluring aspects of body attractiveness.[31] However, the thrust of this chapter is more specifically about female facial beauty and the role of volume in that beauty, and here we see volume-expanded ogee curves (Fig. 3.2) as clues to sexual maturity in the curve of the high cheekbones, eyelid–cheek junction, lips, and eyebrow[32–34]

## The role of volume in the appreciation of facial beauty

Facial volume gives the face its characteristic shape and is a prominent aspect of beauty. It is the concept that

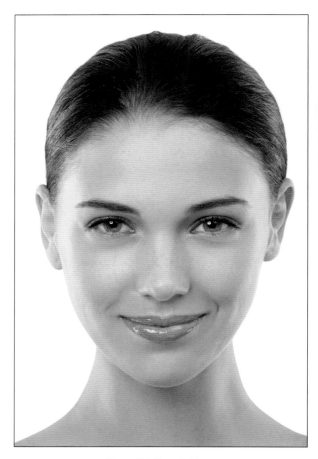

Figure 3.1 Beautiful face.

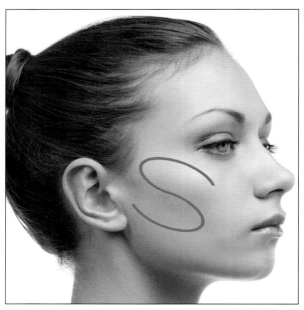

Figure 3.2 Diagram of ogee curve taking in the eyelid–cheek junction, high cheek bone and the concavity inferior to this.

**Pearl 4**

Bone and dentition support the facial form and structure of overlying muscles and resorb with age periorificially and in the bones supporting mastication.

underpins much of what we perceive as the symmetry and geometry of facial attractiveness. This shape fluctuates with weight gain and loss and with age as tissues lose volume in some areas and appear to add volume in others, thus contributing to the rounding of a more youthful face (Fig. 3.3) or squaring of an aging face.

**Pearl 3**

Volume is important in many of the indicators of youth, maturity, attractiveness, symmetry, and gender differentiation.

Volume is important in all facial layers from the base presented by the bone and teeth through to muscle, fat, and the superficial layers of the skin. Most volume loss occurs deeply with resorption around and within major facial orifices. The orbits expand, and the piriform aperture (Fig. 3.4)[35] widens, allowing posterior displacement of the nasal base with drooping of the nose and deepening of the nasolabial fold.

Dentition volume decreases and the mandible and maxilla volume diminishes. Anterior projection of the periorbital zone, midface, nose, perioral area, and chin all suffer as a result. The decrease in volume of the large muscles of mastication (especially the masseter muscle) and changes in the mandible, particularly shortening in the posterior ramus height and the body length, also contribute to an increasingly obtuse mandibular angle.[36] This has significant ramifications for the fading of beauty in older age with the facial shape changing and the support for the lower face waning.

**Pearl 5**

The muscles of mastication (masseter and temporalis particularly) lose volume in the aging process.

There have been separate facial fat compartments (Fig. 3.5) described in both the superficial and deep layers of the face, each with their defined pockets of fat separated by retaining ligaments.[37,38] The major retaining ligaments, such as the mandibular and zygomatic ligaments, do not

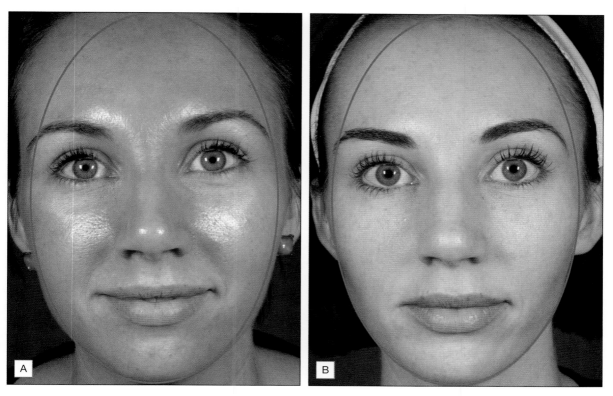

**Figure 3.3** Facial shape before **(A)** and after **(B)** weight loss, showing a change from round to oval.

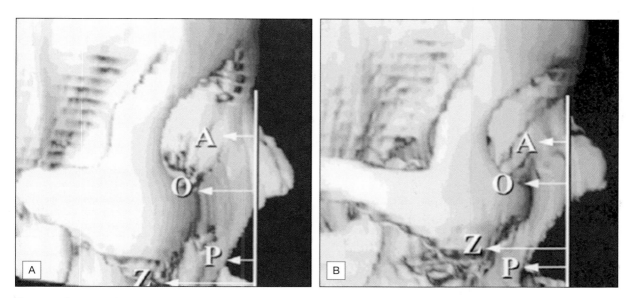

**Figure 3.4** The areas of the facial skeleton that selectively resorb with aging with the size of the *arrows* indicating relative tendency for bone loss. *From Mendelson B, Wong C. Changes in the facial skeleton with aging: implications and clinical applications in facial rejuvenation.* Aesth Plast Surg. *2012;36:4:753–760.*

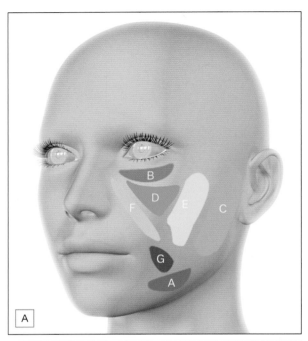

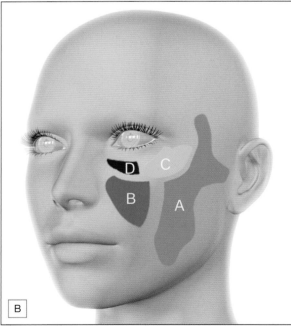

**Figure 3.5** Diagram of facial fat compartments. **(A) Superficial fat compartments**: *A*, Inferior jowl fat. *B*, Infraorbital fat. *C*, Lateral cheek fat. *D*, Medial cheek fat. *E*, Middle cheek fat. *F*, Nasolabial fat. *G*, Superior jowl fat. **(B) Deep fat compartments**: *A*, Buccal fat. *B*, Deep medial cheek fat. *C*, Lateral suborbicularis oculi fat. *D*, Medial suborbicularis oculi fat.

**Table 3.1** Superficial and corresponding deep fat compartments of the face. Deep compartments may be more prone to atrophy with age whereas superficial ones tend to hypertrophy

| Superficial fat compartments | Deep fat compartments |
| --- | --- |
| Nasolabial | Deep medial cheek (medial component) |
| Superficial medial cheek | Deep medial cheek (lateral component) |
| Middle cheek | Buccal |
| Lateral temporal cheek | Lateral suborbicularis oculi (SOOF) |
| Infraorbital | Medial suborbicularis oculi (SOOF) |

significantly change in length over time. The zones of the face and its proportions are an effortless balance in youth and when optimal features are at work. With age or poorly developed features comes a burden on retaining ligaments as volume shifts or sags, exaggerating the deep folds of the face.

**Pearl 6**

Most major retaining ligaments induce deep facial grooves as the face cascades forwards and inwards with age.

The facial fat compartments appear to be bilayered, with a superficial and deeper set of compartments (Table 3.1).[39] The deeper fat pads allow sliding of mimetic muscles and muscles of mastication, but with aging it appears that the midfacial fat compartments migrate medially with an inferior shift within the individual compartments.[40] This has led to the popularization of a deeper injection augmenting the deep system and reinflating the superficial fat pads, allowing better support and projection.[41]

**Pearl 7**

Facial fat compartments appear to have deep and superficial elements with the deeper ones particularly prone to atrophy with aging.

Replenishing atrophic compartments may aid facial rejuvenation.[42,43] For example, deflation of the deep periorbital fat pad with age induces a V-shaped concavity between the medial eyelid and cheek area, opening up the inferior orbital hollows, and a more obvious transition between the lid and cheek. Hence deep augmentation of the medial suborbicularis fat pads or deep medial cheek fat pad using a deep supraperiosteal injection may improve this tear trough deformity.

---

**Pearl 8**

The facial shape seen from the front should be an oval in youth, independent of ethnicity in females, and a sharp angular shape, more base-heavy in males.

---

## Facial shapes

There are many facial shapes which should be pleasing, even at times arresting from any angle; for example, the sweep of the cheek may be best appreciated from an oblique pose and the projected aspects from a lateral one.

We will start from the anteroposterior (AP) view because this is the view we see mostly in the mirror and when in conversation. It should not be forgotten that photographic capture and posing is not usually front-on but various shades of a side-on pose. Looking at the face front-on, volume is important for the outline, shape, symmetry, and width of the features.

Facial shape is an essential aspect underpinning attractiveness, the appearance of youth, and gender identification. In the female, looking at the face front-on, the facial outline should approximate a smooth oval. This oval is a combination of bony skeleton overlain by soft tissues. The oval line should begin at the forehead and curve rather seamlessly around the outside of the face through the temples, outer cheeks, preauricular area, angle of the jaw, jawline, and all the way to the chin.[44] The edge of the features it passes on its way around the face from forehead to chin should sit on the line, neither falling far short of nor projecting past the oval's edge (Fig. 3.6).

---

**Pearl 9**

The oval outline of the attractive female face should pass seamlessly touching on the temples, cheeks, jaw angle, and jawline through to the chin.

---

This facial shape is a very similar beauty consideration across all ethnicities and is a strong determinant of age perception. Variations have been termed heart-shaped or betel leaf, but these may be variations in the upper half of the oval rather than different to the intrinsic oval face. However, not all agree with this stance,[45] but all would agree the female facial shape should be wider in the upper half, tapering to a point at the chin, with no angular sharpness. Squaring of the face begins soon after a female's peak of maturation, around the age of 25, with a more rapid progression into middle age and older years.[46] This masculinizes the face, making it less attractive.

In youth a fatter face is acceptable with an evening out of the fat compartments and support provided by

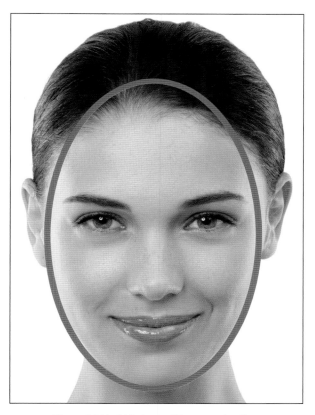

**Figure 3.6** Facial features sitting on oval outline.

retaining ligaments. However, further weight gain may affect these compartments prone to age-related hypertrophy resulting in facial squaring and plentiful folds, which are not aesthetically ideal.

A square male face is acceptable, even desirable, but this squareness must have certain characteristics.[47–50] In the upper face, adequate bi-zigonial distance is required, with the male facial shape most defined in the lower half, requiring strong masseteric volume and jaw angle (Fig. 3.7). What is not desirable is jowls or excess volume posterior to the masseters overlying the parotids.

A strong, defined jawline and strong square chin are the masculinizing facial shape and attractiveness requirements.

---

**Pearl 10**

Attractive female faces are much wider in the mid and upper face than the lower face, whereas attractive males tend to possess greater lower face volume.

---

## Symmetry

Symmetry appears to be our visual clue to the outward show of ideal genetics.

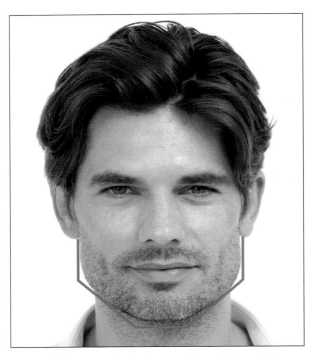

**Figure 3.7** Strong masseteric volume and jaw angle in a male face.

Although symmetry may refer to any aspect of beauty, such as surface irregularities or facial movement peculiarities, it is the differential volume effects that detract most from the beauty of an individual's face.

In one study, only 6 of the 21 subjects were symmetrical across their upper face (bi-zigonial distance) and only 4 symmetrical across the lower face (angle of the jaws). Only 3 out of 21 appeared symmetrical across both the upper and lower face. These subjects were taken from some of the objectively most beautiful females in current and past history—film stars, models, and pageant winners.[45]

**Pearl 11**

Very few people, even beautiful people are symmetrical.

### Ideal proportions of beauty

We now understand that to have a well-proportioned face is a major step towards beauty. The ancient Greeks believed that all beauty was mathematical, and one of the more robust concepts is the golden ratio. This ratio is a mathematical construct fixed at 1.618:1.

In geometry it is a linear relation in which the smaller length is to the larger length as the larger length is to the complete line. It defines ratios we find appealing in nature, architecture, the human body, and faces. This ratio has

been applied to the many aspects making up the attractive face and has helped us to understand what defines facial beauty.

Swift and Remington explored these Phi concepts to illustrate how best to rejuvenate the face in a concept they term "beautiphication."[51]

It is odd that a two-dimensional line has been so extensively used to assess facial beauty and correct proportionality, as the proportions really represent a three dimensionality. The vertical height of the upper and lower lips, the relationship of eye width to the width across the malar ridges, and the proportions of the nose and the teeth are measured by this two-dimensional line but represent volume, a three-dimensional concept.

Divisions of the face into thirds horizontally and fifths vertically are other useful constructs for facial assessment and treatment planning. It is most likely that an inbuilt sense of mathematical analysis and concepts is at work in all of us when assessing beauty.

### Maturity indicators

Gender selection is a hardwired, innate attraction to a particular gender. It is based on sexual dimorphism, or what makes a person obviously one gender or the other.

The soft sloping ogee curves in females and the strong angles of males are volume indicators of the attainment of sexual maturity associated with estrogen and testosterone, respectively.

On a more localized level the human face is meant to be predictable, devoid of volume imperfections. One of the most common local volume abnormalities dermatologists and their patients face is atrophic scars. This is so disfiguring to patients that it is a source of depression and suicidal ideation.[52] It deeply offends the patient cosmetically and is a common reason for seeking treatment. Volume correction in this instance of atrophic scarring has been a neglected aspect in treatment (Fig. 3.8).[53,54]

**Pearl 12**

The oval facial shape transcends ethnicity and is the cornerstone of universal beauty, with differences lying more in an individual's internal features.

### Facial volume, beauty, and ethnicity

Initially researchers believed that different cultures adhere to different styles of beauty, but this may not be correct. Darwin espoused that there is no universal standard of beauty. However, much of the research since the 1970s contradicts this and suggests a more universal standard of beauty.[55–57]

Does our ideal face shape vary with ethnicity? Is an oval facial shape something females of any ethnicity can and should aspire to? It is probable that a smoothly contoured oval-shaped perimeter to a woman's face is the cornerstone of universal beauty and that an angular face

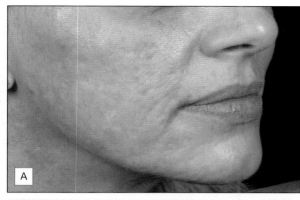

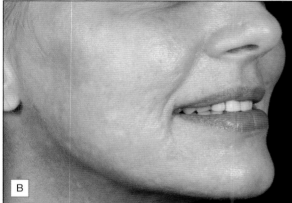

**Figure 3.8** Acne scarring before **(A)** and after **(B)** volume treatment.

with lower facial prominence, defined jawline, square strong chin, large nose, and heavy horizontal brows are similar cornerstones in men.

## So where do the differences lie?

The strength and weaknesses of the ethnicities are more obvious in the internal features of the face—the nose, lips, cheeks, eyes, brows, and chin—and how they project from the face.

These structures are emphasized in Caucasians and Indians but poorly projected in East Asians and Africans. Lip projection varies between ethnicities. Although the upper lip is often quite full in East Asian females, the lower lip tends to be a little less developed. Lips of Caucasians may be more volume-deficient, whereas in West Asians, Africans, and Hispanics the proportions and size more often conform to optimal ratios and size.

A consensus group issued a number of consensus statements with regard to East Asian versus Caucasian aesthetics.[58] Quoting from that paper:

• "Beautiful people of all races show similarity in facial characteristics while retaining distinct ethnic features.

• Asians are not a homogeneous group but rather comprise many varied ethnic origins, with each group having its own unique facial characteristics.

• Treatment to achieve esthetic changes in Asians should not be viewed as an attempt at Westernization, but rather the optimization of Asian ethnic features, in the same way that Westerners who receive lip enhancement, lateral malar enhancement, or skin tanning are not trying to 'Easternize' their appearance as they attempt to make up for their intrinsic ethnicity-associated structural weaknesses."

These statements may be extrapolated to describe the universality of beauty, with each racial or ethnic group exhibiting greater strength in certain volume-related characteristics than other groups. Caucasians may have more anterior projection of facial features, the midface, and lower face, whereas East Asian and African populations may have more facial width intrinsically. In each group, benefit can be sought by maximizing good structural characteristics, while improving common structural deficiencies typical of their ethnicity. Truly beautiful people of any ethnicity show the strong points of the group but may be outliers with regard to that group's deficiencies. So in terms of volume, an oval facial shape in females and a square, angular face in men are truly youthful and attractive in any race.

## Conclusion

Returning to the questions posed at the beginning of this chapter, namely:

1. The very existence of beauty.

Why does beauty exist in nature and in human beings? Why do we strive to achieve a goal of increased beauty? Why do people wish to attain it? What is in it for them?

The answers appear to be that beauty is a basic appreciative skill we all have, which may have survival value. The survival value is to keep us safe and our current gene pool safe.

2. The principles upon which we judge facial beauty.

A major principle is the selective placement of volume. It allows recognition of each other and to distinguish age and gender for mate selection. The different distribution between males and females and the volume shifts occurring from childhood to maturity are our indicators of sexual maturity.

Beauty in the guise of optimal facial shape, symmetry, sweeping curves in a young adult female, angles and sharpness in a young male, proportions of the face, and the relationship between the features all rely on volume distribution. Aging distorts the flow of this volume, creating compartmentalization cascading volume shifts caught up by the retaining ligaments of the face. Volume is utterly instrumental in every aspect of our understanding of facial beauty.

## References

1. Baig MA. Surgical enhancement of facial beauty and its psychological significance. *Ann R Australas Coll Dent Surg.* 2004;17:64–67.

2. Smith CU. Evolutionary neurobiology and aesthetics. *Perspect Biol Med.* 2005;48:17–30.

3. Dutton D. *TED talk.* <http://www.ted.com/talks/denis_dutton_a_darwinian_theory_of_beauty.html>; 2010. Accessed 29.07.16.

4. Rhodes G. The evolution of facial attractiveness. *Annu Rev Psychol.* 2006;57:199–226.

5. Little AC, Jones BC, DeBruine LM. Facial attractiveness: evolutionary based research. *Philos Trans Roy Soc B.* 2011;366:1638–1659.

6. Little AC, Perrett DI. Facial attractiveness. In: Adams RA Jr, Ambady N, Nakayama K, Shimojo S, eds. The Science of Social Vision. Oxford: Oxford University Press; 2011:164–185.

7. Whitehead RD, Ozakinci G, Perrett DI. Attractive skin coloration: harnessing sexual selection to improve diet and health. *Evol Psychol.* 2012;10:842–854.

8. Fink B, Neave N. The biology of facial beauty. *Int J Cosmet Sci.* 2005;27:317–325.

9. Penton-Voak IS, Morrison ER. Structure, expression and motion in facial attractiveness. In: Calder AJ, Rhodes G, Johnson MH, Haxby JV, eds. The Oxford Handbook of Face Perception. New York, NY: Oxford University Press; 2011:653–672.

10. Hogan PC. Literary aesthetics: beauty, the brain, and Mrs. Dalloway. *Prog Brain Res.* 2013;205:319–337.

11. Samson N, Fink B, Matts PJ. Visible skin condition and perception of human facial appearance. *Int J Cosmet Sci.* 2010;32:167–184.

12. Baig MA. Surgical enhancement of facial beauty and its psychological significance. *Ann R Australas Coll Dent Surg.* 2004;17:64–67.

13. Swift A, Remington K. BeautiPHIcation™: a global approach to facial beauty. *Clin Plast Surg.* 2011;38:347–377.

14. Borelli C, Berneburg M. "Beauty lies in the eye of the beholder"? Aspects of beauty and attractiveness. *J Dtsch Dermatol Ges.* 2010;8:326–330.

15. Patel U, Fitzgerald R. Facial shaping: beyond lines and folds with fillers. *Drugs Dermatol.* 2010;9(8 suppl ODAC Conf Pt 2):s129–s137.

16. Buggio L, Vercellini P, Somigliana E, Viganò P, Frattaruolo MP, Fedele L. "You are so beautiful": behind women's attractiveness towards the biology of reproduction: a narrative review. *Gynecol Endocrinol.* 2012;28:753–757.

17. Eagly AH, Ashmore RD, Makhijani MG, Longo LC. What is beautiful is good, but…: a meta-analytic review of research on the physical attractiveness stereotype. *Psychol Bull.* 1991;110:109–128.

18. Dion K, Berscheid E, Walster E. What is beautiful is good. *J Pers Soc Psychol.* 1972;24:285–290.

19. Yokoyama T, Noguchi Y, Tachibana R, Mukaida S, Kita S. A critical role of holistic processing in face gender perception. *Front Hum Neurosci.* 2014;8:477(1–10).

20. Zhao M, Hayward WG. Holistic processing underlies gender judgments of faces. *Atten Percept Psychophys.* 2010;72:591–596.

21. Werheid K, Schacht A, Sommer W. Facial attractiveness modulates early and late event-related brain potentials. *Biol Psychol.* 2007;76:100–108. Epub 2007 Jul 4.

22. Schacht A, Werheid K, Sommer W. The appraisal of facial beauty is rapid but not mandatory. *Cogn Affect Behav Neurosci.* 2008;8(2):132–142.

23. Lu Y, Wang J, Wang L, Wang J, Qin J. Neural responses to cartoon facial attractiveness: An event-related potential study. *Neurosci Bull.* 2014;30:441–450.

24. Chatterjee A, Thomas A, Smith SE, Aguirre GK. The neural response to facial attractiveness. *Neuropsychology.* 2009;23:135–143.

25. Sui J, Liu CH. Can beauty be ignored? Effects of facial attractiveness on covert attention. *Psychon Bull Rev.* 2009;16:276–281.

26. Cappelle T, Fink B. Changes in women's attractiveness perception of masculine men's dances across the ovulatory cycle: preliminary data. *Evol Psychol.* 2013;11:965–972.

27. Postma E. A relationship between attractiveness and performance in professional cyclists. *Biol Lett.* 2014;10:20130966.

28. Golle J, Mast FW, Lobmaier JS. Something to smile about: the interrelationship between attractiveness and emotional expression. *Cogn Emot.* 2014;28:298–310.

29. Xu Y, Lee A, Wu WL, Liu X, Birkholz P. Human vocal attractiveness as signaled by body size projection. *PLoS One.* 2013;8:e62397.

30. Zhang H, Teng F, Chan DK, Zhang D. Physical attractiveness, attitudes toward career, and mate preferences among young Chinese women. *Evol Psychol.* 2014;12:97–114.

31. Fisher ML, Voracek M. The shape of beauty: determinants of female physical attractiveness. *J Cosmet Dermatol.* 2006;5:190–194.

32. Shetty R. Outer Circle Versus Inner Circle: Special Considerations While Rejuvenating an Indian Face Using Fillers. *J Cutan Aesthet Surg.* 2015;8:169–172.

33. Little JW. Volumetric perceptions in midfacial aging with altered priorities for rejuvenation. *Plast Reconstr Surg.* 2000;105:252–266; discussion 286–289.

34. Shetty R. Under eye infraorbital injection technique: the best value in facial rejuvenation. *J Cosmet Dermatol.* 2014;13:79–84.

35. Mendelson B. Wong C. Changes in the facial skeleton with aging: implications and clinical applications in facial rejuvenation. *Aesth Plast Surg.* 2012;36:4:753–760.

36. Wong CH, Mendelson B. Newer understanding of specific anatomic targets in the aging face as applied to injectables: aging changes in the craniofacial skeleton and facial ligaments. *Plast Reconstr Surg.* 2015;136(5 suppl):44S–48S. doi:10.1097/PRS.0000000000001752.

37. Wan D, Amirlak B, Rohrich R, Davis K. The clinical importance of the fat compartments in midfacial aging. *Plast Reconstr Surg Glob Open.* 2014;1(9):e92. doi:10.1097/GOX.0000000000000035 [eCollection 2013].

38. Alghoul M, Codner MA. Retaining ligaments of the face: review of anatomy and clinical applications. *Aesthet Surg J.* 2013;33(6):769–782.

39. Ramanadham SR, Rohrich RJ. Newer understanding of specific anatomic targets in the aging face as applied to injectables: superficial and deep facial fat compartments—an evolving target for site-specific facial augmentation. *Plast Reconstr Surg.* 2015;136(5 suppl):49S–55S. doi:10.1097/PRS.0000000000001730.

40. Gierloff M, Stöhring C, Buder T, Gassling V, Açil Y, Wiltfang J. Aging changes of the midfacial fat compartments: a computed tomographic study. *Plast Reconstr Surg.* 2012;129:263–273.

41. Wan D, Amirlak B, Rohrich R, Davis K. The clinical importance of the fat compartments in midfacial aging. *Plast Reconstr Surg Glob Open.* 2013;1(9):e92. doi:10.1097/GOX.0000000000000035.

42. Rohrich RJ, Ghavami A, Constantine FC, Unger J, Mojallal A. Lift-and-fill face lift: integrating the fat compartments. *Plast*

*Reconstr Surg.* 2014;133(6):756e–767e. doi:10.1097/01. prs.0000436817.96214.7e.

43. Fitzgerald R, Rubin AG. Filler placement and the fat compartments. *Dermatol Clin.* 2014;32(1):37–50. doi:10.1016/j.det.2013.09.007.

44. Goodman GJ. The oval female facial shape—a study in beauty. *Dermatol Surg.* 2015;41:1374–1382.

45. Kane M. Commentary on the Oval Female Facial Shape—A Study in Beauty. *Dermatol Surg.* 2015;41:1384–1388.

46. Goodman GJ, Halstead MB, Rogers JD, et al. A software program designed to educate patients on age-related skin changes of facial and exposed extrafacial regions: the results of a validation study. *Clin Cosmet Investig Dermatol.* 2012;5:23–31.

47. Conway CA, Jones BC, DeBruine LM, Little AC. Sexual dimorphism of male face shape, partnership status and the temporal context of relationship sought modulate women's preferences for direct gaze. *Br J Psychol.* 2010;101:109–121.

48. Claes P, Walters M, Shriver MD, et al. Sexual dimorphism in multiple aspects of 3D facial symmetry and asymmetry defined by spatially dense geometric morphometrics. *J Anat.* 2012;221:97–114.

49. Thayer ZM, Dobson SD. Sexual dimorphism in chin shape: implications for adaptive hypotheses. *Am J Phys Anthropol.* 2010;143:417–425.

50. Glassenberg AN, Feinberg DR, Jones BC, Little AC, Debruine LM. Sex-dimorphic face shape preference in heterosexual and homosexual men and women. *Arch Sex Behav.* 2010;39:1289–1296.

51. Swift A, Remington K. BeautiPHIcation™: a global approach to facial beauty. *Clin Plast Surg.* 2011;38:347–377.

52. Goodman GJ. Acne and acne scarring—the case for active and early intervention. *Aust Fam Phys.* 2006;35:503–504.

53. Goodman GJ. Treating scars: addressing surface, volume and movement to optimize results: Part 1. Mild grades of scarring. *Dermatol Surg.* 2012. doi:10.1111/j.1524-4725.2012.02434.x.

54. Goodman GJ. Treating scars: addressing surface, volume and movement to optimize results: part 2. More severe grades of scarring. *Dermatol Surg.* 2012;doi:10.1111/j.1524-4725 .2012.02439.x.

55. Rhodes G, Yoshikawa S, Clark A, Lee K, McKay R, Akamatsu S. Attractiveness of facial averageness and symmetry in non-western cultures: in search of biologically based standards of beauty. *Perception.* 2001;3:611–625.

56. Magro AM. Evolutionary-derived anatomical characteristics and universal attractiveness. *Percept Mot Skills.* 1999;88(1):147–166.

57. Jefferson Y. Facial beauty—establishing a universal standard. *Int J Orthod Milwaukee.* 2004;15:9–22.

58. Liew S, Wu WT, Chan HH, et al. Consensus on changing trends, attitudes, and concepts of Asian beauty. *Aesthetic Plast Surg.* 2015, Sep 25 [Epub ahead of print].

# 4

# NASHA family

Rhoda S. Narins, Kavita Mariwalla

## Summary and Key Features

- NASHAs (non-animal stabilized hyaluronic acids) are a safe, reliable class of dermal fillers that have low potential for allergic response.

- NASHA fillers are nonpermanent and thus ideal to use for treatment-naïve patients and for beginning injectors because they can be easily dissolved with hyaluronidase.

- The type of injection technique selected (serial puncture, linear, fanning, depot, or cross-hatching) should be based on anatomic site and on injector skill.

- Common areas for injection include the cheeks, followed by the nasolabial folds, melolabial folds, chin, and lips. Injection into the glabella is contraindicated unless it is intradermal, due to the risk of necrosis and reported cases of blindness. Nonetheless, some physicians inject in this area and do so using a small-gauge needle and inject superficially, pulling back on the plunger before injection.

- Depth of the fold and amount of volume replacement required are the key components to consider prior to product brand selection.

- NASHA fillers can be layered on top of each other or on top of other semipermanent fillers.

- Hyaluronic acid (HA) fillers can last from 3 to 18 months, depending on location and amount of product previously injected; they last for longer in areas of low mobility and shorter in areas of greater movement.

- Postoperative sequelae are usually edema and bruising lasting only a few days.

- Cannulas can be used to injected HA fillers and result in decreased bruising.

## Introduction

The use of an exogenous material to augment soft tissue can be traced back to Neuber in 1893, who used fat transplanted from the arms to correct facial defects. Since that time, substances used to volumize the face have changed rapidly and include both biodegradable and nonbiodegradable products. The class of compounds known as non-animal stabilized hyaluronic acids (NASHAs) is composed of biodegradable fillers with an average duration of action of 6 to 12 months. This chapter will review the current NASHA products available in the United States marketplace and provide injection tips for the most common facial areas injected. Potential complications will be presented, as will advice on how to manage patient expectations.

## Background

NASHAs are commonly used to correct moderate-to-severe facial lines and restore volume loss that occurs during the natural course of aging. Since the US Food and Drug Administration (FDA) approval of Restylane in December 2003 the NASHA injectable market has continued to expand. According to the American Society for Dermatologic Surgery, there were approximately 1.01 million hyaluronic acid (HA) injections performed in 2014 alone. This does not include procedures performed by plastic surgeons or other aesthetic practitioners.

Knowing where to place these fillers is as important as understanding the subtle differences between them. In general, NASHA injectables are safe, confer a soft look, and are predictable in their volumizing capacity.

## Basic science

HA, or hyaluronan, is an anionic, hydrophilic, nonsulfated glycosaminoglycan that is abundant in human connective tissue. The chemical structure of this substance is uniform throughout nature and lacks a protein component allowing it to have little to no potential for immunologic reaction in humans when injected. As one of the chief components of the extracellular matrix, HA stabilizes intercellular structures and forms part of the fluid matrix in which collagen and elastic fibers become embedded. The average 70-kg person has approximately 15 g of hyaluronan in the body, of which one-third is degraded and synthesized daily.

HA contributes to cell proliferation and migration, as well as tissue repair. With age, HA concentration in the skin decreases, resulting in reduced dermal hydration, which manifests as an increase in lines and folds. In addition, excessive exposure to ultraviolet B rays causes cells in the dermis to stop producing HA. In its natural form

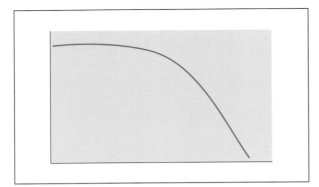

**Figure 4.1** Conceptual degradation curve of NASHA fillers. Note that the line is not linear, which correlates to the cross-linking agents used to stabilize the filler in the skin. Free hyaluronic acid has a half-life of 1 to 2 days in human skin.

**Table 4.1** Hyaluronic acid concentration of commercially available NASHA products

| Trade name | Hyaluronic acid concentration (mg/mL) | Particle size (µm)* |
|---|---|---|
| Restylane Silk | 20 | ~260 |
| Restylane Lyft | 20 | ~1000 |

*Even very cohesive products are particulate. The particle sizes of commercially available NASHA fillers are shown. In comparison, the particulate sizes of non-NASHA products are as follows: Radiesse (25–45 µm), Artefill (over 30–50 µm), Sculptra (40–60 µm), and Dermalive (20–120 µm).

**Box 4.1**
**NASHA products currently available premixed with lidocaine**

- Restylane
- Restylane Silk
- Restylane Lyft

the half-life of HA is 1 to 2 days and is metabolized by the liver to carbon dioxide and water. As a compound, it can absorb up to 1000 times its molecular weight in water; its mechanism of action as a filler is mainly through hydration.

The HA molecule is stabilized with cross-linked hydroxyl groups. It is this cross-linking that confers longevity to the product in the skin, and the degree of cross-linking is one of the distinguishing features of NASHA products. Because of this structural matrix, the degradation curve of implanted HA is not linear. Rather, the product retains its effect until the structural complex around the HA molecule is broken down. Once the unbound HA is exposed, efficacy is then lost (Fig. 4.1). As a result, patients will often suddenly notice a change in their appearance rather than experience a gradual loss over time. In addition, patients sometimes feel they look worse after HA injection than they did prior to it; however, this is more of a function of selective memory. For this reason, taking pre-injection photographs is important. As with natural hyaluronan, HA fillers can be instantly dissolved with the enzyme, hyaluronidase.

## Choosing the right NASHA

The main difference between commercially available NASHA products on the current US market is the viscosity of the product. The higher the concentration of HA, the stiffer the product and the longer it lasts in tissue (Table 4.1). The larger the particle and the greater the concentration of the filler, the greater the lift you get. However, it should be noted that not all of the HA in a given filler is cross-linked. Some is free, fragmented, or only lightly cross-linked so that the gel can actually flow out of the syringe with ease. As discussed above, the cross-linking is what confers longevity to the product, and this does vary between brands. In Restylane, Juvéderm, Voluma, and Belotero, 1,4-butanediol diglycidyl ether is the cross-linking agent, which forms ether linkages in the HA chain. In addition to cross-linking, it is worth mentioning that not all HA products are packaged in the fully hydrated state. As mentioned earlier, NASHA fillers create volume via hydration and, for this reason, patients will often look better or more filled 24 hours after treatment with products like Restylane, which are not completely saturated in the syringe. With that in mind, it is prudent not to overcorrect when using NASHA products.

## Patient evaluation

Prior to injection with any dermal filler, a careful patient history should be obtained. Pertinent items to note in this history include a history of herpes simplex virus, pregnancy or breastfeeding, history of keloid formation, presence of any autoimmune disease, and allergy to lidocaine because most of the fillers now come premixed with lidocaine (Box 4.1). A medication history should include use of multivitamins, fish oil, vitamin E, blood thinners, aspirin, ibuprofen, and *Gingko biloba* because all of these can predispose the patient to bruising. Unless medically necessary, the patient should be advised to discontinue these medications 14 days prior to treatment. In addition, alcohol use within 48 hours of injection can cause an increase in bruising tendency.

If the patient has had fillers in the past, it is recommended that the physician document how long ago, where the fillers were placed, and if the patient was satisfied with the results. In addition to history, preinjection photography is a must. These authors prefer at least three views:

frontal, left side at an oblique angle, and right side at an oblique angle. If a patient is having a specific area corrected, a close-up picture of that area is also advisable. Informed consent must be obtained, and the patient should be aware of the financial cost of the procedure prior to opening the first syringe. We also advise that baseline facial asymmetry be discussed with the patient and noted in the chart. From a physician standpoint, it is important to inform your malpractice coverage carrier of your intention to use fillers because many uses are considered off-label.

## Patient preparation

Patients should be asked to remove their makeup, and the areas to be injected should be cleansed with alcohol or a skin-cleansing solution that does not stain the skin. If there are any areas of infection, injection should be deferred. If the area is to be marked, these authors recommend using a white eyeliner pencil or an erasable marker. Use of gentian violet can create a tattoo if the needle is inserted through the marked line. Patients should be in a seated or reclined position to maximize comfort, while allowing the skin to drape naturally. For this reason, it is not advisable to have the patient lie down because this can distort the natural contours of the face. Hair should be pulled back with a headband or covered and pulled back with a surgical bonnet. The physician may decide to use a topical or local anesthetic prior to injection. If a topical anesthetic is used, this should be completely removed prior to injection and the area cleansed. Depending on the topical anesthetic and duration of application, hyperemia of the skin can occur and may lead to increased bleeding at injection sites.

### Pearl 1

If using a custom-formulated topical anesthetic, such as Betacaine Lidocaine Tetracaine (BLT) (7% betacaine, 7% lidocaine, and 7% tetracaine) be sure to monitor the amount of surface area that is covered with the medication because toxicity can result with high concentrations of anesthetic over large surface areas.

## Physician preparation

A note that includes a detailed facial diagram is helpful to document precisely where filler is placed, and labels from each syringe used should be put in the patient chart for traceability. One should also anticipate adverse events, so we recommend that any physician who is using NASHA products carry hyaluronidase in case of arterial occlusion or if the product needs to be dissolved rapidly, nitropaste in the event of purple dusky discoloration upon injection, and juice and crackers in the event a patient has a vasovagal episode. An emergency plan of action should be in place, especially if occlusion happens in an area that could affect

vision. If the decision is made to use a topical numbing medication prior to injection, topical steroids should also be kept on hand in the event of an allergic contact reaction. Lastly, it is helpful to have aluminum chloride at concentrations of 20% or higher available in the event of excessive bleeding at a needle insertion point, although most bleeding can be stopped with pressure alone.

## Treatment techniques

Several injection techniques exist for the addition of HA fillers to the face and depend mainly on the area of the face that is to be augmented. The five main techniques are illustrated in **Fig. 4.2**. Each has its own advantages and disadvantages, and all are based upon a transcutaneous approach.

### Serial puncture

In this method (see **Fig. 4.2A**) the bevel of the needle is pointed up and the product is dispensed in a droplet-like fashion along the fold that is to be lifted. Depending on the size of the aliquot, the physician may have to massage the area to prevent nodule formation. A disadvantage of this technique is that the patient will experience multiple needle sticks. Examples of areas to use this method include: depot in the infraorbital area with massage into the medial canthal region, acne scarring, and droplet into the lip tubercles (**Table 4.2**). Serial puncture is common for superficial dermal injections.

### Linear threading

The physician points the bevel of the needle up and through one insertion point that is usually at the inferior pole of the fold, the needle is advanced forward, and the

**Table 4.2** Recommended injection technique by facial area

| Area | Technique |
|---|---|
| Nasolabial folds | Serial puncture, threading, fanning or cross-hatching; sharp needle or blunt-tipped cannula can be used |
| Melolabial folds | Fanning, cross-hatching or depot; sharp needle or blunt-tipped cannula can be used |
| Jowls (prejowl sulcus and chin) | Serial puncture, depot or linear threading |
| Cheeks | Fanning, depot or cross-hatching; blunt-tipped cannula can be used |
| Lips—vermilion border | Linear threading |
| Lips—tubercles | Serial puncture |

**Figure 4.2** Filler techniques: (A) serial puncture technique from a side view; (B) linear-threading technique from a side view; (C) fanning technique from a frontal view; (D) cross-hatching technique from a frontal view. Key: *Orange line* is the skin fold.

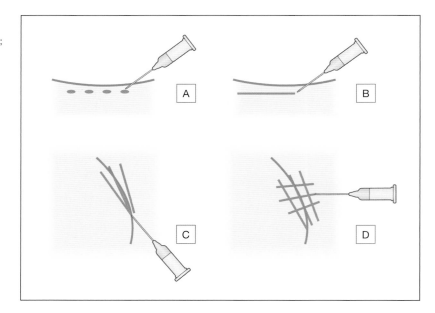

product is dispensed in a retrograde fashion as if laying down a cord (see Fig. 4.2B). This technique is suboptimal in deeper folds as it does not address the underlying structural support needed to lift certain areas of the face. Examples of areas to use this method include nasolabial folds and jawline (see Table 4.2). This can also be done using a blunt-tipped cannula.

## Fanning

Though the insertion point is similar to the linear-threading technique, in this method the needle is not removed from the skin but rather redirected in various directions in a fan-like motion, laying down product underneath the fold (see Fig. 4.2C). A blunt-tipped cannula can be used for this technique, which is excellent to help to prop up deep folds by addressing the overhang that occurs from adjacent skin. Examples of areas to use this method include: nasolabial folds, corners of the mouth, and temples (see Table 4.2). A combination of linear threading and fanning are commonly used together for volume correction.

## Cross-hatching

Several parallel cords are placed in one direction and then overlapped with cords placed perpendicularly creating a strutlike scaffold beneath the fold (see Fig. 4.2D). Though the patient will experience several needle sticks and the placement of filler in multiple planes can lead to more bruising, this method is ideal for treatment areas that require significant volume. Examples of areas to use this method include: cheeks, jowls, and marionette lines (see Table 4.2). Like the other techniques, this can also be performed with a blunt-tipped cannula.

## Depot

Through a single insertion point, NASHA filler is deposited in a single bolus with the needle tip pointing upwards. Massage is required afterwards to ensure that this bolus functions properly as a support rather than creating a nodule. Depth of this depot should be deep to prevent Tyndall effect. Examples of areas to use this technique include: cheeks, prejowl sulcus, chin, lip tubercle, and junction of the submental crease and melolabial fold (see Table 4.2).

---

**Pearl 2**

Injection technique should vary according to the region of the face, the depth and tissue plane of the injection and also on the thickness of the NASHA filler being used. Whereas fanning and cross-hatching provide excellent structural support and enhance volume, they can lead to increased bruising. Similarly, the serial puncture technique allows for more precise microdroplet placement of filler but can be painful for the patient. A blunt-tipped cannula minimizes bruising.

---

## Site-specific treatment strategies

### Nasolabial folds

Correction of the nasolabial fold is an FDA-approved on-label indication for all NASHA products and is the most common site for correction with NASHA fillers. The folds, or "laughter lines," occur as a result of movement of the malar fat pads medially and inferiorly with age, along with a generalized loss of skin elasticity. Fine lines can appear in this area as early as the third decade of life. It is important when assessing the nasolabial fold to note the presence or absence of a heavy cheek. If the cheek has dropped substantially, or if the patient is overweight with substantial contribution to the fold from the inferomedial cheek, the fold will be very deep and several syringes of NASHA will be required before a noticeable result is achieved. If this is the case, consider volumizing the cheek in the area of the zygoma prior to any filler in the fold. This will result in an overall lifting and pulling of the skin back to its original physiologic position. For the deep fold itself, the cross-hatch technique is the best one to use, or one may consider layering a NASHA product over another product that is placed in deeper tissue (e.g., Restylane Silk over Restylane Lyft). For shallow-to-medium folds, a NASHA product alone can suffice and the fanning technique can be used, starting at the inferior pole. In this case, cheek augmentation is not necessary. Whether to start from the superior or inferior portion of the pole is a matter of physician preference. At the completion of injection, place a gloved thumb on top of the fold and two fingers on the inside of the mouth on the other side of the fold. Gently mold the product to make sure that no nodules or bumps are present. HA fillers are malleable and can be molded after injection.

---

**CASE STUDY 1**
**Intraarterial Occlusion?**

A patient presents for correction of medium-depth nasolabial folds. She has no notable medical history, takes no medications, and is treatment-naïve. After injection of a total of 1 mL of HA filler into each nasolabial fold, the patient seems pleased with the results. She is told to ice the area for 10 minutes of every hour for the next 3 hours and to expect some mild discomfort the following day, with some temporary edema. The following morning the patient calls the office to report a patchy red and blue hue of her nasal tip. She denies any pain.

She comes to the office, and on examination she has a livedo pattern on the nasal tip that is dark red with a mild dusky hue.

Although one may suspect accidental intraarterial injection, the delayed discoloration indicates that the cause may be compression of the artery due to edema and product placement rather than overt injection of material into the arterial lumen and embolism, which would be seen by an immediate tissue reaction blanching and then discoloration. Using 12 to 20 units of hyaluronidase, inject slowly into the nasofacial sulcus, making sure to pull back on the syringe prior to injection. Massage gently to enhance dissolution of any HA gel in the area. In addition, apply a small amount of nitrous paste to the nose and advise the patient to use warm compresses to the area for the next 24 hours. The patient should be reevaluated daily until color returns to normal. Do not replace the HA in the area until full resolution of symptoms is achieved.

---

**Pearl 3**

If you see multiple lines lateral to the nasolabial fold, resist the urge to fill them because they are usually due to dynamic movement. Filling each line may improve their appearance at rest, but they will appear as cords upon animation.

---

It is important to remember basic anatomy when injecting the nasolabial folds. The nasal artery runs near the ala, so it is critical when injecting the superior portion of the nasolabial fold that one pulls back on the syringe plunger to make sure no flash of blood is seen. Injecting slowly with small aliquots helps to avoid this problem. This will prevent accidental intraarterial injection. One author uses a cannula 90% of the time.

## Melolabial folds

With time, the area below the oral commissure hollows, pulling down the corners of the mouth, creating melolabial lines, and contributing to jowls. The loss of volume is due to structural bone changes that occur with age; principally, as a person ages, the maxilla and chin grow away from the face and bone resorption decreases maxillary and mandibular height. Along with skin laxity, the result is a sagging appearance of the lower face that responds well to filler use. This location is especially susceptible to bruising after filler injection, and it is important to massage the area after injection to prevent lumps. Because of the need for structural support, the fanning or cross-hatch technique is recommended, as is the use of a thicker HA, such as Perlane. Typically 0.5 mL is adequate to volumize each melolabial fold, though larger amounts are needed to volumize the lower face.

---

**Pearl 4**

Although most patients can tolerate injection into the nasolabial folds, the melolabial fold tends to be more sensitive. Consider a mental nerve block, which will anesthetize not only this area but also portions of the lower lip. Use 0.2 mL of plain lidocaine 1% and inject in the sulcus next to the second premolar. This injection pain can be reduced with a 15-s application of benzocaine 20% (Hurricane gel) to the mucosa prior to injection.

---

## Jowls

Fat and soft tissue descent along the mandible obscures the bony definition of the jaw, which is considered a hallmark of the youthful face. HA fillers can be used to fill in the prejowl sulcus, thereby minimizing the appearance of the jowls. Filler is placed directly against the mandible and molded in a downward sweeping motion with the fingers around the jawline. The best technique to use for this is either a depot or linear threading. Placement of filler in the jowl area not only gives the illusion of a stronger bone line but also creates a relative tucking of the excess skin in the submental area. Be careful not to make a squared, manly looking jaw in a woman. Of the available HA products, Restylane Lyft is recommended for treatment.

---

### Pearl 5

In elderly patients the mental nerve is particularly exposed in this area of the face because it is covered only by thin platysma and skin. Therefore, to prevent nerve injury from the needle tip, be sure to stay in the upper subcutaneous or dermis, which is higher than in other parts of the face, owing to the thin skin in the jowl area.

---

## Cheeks

With age, the orbicularis oculi muscle loses both its tone and ability to act as a sling around the orbital rim. Subsequently, descent of the orbicularis and malar soft tissue complex prevails. Aging of the mid-face is dominated by descent of these malar fat pads (of which there are a total of seven), resulting in a loss of convexity and a flattened or even concave appearance of the cheeks. Filling the cheeks may result in softening of the nasolabial folds but requires injection in a deep subcutaneous or fascial plane. If using NASHA products, more than one syringe may be needed. It is important when injecting in this area that the patient be asked to smile so that the physician does not inadvertently create a chipmunk appearance in the patient. It is important to fan or cross-hatch injections and blend the cheeks back towards the temple so that the person does not appear to have implants at rest.

Anatomically one must keep in mind bony structure and face shape as related to race and gender. It is also important to have a discussion with the patient with regard to the hollow below the zygoma because many people want fuller cheeks but do not want to lose this line of definition on the face. Layering filler in this area is successful, as is use of more viscous HA products. If injecting in the upper part of the cheek near the infraorbital region, a thinner filler, such as Restylane Silk, should be used. The tear trough or infraorbital hollow is a special area most responsive to a HA filler. Small aliquots are placed deeply below the obicularis muscle, along the orbital rim with a linear threading technique. Care must be taken not to overfill this area because it may lead to eyelid edema and nodularity. Never use more than 1 mL of product in the infraorbital area.

---

### Pearl 6

Though it is possible to fill the cheeks through an intraoral approach, caution should be used, owing to the resident bacteria present in oral flora. A biofilm can be created, which can lead to severe complications. These authors recommend a transcutaneous approach when using HA or any other filler products.

---

## Lips

By the second decade of life, lip volume has reached full thickness in both men and women and starts decreasing by the mid-30s. In addition to the lips themselves, the vermilion border tends to thin, the corners of the mouth begin to slope downwards, and fine lines appear on the upper and lower cutaneous lip, which over time elicit the complaint of "lipstick bleeding." The philtral ridge should not be overlooked either because this flattens with the elongation of the cutaneous upper lip. Keep in mind that the philtral ridge is not a vertical ridge but rather angles slightly towards the columella from each apex of the cupid's bow, so restoration should be shaped accordingly. Injection of the lips is a staged process and should be performed with Restylane Silk rather than the more viscous HA products. Usually an infraorbital nerve block and mental nerve block are required for patient comfort, but it should be noted that it is important to work quickly after these blocks because the numbing will distort the position of the patient's lips. In addition, expect significant swelling and more bleeding in this area than in other parts of the face, which can cause a physician to overcorrect one area in response to edema rather than actual volume change. It is important to note any baseline asymmetry in the lips, as well as the presence of any scars, which can make filling more difficult. Lip injections of HA are placed in three planes: (1) volume filling within the lip muscle, (2) linear threading of the vermilion line, and (3) superficial injection of rhytides. The vermillion injection gives contour, shape, and lift to the lip. Identify the white roll at the border of the lip, and, starting at the corner of the mouth, insert the needle and use a linear-threading technique to inject into the white roll in an anterograde

---

### CASE STUDY 2
#### I Only Want to Fill My Upper Lip

A 56-year-old woman presents for filler of the lips. She is most bothered by her upper lip, which she feels has grown increasingly thin with time. She is insistent that she does not want to fill her lower lip because she is happy with the shape of it.

On examination, she has a flattened philtrum consistent with normal aging changes and has significant volume loss of the upper lip compared with the lower lip.

Although one must be considerate of a patient's request, it is appropriate to offer expert guidance so that the patient is not disappointed with the end result. Though patients may insist that filler be placed in only the top or bottom lip, it is important to maintain the lip ratio so that the result looks as natural as possible. The lower lip should always be more full than the upper lip. The ideal ratio of upper lip to lower lip is 1 : 1.6, which is based on the concept of the Fibonacci proportion. It is important to mention this to the patient so that, once filling of the upper lip is complete, the patient understands if some product must be added to the lower lip to maintain this ratio.

fashion. Repeat on the other side, making sure to fill to the apex of cupid's bow. Overfilling of the border will result in a platypus-like appearance of the lips. After crisping of the vermilion border (which by default will evert the lip and create the appearance of fullness) consider a droplet injection into each of the two tubercles of the upper and lower lips to give a more pronounced pout.

## Postoperative care and complication management

In general, NASHA fillers are safe, effective, and easy to use. Complications are generally limited to edema and bruising. After injection, patients are advised to ice the area for up to 10 minutes in every hour. Reusable ice packs can be given to the patient or they can use a bag of frozen peas, which is easy to mold over the area. In the lips, patients are encouraged not to purse their lips or fold them on top of each other, which may cause product movement in the first 6 hours. The following day, patients are advised to expect additional edema as hydration occurs. This may result in a feeling of soreness, which can be relieved with acetaminophen. Bruising can occur up to 72 hours after treatment. Anecdotally, *Arnica forte* can be used to prevent bruising, but no definitive evidence exists to suggest that this is always successful. The Tyndall effect is possible if the product is placed too superficially, as are nodules or lumps. The only way to correct this is to dissolve the product with hyaluronidase, keeping in mind that this will deplete some native HA in the epidermal matrix as well. Repeat injection should be delayed for 1 week after use of hyaluronidase. Complications, such as intraarterial injection, are possible though rare. Extra care is needed in the glabella where the risk of intraarterial injection is high and cases of blindness have been reported. If an entire syringe of product is not used on a patient, some physicians store the product for up to 6 months, carefully labeling the product with the patient's name. Because a physician cannot guarantee sterility of the product after it has been injected, we do not recommend this approach.

## Conclusion

The NASHA family of dermal fillers is a good choice for novice injectors, treatment-naïve patients, and for patients with moderate aging changes. The range of products available in the marketplace is fairly diverse and, once implanted into the mid-to-deep dermis, creates reproducible results with ease. The success of NASHA is as dependent on the injectable as it is on the injector and proper technique.

## Further reading

Bachmann F, Erdmann R, Hartmann V. Adverse reactions caused by consecutive injections of different fillers in the same facial region: risk assessment based on the results from the injectable filler safety study. *J Eur Acad Dermatol Venereol.* 2011;25:902–912.

Bellew SG, Carroll KC, Weiss MA, Weiss RA. Sterility of stored nonanimal, stabilized hyaluronic acid gel syringes after patient injection. *J Am Acad Dermatol.* 2005;52: 988–990.

Brody HJ. Use of hyaluronidase in the treatment of granulomatous hyaluronic acid reactions or unwanted hyaluronic acid misplacement. *Dermatol Surg.* 2005;31:893–897.

Carruthers J, Carruthers A. A prospective, randomized, parallel group study analyzing the effect of BTX-A (Botox) and nonanimal sourced hyaluronic acid (NASHA, Restylane) in combination compared with NASHA (Restylane) alone in severe glabellar rhytides in adult female subjects: treatment of severe glabellar rhytides with a hyaluronic acid derivative compared with the derivative and BTX-A. *Dermatol Surg.* 2003;29:802–809.

Carruthers A, Carey W, De Lorenzi C, Remington K, Schachter D, Sapra S. Randomized, double-blind comparison of efficacy of two hyaluronic acid derivatives, restylane perlane and hylaform, in the treatment of nasolabial folds. *Dermatol Surg.* 2005;31:1591–1598.

Cohen J, Strobos J, Narins, RS, Brandt, FS, Dayan SH, Hornfeldt, CS. Persistence of nasolabial fold correction with a hyaluronic acid dermal filler with retreatment: results of an 18 month extension study. *Dermatol Surg.* 2011, doi:10.1111/j.1524-4725.2010.01863.x.

Day DJ, Littler CM, Swift RW, Gottlieb S. The wrinkle severity rating scale: a validation study. *Am J Clin Dermatol.* 2004;5:49–52.

Hamilton RG, Strobos J, Adkinson NF. Immunogenicity studies of cosmetically administered nonanimal-stabilized hyaluronic acid particles. *Dermatol Surg.* 2007;33:S176–S185.

Hanke CW, Rohrich RJ, Busso M, et al. Facial soft-tissue fillers conference: assessing the state of the science. *J Am Acad Dermatol.* 2011;64:S66–S85.

Hexsel D, Brum C, Schilling de Souza J, Soirefmann M. A phase II, randomized, double-blind clinical trial comparing safety and efficacy of a metallic cannula versus a standard needle for dermal filler injections (hyaluronic acid gel) for the treatment of nasogenian folds. *J Am Acad Dermatol.* 2011;64:AB164.

Hirsch RJ, Cohen JL, Carruthers JD. Successful management of an unusual presentation of impending necrosis following a hyaluronic acid injection embolus and a proposed algorithm for management with hyaluronidase. *Dermatol Surg.* 2007;33:357–360.

Kablik J, Monheit GD, Yu L, Chang G, Gershkovich J. Comparative physical properties of hyaluronic acid dermal fillers. *Dermatol Surg.* 2009;35:302–312.

Leonhardt JM, Lawrence N, Narins RS. Angioedema acute hypersensitivity reaction to injectable hyaluronic acid. *Dermatol Surg.* 2005;31:577–579.

Lupo MP, Smith SR, Thomas JA, Murphy DK, Beddingfield FC 3rd. Effectiveness of Juvéderm Ultra Plus dermal filler in the treatment of severe nasolabial folds. *Plast Reconstr Surg.* 2008;121:289–297.

Matarasso SL, Carruthers JD, Jewell ML, Restylane Consensus Group. Consensus recommendations for soft-tissue augmentation with nonanimal stabilized hyaluronic acid (Restylane). *Plast Reconstr Surg.* 2006;117:S3–S43.

Monheit GD, Baumann LS, Gold MH, et al. Novel hyaluronic acid derm filler: dermal gel extra physical properties and clinical outcomes. *Dermatol Surg.* 2010;36:1833–1841.

Monheit GD, Davis B. Nasolabial folds. In: Carruthers J, Carruthers A, eds. Soft Tissue Augmentation. ed 2. Philadelphia, PA: Elsevier; 2008:105–126.

Narins RS, Bowman PH. Injectable skin fillers. *Clin Plast Surg.* 2005;32:151–162.

Narins RS, Coleman WP, Donofrio LM, et al. Improvement in nasolabial folds with a hyaluronic acid filler using a cohesive polydensified matrix technology: results from an 18-month open-label extension trial. *Dermatol Surg.* 2010;36:1800–1808.

Narins RS, Jewell M, Rubin M, Cohen J, Strobos J. Clinical conference: management of rare events following dermal fillers—focal necrosis and angry red bumps. *Dermatol Surg.* 2006;32:426–434.

Remington K, Schachter D, Sapra S Cohen JL. Understanding, avoiding and managing dermal filler complications. *Dermatol Surg.* 2008;34:S92–S99.

# 5

# Juvéderm family

## Shannon Humphrey, Rebecca Fitzgerald

### Summary and Key Features

- Hyaluronic acid (HA) injectable fillers are the most widely used fillers because they are a safe, effective, and reversible treatment that provides natural-looking, long-term results with little downtime.

- The Juvéderm family of HA fillers represents innovative advances in cross-linking technology (termed Hylacross and Vycross technology) and are currently the most widely used commercially available injectable HA product globally.

- The (newer) Vycross range of fillers are homogeneous smooth gels that are easy to inject and mold and offer products well suited for both lift and lines.

## Introduction

Injectable dermal fillers are commonly used to treat signs of facial aging and provide facial enhancement. According to the American Society of Plastic Surgeons (ASPS)[1] more than 2.4 million soft tissue injections were performed in the United States in 2015, of which 80% used hyaluronic acid (HA)-based fillers.

The Juvéderm family of HA fillers demonstrates innovative advances in design and development using a proprietary cross-linking technology. They are currently the most widely used commercially available inject-able HA product globally. This chapter will review the clinically relevant biophysical properties of this family of fillers (which includes Juvéderm, Juvéderm Plus, Voluma, Vollure, and Volbella; Allergan, Pringy, France) and discuss their clinical use.

## Basic science of hyaluronic acid

HA is extremely abundant in the dermis and consists of a simple nonsulfated two-sugar subunit, glucuronic acid and N-acetylglucosamine, which is repeated thousands of times. Highly charged residues on the sugar moieties confer hydrophilic properties, and the very large molecular size provides a domain that retains large amounts of water. This helps to explain why injected HA-based fillers excel at "plumping up" the dermis. Unlike the highly allergenic collagens, HA is a nonimmunogenic molecule, a "pristine" polysaccharide polymer completely devoid of protein epitopes. Another advantage of HA is that if problems arise, it can be easily removed by digestion with an enzyme, hyaluronidase.

### Pearl 1

All HA fillers can be reversed with the use of hyaluronidase. Longer-lasting HA fillers may require a higher dose or more frequent injections of hyaluronidase to clear completely.

Modern HA-based fillers are created typically by cross-linking the HA chains by conjugation with butanediol diglycidyl ether (BDDE). This cross-linked HA can be processed in different ways to yield homogeneous gels (the Juvéderm family) or suspensions of particles in gel carriers (NASHA Restylane). Each type of HA filler has a different amount of HA and is developed using different cross-linking processes, both of which significantly affect the properties of the gel that contribute to the aesthetic outcome, as well as slow its degradation in tissue.

Finally, although HA fillers were originally thought to act solely by passively adding volume, other possible mechanisms of action were recognized in 2007 when Wang et al. performed the first experiments showing an HA filler indirectly led to neocollagenesis through mechanical stretching of fibroblasts.

## Understanding rheology and its clinical implications

To understand and predict how fillers will behave clinically, quite a bit of attention since 2006 has been given to the various aspects of filler rheology, which is the study of how a material deforms and reacts under mechanical stress. An understanding of some basic terms like viscoelasticity, cohesivity, and viscosity is clinically relevant because it facilitates a better understanding of which fillers are best suited for specific indications.

An excellent summary of this information was published by Pierre et al.[2] and is included here in Table 5.1.

The four main fundamental rheologic parameters that describe viscoelastic properties are $G^*$ (complex modulus), $G'$ (elastic modulus), $G''$ (viscous modulus),

**Table 5.1** Definition and clinical relevance of rheological terms related to hyaluronic acid-based dermal fillers

| Term | Definitions applied to fillers | Clinical relevance |
|---|---|---|
| Viscoelasticity | Elastic and viscous properties of fillers | Elasticity provides a lasting filling effect; the filler must be viscous to be injectable |
| Complex modulus (G*) | Energy needed to deform a filler through shear stress (gel firmness or hardness) | Low G* fillers are better suited for superficial filling because they cannot be felt after implantation; high G* fillers are better suited for volumization (but optimal volumization also requires medium to high cohesivity) |
| Elastic modulus (G′) | Energy stored and given back after shear stress | Shear stress (lateral gliding) causes low G′ fillers to spread; higher G′ fillers will recover their shape better |
| Viscous modulus (G″) | Dissipated energy during shear stress due to friction | Not a measure of viscosity |
| Elasticity (tan $\delta$) | Division of G″ by G; measures whether a filler is more elastic or more viscous | When tan $\delta$ > 1, the filler is mostly viscous (uncommon for cross-linked HA fillers); when tan $\delta$ < 1, the filler is mostly elastic (common for cross-linked HA fillers); lower tan $\delta$ is usually associated with a tighter HA network* |
| Viscosity | Ability of a filler to resist flow (filler thickness) | Low relevance for clinical performance; high relevance for ease of injection |
| Shear stress | External force applied parallel to the surface; can be linear (gliding) or rotational (torsion) | Occurs when the filler is placed between two different tissue planes* |
| Torsion | Rotational version of shear stress | Uncommon in vivo but used with rheometers because this form of stress is easier to control than lateral shear; torsion and linear shear affect fillers similarly |
| Cohesivity | Adhesion between cross-linked HA domains caused by weak (noncovalent) interactions | High cohesivity helps fillers to maintain vertical projection while soft tissues apply vertical stress*; medium cohesivity provides versatility by keeping a balance between vertical projection and relatively easy moldability*; low cohesivity helps the filler to form a sheet by spreading evenly on injection and makes the implant easy to mold initially* |
| Compression force | Force applied perpendicularly to the gel surface | Used to assess filler cohesivity; caused by soft tissues applying pressure over the implant; these forces increase when the filler is placed deep in the dermis |
| Spreading | Lateral distribution of the filler caused by shear and compression stress | Filler hardness influences spreading caused by lateral gliding; filler cohesivity influences spreading caused by compression and stretching forces |
| Extrusion force | Force needed to eject filler from a syringe through a needle/cannula at a certain rate | Highly dependent on syringe geometry and type of needle or cannula |

*May contain assumptions.
HA, Hyaluronic acid.
*Reproduced with permission from Pierre S, Liew S, Bernardin A. Basics of dermal filler rheology. Dermatol Surg. 2015;41(suppl 1):S125.*

and tan $\delta$ (material elasticity). The viscoelastic properties of fillers are determined during the design and manufacturing process and are critically important because they need to allow for deformation when the filler is injected and initially molded, yet also allow for it to be elastic enough to resist deformation forces after being implanted (to provide longstanding correction). Some rheologic properties help to determine "what's used where." For example, a higher resistance to deformation over time is desired in volumizing fillers placed in the supraperiosteal or subcutaneous planes but not in a filler meant to be placed superficially where this property may lead to implant visibility. Softer fillers are easier to spread, a desirable quality for more superficial placement; however, one that would lead to an undesirable loss of projection in a deep plane.

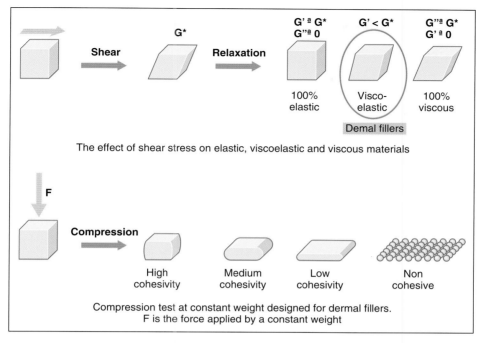

**Figure 5.1 A**, The effect of shear stress on elastic, visoelastic, and viscous materials. **B**, Compression test at constant weight designed for dermal fillers. *F* is the force applied by a constant weight. *Reproduced with permission from Pierre S, Liew S, Bernardin A. Basics of dermal filler rheology. Dermatol Surg. 2015;41(suppl 1):S122-S123.*

G′ is a measured value that describes the elastic behavior of a gel and its ability to recover its shape after lateral shear deformation (such as between tissue planes). G″ is a measured value of viscous properties and describes the proportion of energy lost due to internal friction from shear deformation. It reflects a gel's inability to recover its shape after the stress is removed. These values are measured under standardized conditions and are then used to calculate G*, which represents the energy needed to alter the shape of an individual cross-linked unit of filler. It is a calculation of "hardness," or <u>overall viscoelastic</u> properties, and is defined as $|G^*| = \sqrt{((G')^2 + (G'')^2)}$. In fillers with a high elastic modulus, G′ is nearly equal to G* (gel hardness) because cross-linked HA fillers have lower G″ at the shear rates found in facial tissues. For a given manufacturing process the gel hardness (G*) and elastic modulus (G′) are proportional to the level of cross-linking when all other factors are equal. Tan $\delta$ is simply a ratio of the two measured values defined as G″/G′ and represents the relative elasticity of a material. The lower the tan $\delta$, the more elastic the material.

Cohesivity characterizes filler behavior after it is implanted into the tissue. It describes the internal adhesion forces that hold individual cross-linked HA units together and is a measurement of the resistance to vertical compression and stretching. High cohesivity helps fillers to maintain vertical projection while soft tissues apply vertical stress, and this contributes to lift. Fillers with low cohesivity are easy to mold and form thin uniform layers in the skin (allowing for natural-looking correction of small skin folds; Fig. 5.1).

Rheologic properties of commonly used HA fillers are listed in Table 5.2. Although rheology allows for the comparison of physicochemical properties among different types of fillers, it does not completely translate to clinical performance because the filler's properties likely change upon interaction with tissues and with the impact of the biologic environment over time. As a supplement to rheologic data, animal models have been used to predict in vivo comparative lift capacity, resistance to deformation, and tissue integration of fillers. Hee et al.[3] found that although G′ had a positive correlation in fillers of similar composition and cross-linking technology, lift capacity did not correlate with increasing G′ when comparing different fillers as a group. In addition, evaluation of other physicochemical parameters (G″, compressive forces, HA concentration) did not show a consistent relationship with overall lift. They found that HA fillers had a low resistance to deformation during and immediately after injection and this resistance to deformation significantly increased over time (likely due to water binding and tissue integration). They also noted better tissue integration (related to a natural look and feel clinically) in the homogeneous HA versus particulate HA fillers (Fig. 5.2).

**Table 5.2** Rheologic properties of hyaluronic acid dermal fillers*

| Filler | G′ (Pa) | G″ (Pa) | Tan (δ) | Compression (gmf) |
|---|---|---|---|---|
| Juvéderm Ultra XC | 207 | 80 | 0.39 | 96 |
| Juvéderm Ultra Plus XC | 263 | 79 | 0.30 | 112 |
| Juvéderm Voluma XC | 398 | 41 | 0.10 | 40 |
| Juvéderm Vollure with lidocaine | 340 | 46 | 0.14 | 30 |
| Juvéderm Volbella with lidocaine | 271 | 39 | 0.14 | 19 |
| Restylane-L | 864 | 185 | 0.21 | 29 |
| Restylane Lyft-L | 977 | 198 | 0.20 | 32 |
| Belotero balance | 128 | 82 | 0.64 | 69 |

*Elastic and loss moduli are given at 5 Hz with a 0.8% strain. Compression force is given from a 2-minute linear descent (2.5–0.9 mm). *Reproduced with permission from Pierre S, Liew S, Bernardin A. Basics of dermal filler rheology. Dermatol Surg. 2015;41(suppl 1):S122.*

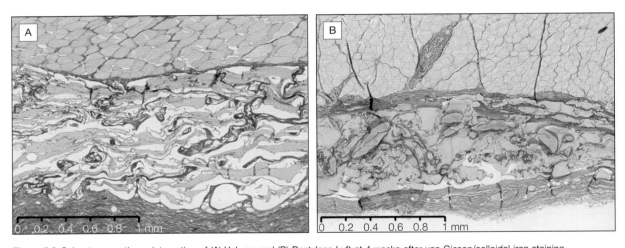

**Figure 5.2** Subcutaneous tissue integration of (A) Voluma and (B) Restylane Lyft at 4 weeks after van Gieson/colloidal iron staining. *Reproduced with permission from Hee CK, Shumate GT, Narurkar V, Bernardin A, Messina DJ. Rheological properties and in vivo performance characteristics of soft tissue fillers. Dermatol Surg. 2015;41(suppl 1):S379.*

## The Juvéderm family of fillers

### Hylacross and Vycross technology

The Juvéderm family of HA fillers began with a proprietary cross-linking technology developed to obtain a smooth homogeneous product with a low extrusion force for easier injection. This method, termed Hylacross, used a higher concentration of HA (24 mg/mL) to obtain a greater duration of effect than that seen with other products available at the time, and is used in Juvéderm Ultra and Juvéderm Ultra Plus, which vary only in the degree of cross-linking (6% vs. 8%, respectively). This product's ability to lift is derived from its high cohesivity (the increased cross-linking in the ultra plus product was done to further increase cohesivity and lift and expand its indications). These products are manufactured from high-molecular-weight (MW) HA and are more than twice as hydrophilic as the Vycross products.

Vycross is also a smooth homogeneous gel. It is differentiated by more efficient cross-linking achieved by mixing both high- and low-MW HA strands in the cross-linking process. This mixture allows for efficient and tight binding using a lower HA concentration, resulting in greater resistance to degradation and longer duration with minimal gel swelling due to low water uptake (**Fig. 5.3**). Vycross includes a range of products, each tailored to optimize gel properties best suited for specific indications, Juvéderm Voluma (20 mg/mL), Juvéderm Vollure (17.5 mg/mL), and Volbella (15 mg/mL).

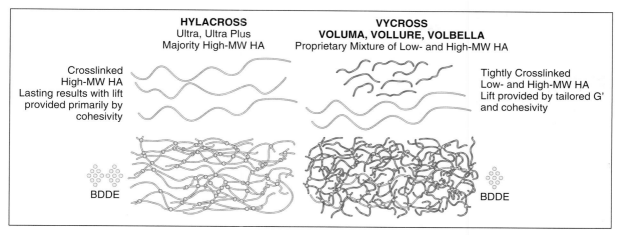

**Figure 5.3** Illustration showing Hylacross versus Vycross technology. *HA,* Hyaluronic acid; *MW,* molecular weight. *Reproduced with permission from Goodman GJ, Swift A, Remington BK. Current concepts in the use of voluma, vollure, and volbella.* Plast Reconstr Surg. *2015;136(suppl 5):140.*

All products in the Juvéderm family of fillers are sterile, biodegradable, nonpyrogenic, viscoelastic, clear, colorless, homogenized gel implants.

## Hylacross: Juvéderm Ultra and Juvéderm Ultra Plus and their clinical use

As mentioned previously, Juvéderm Ultra and Juvéderm Ultra Plus are smooth homogeneous gels with an HA concentration of 24 mg/mL, differing only by their amount of cross-linking (6% vs. 8%, respectively). They are packaged with a 30-gauge and a 27-gauge needle, respectively.

The original US Food and Drug Administration (FDA) Juvéderm approval was in 2006, following a multicenter double-blind, randomized clinical trial by Baumann et al., in which it was compared with bovine collagen: the 24-week study revealed superior persistence in patients injected in the nasolabial areas with Juvéderm. After a subsequent FDA-approved clinical trial by Pinsky et al.[4] demonstrating that after a single treatment the effects could last up to 12 months, the FDA granted a label extension in June 2007. The two XC Juvéderm products contain 0.3% lidocaine for patient comfort but are otherwise identical to the original products and were FDA approved in January 2010. The most recent FDA-approved indication was for lips in October 2015, using a multicenter, single-blind study that randomized 213 subjects to a treatment or delayed treatment group. The responder rate was 79.1% and more than half of the subjects maintained treatment response for 12 months. This is in keeping with subjective findings noted since 2006, as the most common areas of treatment have been the nasolabial folds, lips, commissures, marionette lines, and chin. **Fig. 5.4** shows a young woman treated in the lips with Juvéderm Ultra and in the temples with Juvéderm Ultra Plus, as well as Voluma in the cheeks, chin, and mandible.

## Vycross: Juvéderm Voluma, Volbella, and Vollure and their clinical use

### Juvéderm Voluma

Juvéderm Voluma was the first Vycross product and contains the highest HA concentration (20 mg/mL), the highest G′ (398), and the highest cohesivity (40 gmf) of the Vycross group. It has been used globally for many years and received FDA approval for correction of midfacial volume deficit (MVD) in October 2013 after submission of a multicenter, single-blind, controlled study with 235 patients led by Jones and Murphy.[5] This pivotal study also provided data for a publication focused on patient-reported outcomes by Few et al.[6] and a 24-month follow-up by Baumann et al., showing high patient satisfaction and a duration of at least one point correction (on a five-point scale) in more than half the patients at 24 months. It is packaged with a 27-gauge needle but also approved for use with a 25-gauge needle. This product has a high lift capacity, with little change in the volume of the implant following its deposition(Video 5.1). Voluma should be deposited deeply in the subcutaneous or preperiosteal plane as 0.2 to 0.3 mL boluses to avoid implant visibility. The lower cohesivity of Vycross-based fillers, compared with Hylacross products, is intended to provide appropriate malleability for the intended indication. The lower water uptake of the Vycross products reduces gel swelling.

| **Pearl 2** |
| --- |
| The low water uptake seen in the Vycross line of products means minimal postinjection swelling after treatment with Voluma, Vollure, or Vobella. |

Voluma is a very good volumizer, leaving the challenge with these treatments to deliver appropriate reshape rather than simply volumize or make it fuller. Mauricio

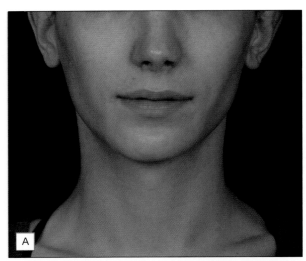

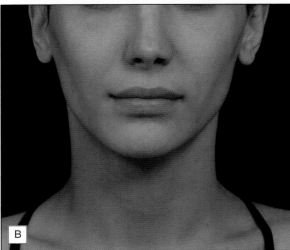

**Figure 5.4** A young woman treated with 1 mL Juvéderm Ultra in the lips and 1 mL of Juvérderm Ultra Plus split between the temples. In addition, a total of 2.5 mL Voluma was used for feature augmentation in her cheeks, chin, and mandible.

de Maio, a Brazilian plastic surgeon who has taught extensively on this subject, suggests that the patients be assessed on animation and in different positions (oblique, profile, head tilting down) and has created a guide with landmarks termed the MD codes. Videos using these MD code landmarks for treatment are included with this chapter (Video 5.2). An additional video using asymmetry and the fat compartments as guide to treatment is also included (Video 5.3).

Fig. 5.4 shows an example of a Voluma treatment for feature augmentation in the cheeks, chin, and jawline of a young woman, using a total of 2.5 mL. Fig. 5.5 shows an antiaging treatment in a much older woman. The older patient is shown in animation in both the before and after

photograph to demonstrate the natural appearance of this correction (as well as the improvement seen in her skin quality).

Juvéderm Voluma has been used with great success for applications requiring structure and volume; however, some practitioners found that blending the product allowed for more even spreading and a softer appearance, believed to be due to better tissue integration and less lift. Blending a filler to reduce its HA concentration can result in a decrease of G*, G′, and G″, making the gel softer, less elastic, and less viscous in addition to possibly reducing the filler's intrinsic duration. Perhaps in response to this, Juvéderm developed Vollure and Volbella, which contain 17.5 and 15 mg/mL HA, respectively, (compared with 20 mg/mL for Voluma). These two products have a lower elastic modulus (G′) and cohesivity than Voluma and are less likely to lead to any irregularities of the skin surface.

> ### Pearl 3
>
> Juvéderm Voluma is well suited to lifting and adding volume and structure to tissue, Juvéderm Vollure is better suited to contouring and filling of lines, and Juvéderm Volbella is ideal for superficial use to smooth fine lines and to add soft volume periorally.

### Juvéderm Vollure

In terms of HA concentration (17.5 mg/mL), elastic modulus (G′ 398 Pa), and cohesivity (30 gmf), Juvéderm Vollure falls between Voluma and Volbella and it has approximately 30% less water uptake than Voluma. There is little published evidence for use of this intermediate formulation, so its suggested use is based on clinical experience and extrapolated from its rheologic properties. Vollure is indicated for implantation in the subdermal plane or into the deep dermis to ameliorate the appearance of nasolabial folds. Vollure can also be injected supraperiosteally for adding volume to the forehead, brow, temporal fossa, and tear trough when volume restoration is required and has been used for contouring of the nasal dorsum and tip. Fig. 5.6 illustrates a tear trough treatment. Vollure is useful for line chasing in the cheek, forehead, and glabella. Vollure's softer nature makes it well suited for perioral use and to restore soft volume to atrophic regions of the vermillion mucosa.

### Juvéderm Volbella

Juvéderm Volbella is the softest (G′ 271 Pa) and has the lowest cohesivity (19 gmf) of the Vycross line and is ideally suited for superficial use where consistent spreading is of utmost importance.

Volbella is a good product for injection into the mucosa of the upper and lower lip for textural enhancement. When used in the lip it provides less volume correction than Juvéderm Vollure. The two can be used together for optimal results, as illustrated in Fig. 5.7. A video of lip treatment is included with this chapter (Video 5.4). Volbella can also be used infraorbitally to correct tear trough

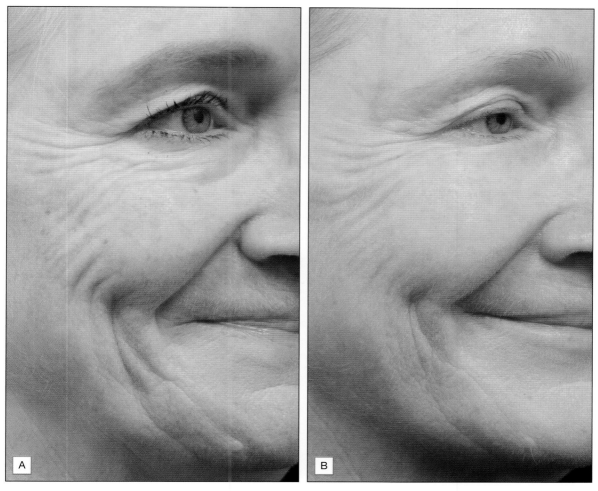

**Figure 5.5** Sixty-four-year old female complained of worsening of her dynamic lines on her lateral orbit and buccal region. She underwent skin restructuring with Vollure placed compositely in the subdermal (superficial subcutaneous) plane with cannula and intradermally with hypodermic needles. She also had Voluma placed in her cheek and Vollure in her lips and lateral eyebrows. Before and after shown in animation to demonstrate the natural look of the correction, as well as improvement in skin quality.

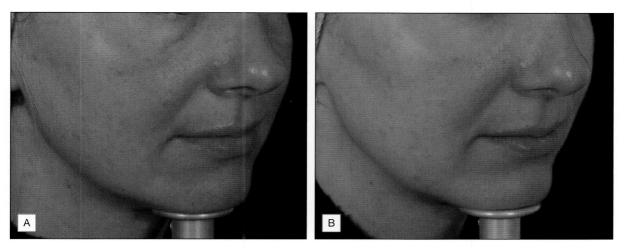

**Figure 5.6** Before and after treatment to the tear trough with 1.2 mL of a 17 mg/mL smooth viscous cohesive hyaluronic acid filler (Juvéderm Vollure).

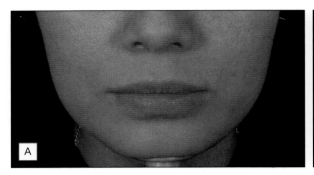 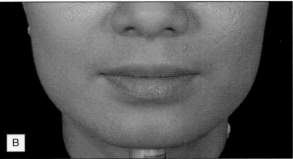

**Figure 5.7** Before and after treatment to the lips with a total of 0.65 mL of a 15 mg/mL smooth viscous cohesive hyaluronic acid filler injected submucosally (Juvéderm Volbella), and 0.4 mL of a 17 mg/mL smooth viscous cohesive hyaluronic acid filler (Juvéderm Vollure) injected intramuscularly along the wet/dry margin of upper lip and 4 units of onabotulinumtoxin A (botox) periorally.

**Table 5.3**  Indications for Vycross products*

| Product | Indications: upper face | Indications: midface | Indications: lower face |
|---------|------------------------|---------------------|------------------------|
| Voluma | **Temples**, forehead, and acne scars (superficial injections). Eyebrow shaping | **All areas of cheek including medial, lateral malar, submalar, cheek apex and preauricular areas, nasolabial fold (deep pyriform fossa injection), acne scars, nose dorsum, nasal projection.** Radix and nasal bridge-lift nasal tip | **Jaw angle, jawline, prejowl sulcus, chin reflation, acne scars. Lateral oral commissures, reflating marionette zone** |
| Vollure | **Forehead volume and lines, eyebrow projection, A frame of upper lid**, temples | **Midcheek accordion lines**, layering for cheek volume with Voluma, nasolabial folds, mid nose contouring (dorsum nasal tip, alar rim contouring) | Marionettes, **perioral cutaneous**, and vermilion; philtral columns |
| Volbella | **Periorbital, tear trough, glabella, forehead lines (intradermal injection)** | **Fine lines cheeks**, and maybe deeper periorbital lines | **Vermilion and perioral areas, fine upper lip lines, ear lobes** |

*When product is the treatment of choice for an area, entries are bolded.

*Reprinted with permission from Goodman GJ, Swift A, Remington BK. Current concepts in the use of Voluma, Vollure, and Volbella. Plast Reconstr Surg. 2015;136(suppl 5):142S.*

and hollowing and has also been used for superficial fine lines of the glabella, forehead, lateral canthus, cheek, and mouth. Accordian lines of the cheek may be treated with injection of Volbella or Vollure, either superficially into the lines themselves or subdermally to provide support to the region.

Off-face uses for Volbella will likely include horizontal neck lines and the décolleté region.

Goodman, Swift, and Remington, three international experts, published an article sharing their extensive experience with all three of these Vycross products, to optimize their use in the upper, mid, and lower face.[7] Their information is included here in Table 5.3.

## Avoiding and managing adverse events

Both Hylacross and Vycross products have been used globally for more than a decade. Published literature supports the use of these products showing consistent efficacy and

an adverse event profile in line with other similar HA fillers. Anecdotally some injectors have reported increased swelling immediately post injection with the use of Juvéderm Volbella. This remains to be substantiated in the literature. In one study, Juvéderm Volbella was reported to be associated with a higher incidence of late inflammatory reactions than previously reported for other HA formulations. Humphrey et al.[8] reviewed their experience with more than 11,000 mL of this product, and noted 23 episodes of inflammatory nodules, an incidence of 0.23%. These authors, along with Beleznay, have also published information on causes and management of late-onset inflammatory nodules.[9]

As with all injectables the face should be cleaned with surgical scrub and alcohol prior to injection. Precautions to avoid vascular occlusion should be taken as with all fillers (slow injections, inject perpendicular to named vessels, stop immediately if any blanching is noted, etc.; this information is presented in greater detail in a chapter in this text dedicated to adverse events.)

## Conclusion

The Juvéderm family of HA fillers represents innovative advances in crosslinking technology (termed Hylacross and Vycross technology) and is currently the most widely used commercially available injectable HA product globally. The products in this family are smooth and easy to inject. Juvéderm Ultra and Ultra Plus have been used for the lips, nasolabial folds, and marionettes for more than a decade. Vycross products can be used to provide lift and volume replacement with initial moldability. Where lift or feature augmentation is desired, Voluma is the product of choice. The more subtle lift from Vollure is an excellent choice in the perioral area, as well as the forehead and brow region. Volbella is soft and spreadable and is the best choice for fine line filling.

## References

1. American Society of Plastic Surgeons. Cosmetic plastic surgery statistics: cosmetic procedure trends. <http://www.plasticsurgery.org/Documents/news-resources/statistics/2015-statistics/cosmetic-procedure-trends-2015>; 2015. Accessed 18.04.16.
2. Pierre S, Liew S, Bernardin A. Basics of dermal filler rheology. *Dermatol Surg.* 2015;41(suppl 1):S120–S126.
3. Hee CK, Shumate GT, Narurkar V, Bernardin A, Messina DJ. Rheological properties and in vivo performance characteristics of soft tissue fillers. *Dermatol Surg.* 2015;41(suppl 1): S373–S381.
4. Pinsky MA, Thomas JA, Murphy DK, et al. Juvederm vs. zyplast nasolabial fold study group. Juvederm injectable gel: a multicenter, double-blind, randomized study of safety and effectiveness. *Aesthet Surg J.* 2008;28:17–23.
5. Jones D, Murphy DK. Volumizing hyaluronic acid filler for midface volume deficit: 2-year results from a pivotal single-blind randomized controlled study. *Dermatol Surg.* 2013;39:1602–1611.
6. Few J, Cox SE, Paradkar-Mitragotri D, Murphy DK. A multicenter, single-blind randomized, controlled study of a volumizing hyaluronic acid filler for midface volume deficit: patient-reported outcomes at 2 years. *Aesthet Surg J.* 2015;35:589–599.
7. Goodman GJ, Swift A, Remington BK. Current concepts in the use of Voluma, Volift, and Volbella. *Plast Reconstr Surg.* 2015;136(suppl 5):139S–148S.
8. Humphrey S, Carruthers J, Carruthers A. Clinical experience with a 11,460 mL of a 20-mg/mL, smooth, highly cohesive, viscous hyaluronic acid filler. *Dermatol Surg.* 2015;41(9):1060–1067.
9. Beleznay K, Carruthers JD, Carruthers A, Mummert ME, Humphrey S. Delayed-onset nodules secondary to a smooth cohesive 20 mg/mL hyaluronic acid filler: cause and management. *Dermatol Surg.* 2015;41(8):929–939.

## Further reading

Artzi O, Loizides C, Verner I, Landau M Resistant and recurrent late reaction to hyaluronic acid-based gel. *Dermatol Surg.* 2016;42(1):31–37.

Baumann L, Narins RS, Beer K et al. Volumizing hyaluronic acid filler for midface volume deficit: results after repeat treatment. *Dermatol Surg.* 2015;41:S284–S292.

Baumann LS, Shamban AT, Lupo MP, et al. Comparison of smooth-gel hyaluronic acid dermal fillers with cross-linked bovine collagen: a multicenter, double-masked, randomized, within-subject study. *Dermatol Surg.* 2007;33:S128–S135.

Dayan S, Bruce S, Kilmer S, et al. Safety and effectiveness of the hyaluronic acid filler, HYC-24L, for lip and perioral augmentation. *Dermatol Surg.* 2015;41:S293–S301.

Eccleston D, Murphy DK. Juvederm® Volbella in the perioral area: a 12-month prospective, multicenter, open-label study. *Clin Cosmet Investig Dermatol.* 2012;5:167–172.

Ho D, Jagdeo J. Biological properties of a new volumizing hyaluronic acid filler: a systematic review. *J Drugs Dermatol.* 2015;14:50–54.

Maytin EV. Hyaluronan: More than just a wrinkle filler. *Glycobiology* 2016;26(6):553–559.

Philipp-Dormston WG, Hilton S, Nathan M. A prospective, open-label, multicenter, observational, postmarket study of the use of a 15 mg/mL hyaluronic acid dermal filler in the lips. *J Cosmet Dermatol.* 2014;13(2):125–134.

Raspaldo H, Chantrey J, Belhaouari L, Saleh R, Murphy DK. Juvederm Volbella with lidocaine for lip and perioral enhancement: a prospective, randomized, controlled trial. *Plast Reconstr Surg.* 2015;3(3):e321.

Wan D, Amirlak B, Rohrich R, Rohrich R, Davis K. The clinical importance of the fat compartments in midfacial aging. *Plast Reconstr Surg.* 2013;1:e92.

# 6

# Belotero and Teosyal

## Berthold Rzany

### Summary and Key Features

- Belotero and Teosyal are two commonly used hyaluronic acid families.
- Belotero and Teosyal come in several products with and without lidocaine.
- Good clinical data (e.g., data from randomized controlled trials) have been published for Belotero Balance (formerly Belotero Basic) and Teosyal Deep Lines.
- After treatment of the nasolabial folds Belotero Balance and Teosyal Deep Lines still show at least a 1-grade difference at 6 months.
- So far the Belotero and the Teosyal family have a good safety profile.

## Introduction

Hyaluronic acid (HA)-based dermal fillers are currently the most popular, nonpermanent injectable materials available for the correction of age-related changes of the face and beyond the face (wrinkles, folds, and volume loss). HA fillers derive from bacterial fermentation from a specific *Streptococcus* strain *(Streptococcus equi)*, a bacterium nonpathogenic for man. Because natural HA does not persist in tissues for more than 24 hours, it needs to be chemically stabilized by cross-linking techniques. Most hyaluronic-based fillers, such as the Belotero and Teosyal brands, are stabilized by 1,4-butanediol diglycidyl ether (BDDE).

## Differentiation of hyaluronic acid fillers

How to differentiate HA fillers? Outside the United States a multitude of injectable fillers, specifically HA fillers, are available. Most of them are not based on good randomized controlled trials (RCTs). With no good RCT as a base it is difficult to give guidance on efficacy and safety for these products. The HA filler families discussed in this chapter are all based on at least one good RCT.

## Methods

For this chapter a Medline search was performed with the aim to identify clinical trials on the fillers discussed in this chapter. To reduce bias, only larger randomized controlled clinical trials and case series were included in this overview.

## The Belotero family

Belotero is produced and distributed by Merz Pharmaceuticals. It was formally produced by the Swiss company Anteis SA, which also distributed the product under the name of Esthelis (NB in some countries it is still available as Esthelis). The stabilizer is BDDE, and according to the manufacturer two cross-linking processes are used, leading to cohesive and polydensified matrix (CPM), which is supposed to ease injection while maintain long-lasting results. Belotero offers several different formulations: Belotero Soft (superficial), Balance (formally known as Basic), Intense, and Volume (deep). The Belotero products come with and without lidocaine.

## Evidence

We could find two randomized controlled clinical trials for Belotero Balance,[1,2] the first of the two with an open extension phase.[3] Furthermore, we were able to detect two large German case series, one focusing on Belotero Balance and one on Belotero Intense.[4,5]

## Randomized controlled trials

The aim of the first trial was to compare the safety and effectiveness of Belotero Balance with that of bovine collagen (probably Zyplast; name not given) in the correction of moderate-to-severe nasolabial folds (NLFs) in a split-face study. This is a standard study design for a filler product when approaching the US market. The study included 118 patients who were randomized to receive Belotero Balance and bovine collagen on contralateral sides of the face. NLF severity was measured using the Wrinkle Severity Rating Scale (WSRS; five points). As expected compared with bovine collagen, Belotero Balance was doing better at weeks 8 ($p = 0.009$), 12 ($p = 0.001$), 16 ($p = 0.001$), and 24 ($p = 0.001$). There were no significant differences between the two groups in the

**Table 6.1** Randomized clinical trials on Belotero products

| Reference | Products | Randomized/blinded | Area assessed | Duration of study | No of patients | Objective outcome criteria | Comments |
|---|---|---|---|---|---|---|---|
| Narins et al.[1] | Belotero compared with bovine collagen | Y/evaluator blinded | NLF | 6 months | 118 (92.6% females) | 5-point WSRS* | Belotero is safe and effective and superior to bovine collagen at 6 months |
| Butterwick et al.[2] | Juvéderm Ultra vs Belotero Balance | Y/evaluator blinded | Perioral lines | 6 months | 132 (99% females) | 4-point Perioral Lines Severity Scale, SGA (Subjects Global Assessment of Change) | Juvéderm Ultra shows pretty very similar effects compared to Belotero (NB the authors see some superiority of Juvéderm Ultra) |

*Wrinkle Severity Rating Scale.

proportion of AEs considered related to the injection site procedure. Most AEs were mild to moderate in severity and resolved within 7 days.[1] The Butterwick trial focused on the upper lip lines.[2] Here Belotero Balance was compared with Juvéderm Ultra. Although the authors saw a better performance of Juvéderm Ultra, the objective Lip Wrinkles Score did show quite similar results between both products (Table 6.1).

## Case series

The Narins RCT was extended by an 18-month open-label extension phase.[3] Ninety-four of the 118 patients were reinjected with Belotero Balance (now both sides, various time points) and followed for a maximum of an additional 72 weeks (96 weeks with the 24 weeks from the RCT included). The severity of the NLFs showed a decrease from baseline on both sides of the face, although the mean change from baseline was greater on the side of the face that had been previously injected with Belotero Balance than on the contralateral side injected with bovine collagen. Mean Global Aesthetic Improvement Scale (GAIS) scores, as assessed by the treating physician, were between two (improved) and three (much improved) at all time points. Only one (2.9%) related adverse event (hematoma on both sides of the face) was documented.[3] A further case series on Belotero Balance on NLFs with a follow-up of 6 months could be found. In this case series by Dirting et al.[4] 114 subjects with moderate-to-severe NLFs (WSRS five points) were treated with Belotero Balance. After 6 months 81% of 109 subjects, who finished the 6-month study, showed at least a one-point improvement on the WSRS for NLFs. Adverse events were mild, with acute erythema and swelling in approximately 70% of patients.[4] In another case series from Hevia et al.[6] on the correction of the infraorbital hollow, a very important indication with certain challenges,[9]

Belotero Balance was demonstrated to be efficacious and safe.

For Belotero Intense a large case series comprising 149 patients can be found.[5] In contrast to the previous trials, patients could be treated in several areas at the same time. However, follow-up was limited to only 3 months. Efficacy was measured by the WSRS (five-point score) and GAIS. Most treated folds were NLFs (83.9%), followed by Marionette lines (32.9%) and mentolabial folds (20.8%). Mean WSRS (all areas involved) improved significantly by 1.9 points from initially 3.98 to 2.07 (12 weeks). Satisfaction was described as excellent or good by 94% of the patients. Most common adverse events were acute erythema (63.8%), swelling (52.3%), and pain (49%) (NB at that time Belotero Intense did not contain lidocaine). These adverse events generally appeared on the treatment day and resolved over time (Table 6.2).[5]

## Rare adverse events

The Belotero family seems to be a rather safe family. Although adverse reactions can occur after every filler, no significant reports have been published.

## Clinical impressions

The nice thing with the Belotero family is that they come in not too many different products. With three products I can nearly treat every indication using Belotero Volume/Intense for deeper injections and Belotero Balance for more superficial indications (Fig. 6.1A to C). Belotero Balance is very soft and integrates nicely in the injected area. Merz does not have a specific lip product. Usually Belotero Balance or Belotero Intense is injected in the lip area. Compared with other products, Belotero Balance is softer but on the other hand might not last as long for this very movable indication.[2]

**Table 6.2** Case series on Belotero products

| Reference | Products | Randomized/ blinded | Area assessed | Duration of study | No of patients | Objective outcome criteria | Comments |
|---|---|---|---|---|---|---|---|
| Dirting et al.[4] | Belotero Balance | No/No | Nasolabial fold | 6 months | 114 (92.4% females) | 5-point WSRS* | This was a multicenter study. Product was assessed as efficacious and safe |
| Narins et al.[3] | Belotero Balance | No/No | Nasolabial fold | 18 months | 95 (92.6% females) | 5-point WSRS* | This is an extension study from the RCT from Narins et al.[3] At baseline all subjects received Belotero Balance |
| Pavicic et al.[5] | Belotero Intense | No/No | Nasolabial folds, marionette lines, mentolabial folds, cheeks, lips and chin | 3 months | 149 (88.9% females) | 5-point WSRS*, GAIS† | A real-life study with multiple areas treated, NLF and marionette lines were treated mostly with 83.9% respectively 32.9% |
| Hevia et al.[6] | Belotero Balance | No/Blinded evaluator, however the sequence of treatment was not blinded | Infraorbital hollow | 10 months | 46 (38 females) | 5-point FWS‡ | Product was efficacious and safe |

*Wrinkle Severity Rating Scale.
†Global Aesthetic Improvement Scale.
‡Facial Wrinkle Scale.

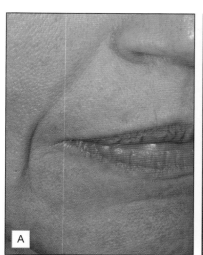 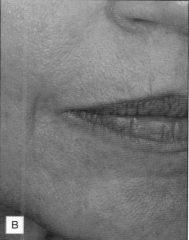 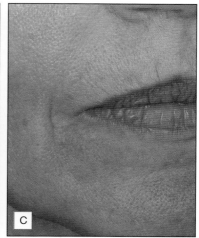

**Figure 6.1 A**, Patient (56 years old) on baseline. **B, C** Fourteen days and 182 days after a single injection of 1 mL Belotero Intense, respectively.

## The Teosyal family

Teoxane, a Swiss company, is the manufacturer of the HA filler family Teosyal. The Teosyal family comes without (the Classic line) and with lidocaine (the PureSense line). In 2015 a new line of Teosyal was launched, the Teosyal RHA family. All Teosyal products are stabilized with BDDE. All lines consist of various products. The Teosyal, as well as the Teosyal Pure sense line (the latter with lidocaine), ranges from Teosyal Redensity II, Global Action (superficial), Deep Lines, Ultra Deep, Ultimate

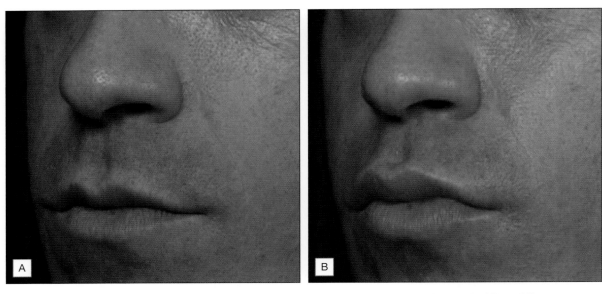

Figure 6.2 Upper lip augmentation in a 45-year-old man: (A) before and (B) 4 months after 1.7 mL of Teosyal Kiss.

(deep) to Kiss (Fig. 6.2A and B). The Teosyal RHA line includes RHA-1 (superficial), RHA-2, RHA-3, RHA-4 (deep). RHA-2 and RHA-3 are indicated for lip treatment.

## Evidence

So far only one good RCT has been published for the Teosyal line.[7] For the RHA line, one trial has been presented at a scientific meeting. However, this trial has not been published so far.[8] No larger case series for this product family could be found.

## Randomized controlled trials

This was a participant- and assessor-blinded, randomized clinical trial involving 60 participants with moderate-to-severe NLFs (three or higher on the five-point WSRS).[7] The study was conducted in a split-face design comparing Teosyal Deep Lines with Restylane Perlane. Wrinkle improvement was measured up to 7 months, using the WSRS and the GAIS. Both products showed immediate, good results after injection and touch-up and demonstrated good durability over time. The initial average WSRS for Teosyal Deep Lines decreased from 3.17 to 1.62 (two injections) and was still 2.23 at the end of 7 months. Participant preference for optional treatment at the end of the study favored Teosyal Deep lines. Both products were well tolerated, without serious adverse events.[7] For the RHA-family we have a 90-patient NLFs trial with three arms and six products among them, Teosyal RHA 2, 3, and 4 showing at 6 months good efficacy and safety for all the tested products (Table 6.3).[3]

## Safety

Despite being available for several years, there are no reports on adverse reactions in the medical literature. Because the RHA Teosyal family has been recently launched, no final conclusion can be at that moment made for this part of the family. However, I would expect not much difference compared with the original Teosyal family.

## Clinical impressions

Teosyal products are very easy to inject, specifically the new modified family Teosyal RH-family. One product, Teosyal Redensity II, is a very smooth product that can be easily injected in small amounts in very critical areas as the infraorbital hollow.

## Conclusions

Both Belotero Balance and Teosyal Deep Lines have been demonstrated to be effective and safe HA products for the correction of NLFs. These two products showed a superior efficacy to their comparators, a collagen for Belotero Balance[1] and Restylane Perlane for Teosyal Deep Lines (here the difference was not so striking).[7] When compared with other products, the new Teosyal RHA line gave at 6 months comparable results to Juvéderm products and the classic Teosyal line.[8] Although comprising 90 patients, this three-arm trial is still a comparably small study, which would have been able to detect large differences only. For the correction of lip lines, Belotero

**Table 6.3** Randomized clinical trials on Tesoyal products

| Reference | Products | Randomized/blinded | Area assessed | Duration of study | No of patients | Objective outcome criteria | Comments |
|---|---|---|---|---|---|---|---|
| Nast et al.[7] | Teosyal Deep vs. Restylane Perlane | Y/Y (evaluator blinded) | NLF | 7 months | 60 (86.7% females) | 5-point WSRS* and GAIS[†] | Teosyal Deep is safe and efficacious |
| Converset-Viethel et al.[8] | Teosyal RHA 2 vs. Juvéderm Volift, Teosyal RHA 3 vs. Juvéderm Ultra 4, Teosyal RHA 4 vs. Teosyal PureSense Ultra Deep | Y/Y (evaluated blinded) | NLF | 9 months | 90 (30 in each sub-study) 83.3% females | 5-point WSRS*, GAIS[†], and other | No clinical significant differences between the fillers could be noted. The final publication of the study is still pending. |

*Wrinkle Severity Rating Scale.
[†]Global Aesthetic Improvement Scale.

Balance seems to be comparable if not a little weaker compared with Juvéderm Ultra Smile.[2]

How far can we go with analogous assumptions? We have, except for one RCT on lip lines, mostly RCTs on NLFs. We do have case series; however, only two went beyond nasolabial lines.[5,6]

Because both product families have been around for several years with no major reports on adverse reactions, they appear to be safe (NB the Teosyal RHA series has not been on the market for long; therefore strictly speaking we need to be cautious here).

What do we want from the companies? I guess we have had our share for NLF trials. Ideally we would like to have more RCTs or at least case series on important indications. Will we get these? This depends if the companies target the US market, where RCTs are required for every member of the line, or if they have a special marketing interest in one indication.

## Acknowledgment

Martina Kerscher, Heike Buntrock, and Vanessa Hartmann contributed to the chapter of the 1st edition of the book, which served as a base for the chapter of the 2nd edition.

## References

1. Narins RS, Coleman W, Donofrio L, et al. Nonanimal sourced hyaluronic acid-based dermal filler using a cohesive polydensified matrix technology is superior to bovine collagen in the correction of moderate to severe nasolabial folds: Results from a 6-month, randomized, blinded, controlled, multicenter study. *Dermatol Surg.* 2010;36(suppl 1):730–740.

2. Butterwick K, Marmur E, Narurkar V, et al. HYC-24L demonstrates greater effectiveness with less pain than CPM-22.5 for treatment of perioral lines in a randomized controlled trial. *Dermatol Surg.* 2015;41(12):1351–1360.

3. Narins RS, Coleman WP, 3rd, Donofrio LM, et al. Improvement in nasolabial folds with a hyaluronic acid filler using a cohesive polydensified matrix technology: results from an 18-month open-label extension trial. *Dermatol Surg.* 2010;36(suppl 3):1800–1808.

4. Dirting K, Lampe H, Wolters M, et al. Hyaluronsäurefiller zur Korrektur der Nasolabialfalten—Ergebnisse einer klinischen Studie. [Hyaluronic acid filler for correction of nasolabial grooves—results of a clinical study.] *J Ger Soc Dermatol.* 2008;6(suppl 2):S10–S14.

5. Pavicic T. Efficacy and tolerability of a new monophasic, double-crosslinked hyaluronic acid filler for correction of deep lines and wrinkles. *J Drugs Dermatol.* 2011;10:134–139.

6. Hevia O, Cohen BH, Howell DJ. Safety and efficacy of a cohesive polydensified matrix hyaluronic acid for the correction of infraorbital hollow: an observational study with results at 40 Weeks. *J Drugs Dermatol.* 2014;13:1030–1036.

7. Nast A, Reytan N, Hartmann V, et al. Efficacy and durability of two hyaluronic acid-based fillers in the correction of nasolabial folds: results of a prospective, randomized, double-blind, actively controlled clinical pilot study. *Dermatol Surg.* 2011;37:768–775.

8. Converset-Viethel S, Larrouy JC, Hartmann M, et al. *Safety and effectiveness of three new commercially available injectable dermal fillers in moderate to severe nasolabial folds treatment.* Poster at the AWMC; 2015.

9. Carruthers J, Rzany B, Sattler G, Carruthers A. Anatomic guidelines for augmentation of the cheek and infraorbital hollow. *Dermatol Surg.* 2012;38(7 Pt 2):1223–1233.

# 7

# Radiesse and Radiesse with lidocaine

Renee C. Sheinin, Bassel H. Mahmoud, David M. Ozog

## Summary and Key Features

- The ideal soft tissue filler for facial augmentation should be nonallergenic and provide a natural look and feel.
- The procedure should require minimal downtime and exhibit few side effects.
- Fillers can be permanent or temporary.
- Calcium hydroxylapatite (CaHA) is well suited for facial augmentation and contouring.
- CaHA has demonstrated a favorable safety profile.
- CaHA longevity is approximately 15 months in active tissues of the face and may approach 24 months in more static locations.
- CaHA is approved by the US Food and Drug Administration for the correction of moderate-to-severe facial lines and folds, correction of soft tissue loss from human immunodeficiency virus lipoatrophy, and hand rejuvenation.
- CaHA injection does not require overcorrection, unlike collagen or hyaluronic acid filler materials.
- CaHA particles become fixed in position over time, do not migrate, and take on the natural characteristics of the soft tissue.
- CaHA filler showed a high overall level of patient satisfaction, a remarkable safety profile, and clinical longevity.

## Introduction

Soft tissue augmentation began in 1893 with free fat grafting and became more popular with the introduction of bovine collagen injections in the late 1970s. Dermal filler injections are the second most common nonsurgical cosmetic treatment performed in the United States, next to neurotoxin injections. The ideal soft tissue filler for facial augmentation should be nonallergenic, durable, and cost-effective and provide a natural look and feel. It should degrade naturally, require no reconstitution or refrigeration, have a long shelf life, evoke minimal pain on injection, require minimal downtime, and exhibit few side effects.

Dermal fillers are injected into the mid- to deep dermis for the correction of moderate-to-severe wrinkles and folds, restoration of age-related facial soft tissue volume loss, augmentation of existing facial structures, and improvement of nasal function. Some have limited indications for correction of facial lipoatrophy in human immunodeficiency virus (HIV) and acne scarring. There are many injectable types of filler on the international market, but only a small number have US Food and Drug Administration (FDA) approval. Fillers can be permanent or temporary and are classified into three categories: collagens, hyaluronic acids (HAs), and biosynthetic polymers.

The effects of biologic products, such as collagen and HA, typically last for less than 1 year post treatment. Semipermanent fillers, such as calcium hydroxylapatite (CaHA), are observed to persist for 1 to 2 years in patients. Poly-L-lactic acid relies upon the patient's granulomatous (collagen-producing) reaction to the injected material and the result can last 1 to 2 years. Nonabsorbable fillers, such as polymethylmethacrylate, silicone oil, and polyacrylamide gel, achieved the longest lasting aesthetic results, persisting for longer than 2 years.

CaHA, also known as Radiesse (BioForm Medical Inc., San Mateo, CA), consists of a 30% concentration of 25- to 45-mm spherical particles suspended in sodium carboxymethylcellulose gel. Its unique profile makes it particularly well suited for facial augmentation and contouring. In particular, its biocompatibility, ease of use, and enhanced durability offer physicians flexibility in both injection and areas of application. CaHA was first used in 2002 and was initially approved for vocal cord augmentation, radiographic soft tissue marking, and maxillofacial defect correction. In these applications, it demonstrated a favorable safety profile and was rapidly adopted for off-label use in facial contouring. On December 22, 2006, CaHA (Radiesse) received FDA approval for soft tissue augmentation in the United States. The product may be stored for 2 years at room temperature. The correction ratio is 1:1 implant to tissue volume. The longevity is reported to be approximately 14 to 15 months in active tissues of the face, may approach 18 to 24 months in more static locations, and is sited up to 30 months in the nasolabial folds. In addition to the site of injection, factors influencing longevity include the patient's age, ability to synthesize soft tissue, and rate of metabolism.

## Indications for calcium hydroxylapatite

On December 22, 2006, CaHA received FDA approval for facial soft tissue augmentation (specifically for the correction of moderate-to-severe facial lines and folds, including nasolabial folds, marionette lines, oral commissures, the prejowl sulcus, and chin wrinkles), as well as for the correction of soft tissue loss from HIV lipoatrophy. It had already received FDA approval as a radiological tissue marker in 2001, for vocal cord augmentation in 2002, for oral/maxillofacial defects in 2003, and for stress urinary incontinence in 2005. Most recently, on June 4, 2015, it became the first FDA-approved injectable filler for hand rejuvenation. In addition, CaHA has been reported for the off-label treatment of the infraorbital rim, periorbital area, forehead, tear troughs, temples, nose, neck, glabella, zygomatic area, internal nasal valve, malar/submalar regions, as well as orbital augmentation to correct post-enucleation enophthalmos, improvement of surgical and acne scars, treatment of a patulous eustachian tube, and treatment of skin flaccidity of the thighs, abdomen, and upper arms.

## Specific characteristics of calcium hydroxylapatite

A conservative approach is best with CaHA injection, with no need for overcorrection, because it naturally provides for a 1:1 correction, unlike collagen or HA fillers. The plastic surgery literature reports the clinical effects lasting 12 to 18 months post injection. Excellent longevity was noted by Bass et al., who demonstrated that CaHA has longevity of up to 30 months after implantation into nasolabial folds. This includes the immediate volume replacement, which lasts up to 12 months, in addition to the long-term corrective effect due to the collagen scaffold that is subsequently produced. In a clinical trial for lipoatrophy by Silvers et al. skin thickness measurements at 12 months remained statistically better than those at baseline. CaHA is highly biocompatible, with minimal acute reactions to injection and no reported serious adverse events. The particles become fixed in position over time, do not migrate, and take on the natural characteristics of the soft tissue as new collagen is deposited. In one study CaHA was successfully used in patients up to 85 years old. However, the results may be limited in this patient population as they have poorer skin elasticity with deeper lines and grooves and a decreased fibroelastic response. Therefore larger volumes of filler with repeat injections are often needed, and patients should be counseled to help to avoid unrealistic expectations.

## Mechanism of action

Following injection of CaHA, the gel carrier is phagocytized, and the CaHA particles act as a scaffold for new tissue formation and collagen deposition. Over time the CaHA particles are broken down into calcium and phosphate ions and are slowly removed via the body's normal metabolic pathways. When CaHA is placed in soft tissue, new collagenous matrix forms at the implant site. Collagen type III is made first and then subsequently replaced by collagen type I. Collagen proliferation and slow degradation of the microspheres lead to a prolonged duration of effect for up to 2.5 years. Imaging studies of patients after CaHA filler implantation showed the corrective effect lasted up to 12 months after the product was no longer visible.

## Injection techniques

In general, for dermal fillers the depth of the defect determines the depth of injection: the deeper the defect, the more viscous the filler. CaHA is typically placed in the mid- to deep dermis or subdermal plane. Deeper periosteal injections are used for tear troughs, temporal depressions, lateral cheek shaping, and mandibular contouring. Four techniques for injection are reported: serial puncture, linear threading, fanning, and cross-hatching (see Video 7.1).

### Serial puncture

In the serial puncture technique the defect is stabilized and multiple boluses of filler are delivered along the defect line. The injection sites should be close enough to form a continuous smooth bead, molding small gaps with massage. This technique is useful for acne scarring, shallow forehead rhytides, the glabellar region, philtrum enhancement, and nonsurgical rhinoplasty. Rolling acne scars may be treated with subcision prior to filler placement to create a receptive pocket for the implant and to prevent "doughnutting," or placement of filler around rather than under the scar.

### Linear threading (Figs. 7.1 and 7.2)

For this method the full length of the needle is advanced along the wrinkle or fold to create a tunnel for filler placement. Injection can be anterograde, with product deposition as the needle is advanced, or retrograde as it is withdrawn. Anterograde delivery has the advantage of displacing small blood vessels and decreased bruising, particularly in marionette lines and the prejowl sulcus. By contrast, retrograde delivery allows more uniform placement for the more novice injector. The preference

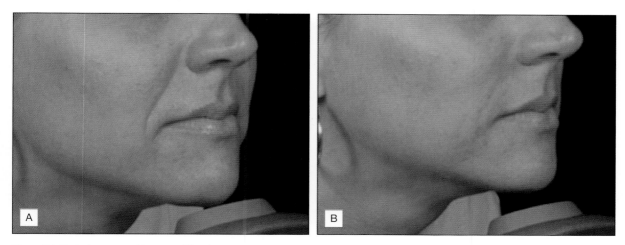

**Figure 7.1** Forty-three-year-old woman **(A)** before and **(B)** after injection of the nasolabial folds using 1.3 mL of Radiesse. *(Courtesy of Dr. David Ozog.)*

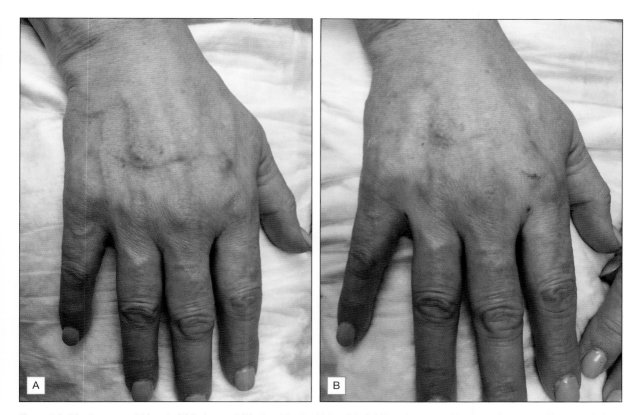

**Figure 7.2** Fifty-four-year-old female **(A)** before and **(B)** after 1.3 mL of injectable CaHA to the dorsal right hand via cannula. Vasoconstriction is due to use of epinephrine. *(Courtesy of Dr. David Ozog.)*

is largely operator-dependent. Linear threading is best for the nasolabial folds and vermilion contour. Serial threading uses elements of both techniques and is useful in wider folds.

### Pearl 3

Anterograde injection decreases bruising, particularly in marionette lines and the prejowl sulcus, whereas retrograde delivery may allow for more uniform placement of product.

### Pearl 4

The linear threading technique is best for the nasolabial folds and vermilion contour.

## Cross-hatching and fanning

The fanning (Fig. 7.3) and cross-hatching techniques are variations of linear threading that allow filling of larger defects or facial contouring. In the fanning technique a single needle puncture allows "fanlike" placement of successive linear threads by radially changing the needle direction through a single puncture site. Cross-hatching delivers linear threads in a predetermined grid by multiple punctures. Both techniques are useful in the malar region and oral commissures to build a scaffold in deeper defects.

### Pearl 5

The cross-hatching technique is useful in the malar region and oral commissures to build a scaffold in deeper defects.

Following administration, the injection site is gently massaged and patients are observed for adverse reactions. Other injection techniques may be preferred for other areas of the face for volumizing and facial contouring.

For temporal augmentation, the plane of injection is deep, immediately over the periosteum. Neurovascular structures are significantly more superficial in the temporal fossa, and a deep plane of injection decreases the possibility of inadvertent intravascular injury or injection. For each temple, start with a bolus of 0.3 to 0.5 mL of product with molding and massage to avoid overcorrection and nodule formation. Due to its high viscosity and elasticity relative to HA fillers, a smaller volume of CaHA produces the same degree of correction. This has the potential to be more cost-effective for the patient.

CaHA has been successfully used to correct volume defects in the periocular region, specifically between the lower eyelid and cheek, otherwise known as the tear trough medially and the infraorbital hollow laterally. Historically, CaHA was considered challenging in this area and thus not indicated. However, Bernardini et al. reported that treatment of this area with CaHA was safe and effective, with a favorable side effect profile and high patient satisfaction. This area does not contain any major blood vessels; the closest vessel of significance is the angular artery, which is relatively far away from the injection site. To avoid superficial nodules, as in temporal augmentation,

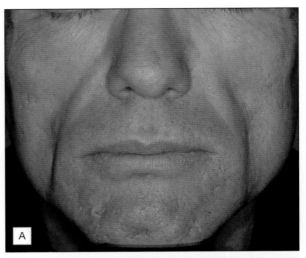

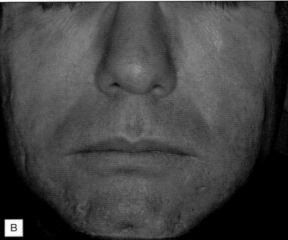

**Figure 7.3** Fifty-two-year-old male with HIV lipoatrophy **(A)** before and **(B)** after treatment with 6.5 mL of Radiesse per side. *(Courtesy of Dr. Alastair Carruthers.)*

the plane of injection is deep, immediately over the periosteum. At all times during injection, the needle should be angled away from the globe or vertically if performing a depot injection. The authors recommend treatment of this area to be performed only by experienced injectors, as well as preinjection and postinjection eye exams to assess for existing visual deficits and to allow for immediate diagnosis and intervention should a complication occur.

### Pearl 6

For augmentation of the temples and the lower eyelid–cheek margin, the plane of injection is deep, immediately over the periosteum, with the needle angled either away from the globe or vertically when performing a depot injection.

CaHA became the first FDA-approved injectable filler for hand rejuvenation in June 2015. In the FDA-approval study, 114 patients were followed for 1 year: 85 patients in the experimental group and 29 patients in the control group. CaHA mixed with lidocaine was used to perform multiple small bolus injections (0.2 to 0.5 mL) between metacarpals using a 27-gauge needle. A maximum of two syringes of CaHA were used per hand. The authors reported that 75% of patients had greater than a one-point improvement on the Merz hand grading scale. The mean injected volume was 2.6 mL per hand.

Prior to injecting, it is important to have an image of the ideal hand in mind to prevent overcorrection. Many injection techniques for hand rejuvenation have been reported, including single bolus, several small boluses between metacarpals, and using a 22- to 27-gauge blunt-tipped cannula through a 21-gauge needle incision. The dorsal skin is first lifted to create a tent for injection away from tendons and vessels, and the hand is then immediately massaged.

Gubanova and Starovatova demonstrated equivalent clinical efficacy and comparable safety profiles when comparing two injection techniques, serial needle puncture, and fanlike cannula, for hand rejuvenation with CaHA. To correct atrophy in each hand, an injection of 2 mL of CaHA mixed with lidocaine is sufficient. The effects of CaHA in the dorsal hand can last 1 to 2 years.

---

**Pearl 7**

For treatment of the aging hand and pedal defects, dorsal skin is first lifted to create a tent for injection away from tendons and vessels.

---

Prior to the introduction of lidocaine into CaHA, pain during injection was a limitation. Methods to minimize pain included application of nerve blocks, tissue infiltration with anesthetics, topical anesthetics, and physical aids, such as vibration, icing, and skin cooling. In 2009 the FDA approved a novel technique using the addition of lidocaine into the CaHA syringe just before injection. First, 0.2 mL of plain 2% lidocaine are drawn into a 3-mL syringe, which is then attached to a 1.3-mL syringe of CaHA through a Luer-Lock connector. The CaHA and lidocaine are pushed from one syringe to the other, back and forth 10 times, to create a homogeneous mixture. In a study by Marmur et al., of the 50 patients who received CaHA in one nasolabial fold and CaHA/lidocaine blend in the other, all patients preferred premixed CaHA with lidocaine compared with CaHA with no anesthetic. Busso and Voigts showed that the CaHA/lidocaine blend exhibited decreased viscosity, elasticity, and extrusion force and did not affect the longevity of the clinical benefits. This results in a product that is more spreadable and moldable, while decreasing the risk of ecchymosis and tissue edema. The addition of lidocaine to CaHA has significantly decreased injection site pain and decreased the need for adjuvant anesthetic techniques. Furthermore, the addition of lidocaine with epinephrine to CaHA has not formally been studied. However, there is anecdotal evidence that it produces less bruising when mixed with CaHA.

## Adverse events

In general, complications tend to be mild and technique- or location-related. Adverse events are classified into immediate (pain, hypersensitivity, anaphylaxis), early (swelling, ecchymosis, erythema, infection, overcorrection, necrosis), late (activation of herpes simplex virus, nodules, granuloma formation), and permanent (scarring). Patients' expectations should be addressed prior to treatment, and informed consent of the risks, alternatives, and aftercare instructions should be extensively reviewed.

The effect of CaHA in the cheek area has been thoroughly studied and has shown improved cosmetic outcomes and minimal adverse events. One study analyzed 100 patients with HIV-associated lipoatrophy who received CaHA injections into the submalar region. All patients were rated as improved or better on the Global Aesthetic Improvement Scale (GAIS) for the first 12 months, and 91% were rated as improved or better at 18 months. In addition, skin thickness measurements were statistically improved at 12 months compared with baseline. Adverse events resulting from the treatment were mild (e.g., ecchymosis, edema, erythema, pain, pruritus) and of short duration. Other clinical trials were performed in healthy patients seeking a fuller appearance to the cheeks and demonstrated similar patient satisfaction and side effect profiles.

Erythema and swelling may sometimes require steroid treatment. Nonsteroidal antiinflammatory drugs and other anticoagulants should be discontinued prior to treatment so as to minimize postprocedural ecchymosis. Use of anterograde injections, icing both before and post injection, and slow injection technique may also decrease postprocedural bruising, particularly in the prejowl sulcus and marionette lines.

Injectors should be aware of facial danger zones, specifically embolization of the supratrochlear (glabella), the angular branch of the facial (alar–peri-alar), and the dorsal nasal arteries. These injections should only be performed by experienced injectors, with a thorough patient understanding and written consent regarding potential risks, as well as easy access to appropriate tools for managing incidental intraarterial injections, such as nitric oxide paste and massage. Unfortunately, there is no reversal agent for CaHA similar to hyaluronidase for HA filler. Large nodules rarely occur when the injector is experienced. They can be treated with an injection of normal saline and lidocaine to break up the overaccumulation of product. Another technique used to disrupt the nodule and reduce its fibroblastic activity involves injecting equal parts 5-fluorouracil with lidocaine or lidocaine with epinephrine directly into the nodule.

**Pearl 8**

Injectors should be aware of facial danger zones, specifically embolization of the supratrochlear (glabella), angular branch of facial, and dorsal nasal arteries.

For hand rejuvenation, CaHA has a similar favorable side effect profile. Most postinjection adverse events are mild to moderate, transient, and self-resolving. No severe adverse events are reported. In the FDA-approval study, swelling, pain, redness, bruising, and pruritus were the most common side effects, reported in 99.1%, 92%, 81.4%, 74.3%, and 46% of patients, respectively. Swelling usually resolves within 2 weeks after injection. Pruritus can be treated with a high-potency topical corticosteroid.

With CaHA, no osteoblast activity (i.e., calcification or ossification) has been observed in soft tissue. CaHA is unlikely to provoke allergic or other adverse reactions. However, patients with a history of anaphylaxis to any substance or multiple severe allergies are contraindicated for CaHA injections for cosmetic indications.

Marmur et al. examined punch biopsies using standard light and electron microscopy techniques in a small number of patients at 1 and 6 months following intradermal injection of CaHA. Biopsies at 1 and 6 months showed CaHA microspheres scattered in the dermal/subcutaneous junction with minimal inflammation and evidence of new fibroelastic fibers surrounding the microspheres, but no apparent migration. No granuloma formation, ossification, or foreign-body reactions were evident.

One potential adverse event is nodule formation after injection. In patients undergoing augmentation of the lip, nodules can occur in up to 12.4% of patients. In the lip, they are an aggregation of material due to the sphincteric action of the orbicularis oris muscle. Regardless of location, nodules are treatable via massage, needle disruption of the nodules, or excision. Jansen and Graivier reported a reduced incidence of lip nodules by using a smaller injection volume in combination with a more conservative threading technique and by injecting at the proper depth (subdermal plane). At present, the authors do not recommend using CaHA for lip augmentation or for injections within the orbital rim.

Adverse events specific to temporal augmentation include bruising of the lower eyelid, headache, local tenderness, and prominence of the superficial vessels the first few days after injection.

Long-term safety has been demonstrated as an extension of the initial FDA-approval study. In 99 patients who received CaHA injection of their nasolabial folds, there were no long-term or delayed-onset adverse events, including no nodules, foreign body granulomas, infections, necrosis, or erosions for up to 3 years.

## Comparative research studies

CaHA has been extensively reviewed; however, the most frequently studied site in the literature was the nasolabial folds, followed by the cheeks. Two multicenter, blinded, split-face, randomized controlled trials by Moers-Carpi et al. determined that CaHA was superior to HA fillers in the treatment of nasolabial folds. The first study (n = 205) compared three HA fillers (Juvéderm 24, Juvéderm 24HV, and Perlane) with CaHA. Investigators found that CaHA showed the largest number of nasolabial folds rated "improved" or better. The authors concluded that the CaHA was more effective and longer-lasting than each HA filler in maintaining nasolabial fold augmentation. There was no serious adverse event requiring intervention for any of the injected materials. The second study (n = 60) compared Restylane and CaHA and again showed that CaHA was significantly more effective than HA, demonstrating greater improvement and longer-lasting effects. Both products were well tolerated, and no serious adverse events were reported with either treatment. Only four adverse events (two hematomas, one nodule, and one extrusion) were reported in 118 folds injected two times each during the course of treatment and were resolved without complications.

A third randomized controlled trial by Smith et al. (n = 117) compared CaHA with human-based collagen for 6 months. Photographs by blinded experts indicated that CaHA achieved superior improvement to collagen. Adverse event rates for both treatments were comparable, with some increase in bruising and edema at CaHA-treated sites.

## Outcomes in subjects with Fitzpatrick skin types IV to VI

An uncontrolled clinical trial (n = 100) by Marmur et al. assessed safety results of CaHA for the treatment of nasolabial folds in Fitzpatrick skin types IV to VI. Results from this study indicated that subjects injected subdermally with CaHA did not show signs of keloid formation, hypertrophic scarring, hyperpigmentation or hypopigmentation, or other clinically significant adverse events 6 months post treatment. Similarly, a case series comparing HA treatment in 40 patients with Fitzpatrick skin types I to III with 20 patients with Fitzpatrick skin types IV to VI concluded that patients with Fitzpatrick skin types IV to VI achieved improved aesthetic outcomes similar to patients with other skin types. No transient or permanent adverse events were reported among patients with Fitzpatrick skin types IV to VI.

## Safety outcome of calcium hydroxylapatite

A study by Carruthers et al. (n = 58) used radiography and computed tomography scans to assess whether CaHA poses radiographic safety concerns. The study determined that CaHA is usually visible and does not obscure underlying structures on computed tomography scans. In addition, the study found no evidence that CaHA migrates or that osteogenesis results from the CaHA being placed in the deep dermis and subcutaneous plane. However, patients should be made aware that this product will be visible on these scans and they should inform physicians to avoid any confusion from the appearance of the calcium.

## Patient satisfaction

A meta-analysis by Fakhre et al. showed that CaHA receives high patient satisfaction ratings. A limitation of this patient-centric data is its retrospective nature that is subject to recall bias. A rolling survey at multiple time intervals would be a potential solution.

CaHA, with all of its desirable attributes, is proving to be a valuable tool in the era of soft tissue augmentation. It has a high overall level of patient satisfaction, a remarkable safety profile, and clinical longevity superior to many other agents. CaHA remains an excellent option for the augmentation of nasolabial folds and other soft tissue structures of the face and is a valuable addition to the limited armamentarium of hand rejuvenation.

## Acknowledgments

**Funding source:** Radiesse materials used to make the photographs and video linked to this chapter were provided, free of charge, by Merz Aesthetics Inc., San Mateo, CA.

## Further reading

Amselem M. Radiesse: a novel rejuvenation treatment for the upper arms. *Clin Cosmet Investig Dermatol.* 2015;9:9–14.

Bass LS, Smith S, Busso M, McClaren M, et al. Calcium hydroxylapatite (Radiesse) for treatment of nasolabial folds: long-term safety and efficacy results. *Aesthet Surg J.* 2010;30(2): 235–238.

Bernardini FP, Cetinkaya A, Devoto MH, Zambelli A. Calcium hydroxyl-apatite (Radiesse) for the correction of periorbital hollows, dark circles, and lower eyelid bags. *Ophthal Plast Reconstr Surg.* 2014;30(1):34–39.

Bray D, Hopkins C, Roberts DN. A review of dermal fillers in facial plastic surgery. *Curr Opin Otolaryngol Head Neck Surg.* 2010;18:295–302.

Breithaupt A, Fitzgerald R. Collagen stimulators: poly-l-lactic acid and calcium hydroxylapatite. *Facial Plast Surg Clin North Am.* 2015;23(4):459–469.

Busso M, Karlsberg P. Cheek augmentation and rejuvenation using injectable calcium hydroxylapatite (Radiesse). *Cosmet Dermatol Surg.* 2006;19:583–588.

Busso M, Voigts R. An investigation of changes in physical properties of injectable calcium hydroxylapatite in a carrier gel when mixed with lidocaine and with lidocaine/ epinephrine. *Dermatol Surg.* 2008;34(suppl 1):s16–s23; discussion s24.

Carruthers A, Liebeskind M, Carruthers J, Forster BB. Radiographic and computed tomographic studies of calcium hydroxylapatite for treatment of HIV-associated facial lipoatrophy and correction of nasolabial folds. *Dermatol Surg.* 2008;34(suppl 1):s78–s84.

Emer J, Sundaram H. Aesthetic applications of calcium hydroxylapatite volumizing filler: an evidence-based review and discussion of current concepts: part 1 of 2. *J Drugs Dermatol.* 2013;12:1345–1354.

Eviatar J, Lo C, Kirszrot J. Radiesse: advanced techniques and applications for a unique and versatile implant. *Plast Recontr Surg.* 2015;136(5s):164s–170s.

Fakhre GP, Perdikis G, Shaddix KK, Terkonda SP, Waldorf JC. An evaluation of calcium hydroxylapatite (Radiesse) for cosmetic nasolabial fold correction: a meta-analysis and patient centric outcomes study. *Ann Plast Surg.* 2009;63:486–489.

Glaich AS, Cohen JL, Goldberg LH. Injection necrosis of the glabella: protocol for prevention and treatment after use of dermal fillers. *Dermatol Surg.* 2006;32:276–281.

Gubanova EI, Starovatova PA. A prospective, comparative, evaluator-blind clinical study investigating efficacy and safety of two injection techniques with Radiesse for the correction of skin changes in aging hands. *J Cutan Aesthet Surg.* 2015;8(3):147–152.

Hanke CW, Rohrich RJ, Busso M, et al. Facial soft-tissue fillers conference: assessing the state of the science. *J Am Acad Dermatol.* 2011;64:s66–s85, e1–e136.

Jansen DA, Graivier MH. Evaluation of a calcium hydroxylapatite-based implant (Radiesse) for facial soft-tissue augmentation. *Plast Reconstr Surg.* 2006;118: s22–s30, discussion s31–s33.

Lemperle G, Morhenn V, Charrier U. Human histology and persistence of various injectable filler substances for soft tissue augmentation. *Aesthet Plast Surg.* 2003;27:354–366; discussion 367.

Marmur ES, Phelps R, Goldberg DJ. Clinical, histologic and electron microscopic findings after injection of a calcium hydroxylapatite filler. *J Cosmet Laser Ther.* 2004;6:223–226.

Marmur ES, Taylor SC, Grimes PE, Boyd CM, Porter JP, Yoo JY. Six-month safety results of calcium hydroxylapatite for treatment of nasolabial folds in Fitzpatrick skin types IV to VI. *Dermatol Surg.* 2009;35(suppl 2):s1641–s1645.

Marmur E, Green L, Busso M. A controlled, randomized study of pain levels in subjects treated with calcium hydroxylapatite (Radiesse) premixed with lidocaine for correction of nasolabial folds. *Dermatol Surg.* 2010;36(3):309–315.

Moers-Carpi MM, Tufet JO. Calcium hydroxylapatite versus nonanimal stabilized hyaluronic acid for the correction of nasolabial folds: a 12-month, multicenter, prospective, randomized, controlled, split-face trial. *Dermatol Surg* 2008;34:210–215.

Moers-Carpi M, Vogt S, Santos BM, Planas J, Vallve SR, Howell DJ. A multicenter, randomized trial comparing calcium hydroxylapatite to two hyaluronic acids for treatment of nasolabial folds. *Dermatol Surg.* 2007;33(suppl 2):s144–s151.

Muti GF, Astolfi G, Renzi M, Rovatti PP. Calcium hydroxylapatite for augmentation of face and hands: a retrospective analysis in Italian subjects. *J Drugs Dermatol.* 2015;14(9):948–954.

Oh SJ, Kang DW, Goh EK, Kong SK. Calcium hydroxylapatite injection for the patulous Eustachian tube. *Am J Otolaryngol.* 2014;35(3):443–444.

Radiesse. Bioform Medical Inc.; 2009 [package insert].

Ridenour B, Kontis TC. Injectable calcium hydroxylapatite microspheres (Radiesse). *Facial Plast Surg.* 2009;25:100–105.

Riyaz FR, Ozog DM. Hand rejuvenation. *Semin Cutan Med Surg.* 2015;34:1–6.

Rose AE, Day D. Esthetic rejuvenation of the temple. *Clin Plast Surg.* 2013;40:77–89.

Silvers SL, Eviatar JA, Echavez MI, Pappas AL. Prospective, open-label, 18-month trial of calcium hydroxylapatite (Radiesse) for facial soft-tissue augmentation in patients with human immunodeficiency virus-associated lipoatrophy: one-year durability. *Plast Reconstr Surg.* 2006;118:s34–s45.

Smith S, Busso M, McClaren M, Bass LS. A randomized, bilateral, prospective comparison of calcium hydroxylapatite microspheres versus human-based collagen for the correction of nasolabial folds. *Dermatol Surg.* 2007;33(suppl 2):s12–s21; discussion s21.

Tzikas TL. A 52-month summary of results using calcium hydroxylapatite for facial soft tissue augmentation. *Dermatol Surg.* 2008;34(suppl 1):s9–s15.

Voigts R, DeVore DP, Grazer JM. Dispersion of calcium hydroxylapatite accumulations in the skin: animal studies and clinical practices. *Dermatol Surg.* 2010;36(suppl 1): s798–s803.

Wasylkowski VC. Body vectoring technique with Radiesse for tightening of the abdomen, thighs, and brachial zone. *Clin Cosmet Investig Dermatol.* 2015;8:267–273.

Yutskovskaya Y, Kogan E, Leshunov E. A randomized, split-face, histomorphologic study comparing a volumetric calcium hydroxylapatite and a hyaluronic acid-based dermal filler. *J Drugs Dermatol.* 2014;13(9):1047–1052.

# 8

# Poly-L-lactic acid

Katie Beleznay, Rebecca Fitzgerald, Shannon Humphrey

## Summary and Key Features

- Gradual, subtle, and natural results with a long duration (>2 years) are achievable with poly-L-lactic acid.
- Thorough facial analysis of changes in all structural tissues will enhance site-specific augmentation of volume loss and enhance outcomes.
- The amount of product used at one session is determined by the amount of surface area to be treated at that session. The final volumetric correction is determined by the number of treatment sessions.
- Proper technique in the preparation and injection of this biostimulatory agent will minimize adverse events.
- As experience has been gained with this product and techniques have evolved it has been found to be a safe and effective product with predictable and reproducible results.

## Introduction

Poly-L-lactic acid (PLLA) is a biocompatible and biodegradable synthetic polymer. The currently commercially available forms, Sculptra and Sculptra Aesthetic (Sinclair Pharmaceuticals, Galderma Laboratories, Fort Worth, TX, USA) are US Food and Drug Administration (FDA)-approved for the treatment of human immunodeficiency virus (HIV)-associated lipoatrophy and correction of shallow to deep nasolabial fold contour deficiencies and other facial wrinkles, respectively. PLLA provides gradual, subtle, and natural results with long duration. The approach to treatment with PLLA involves replacing volume by considering the entire face and its structural foundation from a three-dimensional (3D) perspective rather than focusing on individual lines and folds. Proper patient selection and assessment, as well as attention to technique in the preparation and injection of the material, will minimize adverse events and optimize results.

## Patient selection, expectations, and satisfaction

PLLA is a good choice for patients specifically desiring a gradual improvement or those looking for a subtle yet panfacial improvement. The gradual results may not make this the optimal choice for someone looking for an immediate "quick fix" for an upcoming event. However, it is an excellent choice for those wanting long-lasting results. In the study used to gain FDA aesthetic approval, almost 80% of patients treated still saw full correction at 25 months (the cutoff time for the study).

It is important to recall that the initial global experience with PLLA was in the HIV population, as well as in older cosmetic patients, most of whom required a fair amount of product and multiple treatment sessions to achieve the desired outcome. We now recognize this as an issue of patient selection, not product selection (i.e., older and emptier faces require more product of any kind to achieve correction). Patients who require significant volume need to be corrected with PLLA in a gradual progressive manner over multiple treatment sessions. Treatments are usually administered at 4- to 6-week intervals. Younger or fuller-faced patients may respond well and need less product and fewer treatment sessions. A longer interval between treatment sessions may be appropriate for younger or fuller-faced patients who require less volume. This difference is illustrated in the patient cases seen in Figs. 8.1 to 8.4. The video accompanying this chapter demonstrates treatment of a 41-year-old patient with aging changes superimposed on congenital skeletal hypoplasia (see Fig. 8.1).

## Pathophysiology of the aging face: structural and morphologic

Aging leads to loss or redistribution of volume in the bony substructure and fat compartments of the face. This occurs in conjunction with loss of elasticity of the skin that envelops it. As these structures change, it changes the morphology of the face in terms of its shape, proportions, and 3D topography. Recognizing where these structures are changing enhances our ability to address them with site-specific correction to achieve optimal, natural-looking results. Obviously, this knowledge is in a constant state of evolution. It is now widely accepted that significant

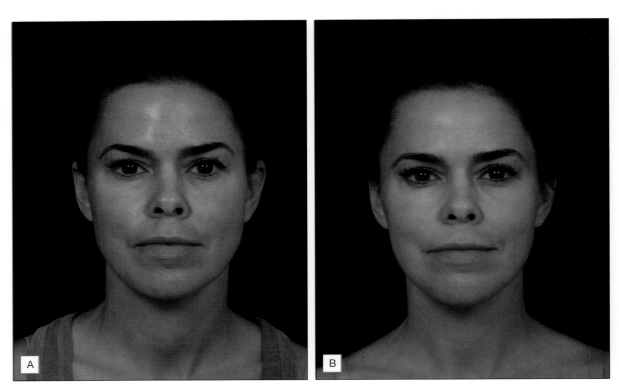

**Figure 8.1** A 41-year-old patient with aging changes superimposed on congenital skeletal hypoplasia before **(A)** and 4 weeks after **(B)** two vials of PLLA used panfacially, as demonstrated with narration in Video 8.1. Neuromodulator was used in the glabella. Note the increased brow projection, bizygomatic width, and improvement in perioral support giving an improved phi ration to the lower third of the face. Note also the ovalization of the facial shape, as well as improvement in skin quality. See the accompanying video for treatment of this patient.

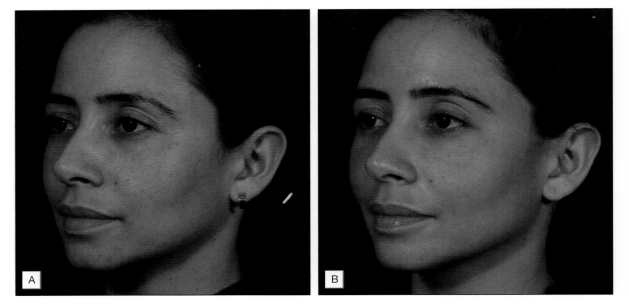

**Figure 8.2** A 38-year-old patient **(A)** before and **(B)** 3 months after post two vials PLLA performed in one session. Product was placed supraperiosteally along the supraorbital rim, medial maxilla, pyriform aperture, zygoma, and mandible. Product was also placed in the temporal lateral cheek, deep medial cheek, and submentalis fat compartments. Note the effacement of the early shadowing in the nasojugal fold and prejowl sulcus, leading to sharper definition of the cheeks and jawline.

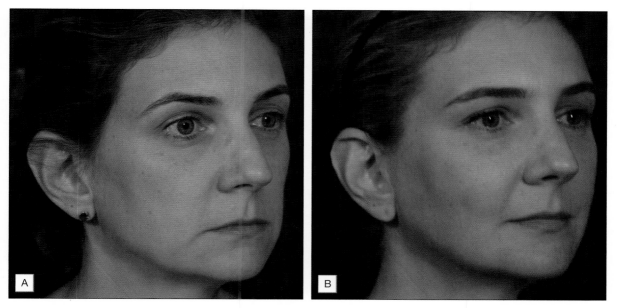

**Figure 8.3** A 38-year-old patient **(A)** before and **(B)** 6 months after post PLLA two vials per session, three sessions spaced 1 month apart. Note the improvement in the anterior projection and convexity of the face, as well as in skin quality. This athletic patient presented with significant loss of volume in her facial fat and therefore required more sessions than most patients her age.

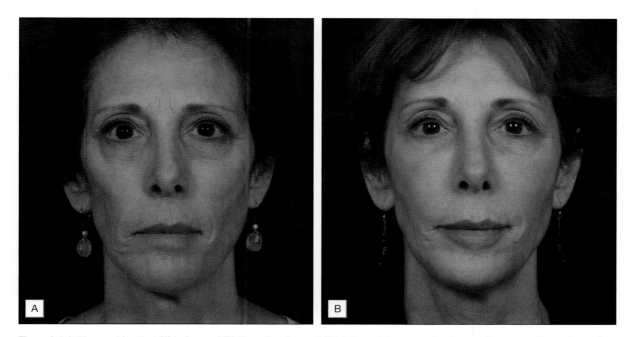

**Figure 8.4** A 59-year-old patient **(A)** before and **(B)** 6 months after post PLLA three vials per session, two sessions spaced 1 month apart. PLLA was placed supraperiosteally along the supraorbital rim, anterior maxilla, pyriform aperture, and mandible, and in fat compartments in the temple, cheek, and chin. Hyaluronic acid and neuromodulator were placed around the eyes and lips with the initial treatment. Note the ovalization and increased anterior convexity of her face, as well as the improvement in skin quality.

changes occur in specific regions of the facial skeleton with advancing age, and these changes in bony structure affect soft tissue position. The most significant changes have been documented in the glabellar, orbital, maxillary, and pyriform angles, as well as in the height and width of the orbital and pyriform aperture, as seen in Fig. 8.5. In 2007 Rohrich and Pessa first performed multiple cadaver studies using dye sequestration to show that subcutaneous fat exists in both superficial and deep compartments. A few years later Geirloff et al. corroborated this finding in 3D using computed tomography and radiopaque dye. These fat compartments are illustrated in Fig. 8.6. We now recognize that changes in volume and position of these fat compartments contribute to the changes in facial contour seen with aging; for example, the contribution of the temporal and lateral superficial fat compartments in the overall oval shape of the face, as well as the role of the midfacial deep cheek compartments in the anterior projection of the midface and the development (or effacement) of nasojugal and nasolabial folds. An older patient often needs augmentation that mimics both bony and soft tissue. However, we all start with our own individualized sizes and shapes. Add to this that, although the sequence of events as we age is somewhat predictable, the pace of these events is individualized. By understanding the role these structures play, as well as the changes seen in them with aging, we are better able to appreciate the 3D picture and rejuvenate the aging face with greater precision.

## Product and mechanism of action

The currently commercially available form of PLLA consists of microparticles of PLLA measuring 40 to 63 μm in diameter. This size means that the particles are large enough to avoid phagocytosis by dermal macrophages and cannot pass through capillary walls but are small enough to be injected with needles as fine as 26 gauge (G).

After being injected, PLLA induces a subclinical inflammatory response, followed by encapsulation of the particles and subsequent fibroblast proliferation and collagen formation. Goldberg et al. showed a statistically significant 33.7% increase in mean level of type I collagen 6 months after PLLA injection ($p = 0.03$). In addition, increases in type I and type III collagen were seen in 79% and 72% of patients, respectively. PLLA acts differently than traditional injectable fillers because new volume is generated in a gradual, progressive manner through fibroplasia. PLLA is gradually degraded and metabolized to $CO_2$ and $H_2O$.

## Poly-L-lactic acid: technical considerations

Proper technique will minimize adverse events and optimize results when using stimulatory agents, such as PLLA. This is outlined below and summarized in Box 8.1.

### Dilution, hydration, and storage

Current reconstitution recommendations are a dilution of more than 5 mL (most experienced practitioners

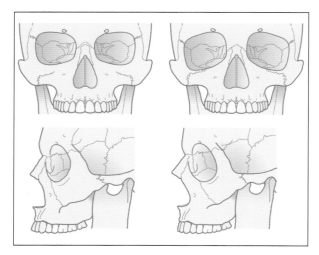

**Figure 8.5** A pictorial summary of age-related changes to the midface skeleton. *(Left)* Features of a youthful skull include a malar eminence, infraorbital rim, and pyriform aperture that are positioned anterior and vertical in the sagittal plane. The orbital aperture is small with a horizontally positioned inferior orbital rim. *(Right)* Older patients have a retroclined malar eminence, infraorbital rim, and pyriform aperture compared with those of young patients. The orbital aperture area is increased secondary to progressive curve distortion of the orbital rim superomedially and inferolaterally.

---

**Box 8.1**
**Strategies to minimize adverse events and optimize results**

- Proper preparation and placement are critical. Most problems with this agent stem from global or focal overcorrection ("too much, too soon")
- Papules and nodules may occur secondary to an issue with reconstitution (i.e., shaking the vial immediately after adding water [crystals on sidewalls of the vial will not hydrate], inadequate hydration time, or poor suspension prior to injection)
- The product should be evenly suspended immediately prior to injection
- Even distribution and appropriate plane of injection of PLLA is key to a desirable outcome
- Superficial placement leads to visible neocollagenesis
- Placement in active muscles can lead to clumping of particles and nodules
- Depositing significant product at one location, such as the apex of the "fan" when using a fanning technique, can lead to focal papules and nodules
- Massage should be performed immediately post injection and may be continued for 5 days

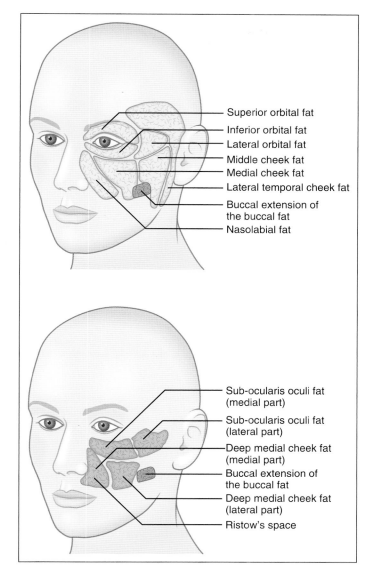

Superior orbital fat
Inferior orbital fat
Lateral orbital fat
Middle cheek fat
Medial cheek fat
Lateral temporal cheek fat
Buccal extension of
the buccal fat
Nasolabial fat

Sub-ocularis oculi fat
(medial part)
Sub-ocularis oculi fat
(lateral part)
Deep medial cheek fat
(medial part)
Buccal extension of
the buccal fat
Deep medial cheek fat
(lateral part)
Ristow's space

**Figure 8.6** Anatomic relationships of the superficial and deep facial fat compartments. The superficial layer *(yellow)* is composed of the nasolabial fat, the medial cheek fat, the middle cheek fat, the lateral temporal cheek compartment, and three orbital compartments. The deep midfacial fat compartments are composed of the suborbicularis oculi fat (medial and lateral parts) and the deep medial cheek fat (medial and lateral parts). Three layers of distinct fat compartments are found laterally to the pyriform aperture, where a deep compartment *(blue)* is located posterior to the medial part of the deep medial cheek fat. The buccal extension of the buccal fat pad extends from the paramaxillary space to the subcutaneous plane. *(Adapted from Geirloff M, Stohring C, Buder T, Gassling V, Acil Y, Wiltfang J. Aging changes of the midfacial fat compartments: a computed tomographic study. Plast Reconstr Surg. 2012;129(1):263–273.)*

recommend an 8 to 9 mL dilution), and a hydration time of at least 2 hours (most injectors recommend at least 24 hours). Sterile water is recommended for dilution, but bacteriostatic saline can be substituted off-label. Lidocaine 1% to 2% with or without epinephrine can also be added at the time of hydration or immediately prior to injection to help to achieve the final dilution (i.e., 7 mL sterile water and 2 mL of anesthetic). The initial fluid should be added gently to the vial, and the vial should not be shaken. This will avoid inadvertent deposition of clumps of dry product on the wall of the vial to ensure proper hydration of all particles (as injection of poorly hydrated product may lead to nodule formation). The vial can be stored at room temperature for 24 to 48 hours or kept refrigerated for up to 3 to 4 weeks prior to use. Adequate dilution and hydration leads to easier injection, more even product distribution, reduced risk of needle clogging, and decreased risk of papules and nodules.

## Preparation prior to use

Prior to injection, topical anesthesia and/or ice can be applied to the target region. In our practice we use 30% lidocaine in a plasticized base. The area should be cleansed thoroughly using topical antiseptics, such as 4% chlorhexidine (Hibiclens) and 70% alcohol. The vial should be rolled in the hands or mixed using a laboratory vortex until a homogeneous suspension results. Check that the bottom of the vial is clear of product to ensure all PLLA is in the suspension. To avoid foaming, do not shake too vigorously. Use an 18G needle to withdraw the suspension into 1 or 3 mL syringes. Before injecting, change the needle. A 25G or 26G 1 to 1½ inch needle or 25G blunt-tip cannula can be used. Needle clogging occurs if there is excessive foam in the syringe. The foam should be expelled from the hub of the syringe prior to placement of a needle or cannula. The needle or cannula should then be primed prior to use.

## Product amount

The amount of product used for any single treatment session should be determined by the surface area to be treated, using approximately 0.1 to 0.3 mL/cm. The final volumetric correction is addressed by the number of treatment sessions. For instance, this means that a very large face with mild volume loss may require three vials injected in only one session, but a small face with severe volume loss may require one to two vials per session over three or more sessions.

## Product placement

PLLA is injected deeply in a supraperiosteal location at the temple and along the zygoma, maxilla, and mandible. It may be placed subcutaneously in the midcheek as well. Injections in the preauricular and lateral cheek are performed subcutaneously just under the dermis because deeper injections in this area may enter the parotid gland or duct. Fig. 8.7 illustrates site-specific recommendations for injection of PLLA. Upon injection there is an immediate volumizing effect due to the presence of liquid used for reconstitution, which dissipates over 1 to 4 days. The subsequent fibroplasia develops over the next 4 weeks.

PLLA has also been used with great success in the treatment of the décolleté area. This is performed with a 16-mL dilution placed in a cross-hatch or fanning pattern over the area and is described in detail by Vanaman and Fabi. The number of sessions needed is contingent upon the initial degree of volume loss.

PLLA has also been used off-label to treat moderate-to-severe scarring from acne or varicella and for postoperative soft tissue loss by injecting under the scar at the dermal–subcutaneous tissue junction.

Treatment of the neck and hands with PLLA has been associated with a relatively high incidence of papules and nodules and is best avoided.

## Aftercare

Massage is performed after every few injections and again at the end of treatment. Some practitioners have the patient massage the area over the next few days, using the "rule of fives" (5 minutes/5 times daily/5 days). Follow the mantra "treat, wait, assess." Patients should receive repeat treatment no sooner than 4 weeks after previous treatment.

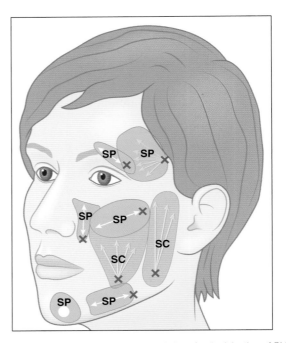

**Figure 8.7** Site-specific recommendations for the injection of PLLA. Potential areas amenable to correction with PLLA are indicated on this model. Recommended points of entry for each anatomic site are marked with a *red* ×. Injectable PLLA should be placed supraperiosteally in the temples, lateral brow, zygomatic area, maxillary area, mandibular area, and mental area *(green areas marked with "SP")*. Injectable PLLA should be placed in the subcutaneous fat in the midcheek regions and preauricular area *(purple areas marked with "SC")*. Depending on the anatomic area, recommended techniques include fanning *(yellow arrows)*, retrograde linear threading *(white arrows)*, or depot *(white circle)* injection. *Adapted with permission from Bartus C, Hanke W, Daro-Kaftan E. A decade of experience with injectable poly-L-lactic acid: a focus on safety.* Dermatol Surg. 2013;39:698–705.

## Complications and management

Potential complications can be secondary to the injection itself, suboptimal preparation or technique, or inflammatory or vascular events. The most common injection-related events are swelling, bruising, erythema, and pain, which resolve spontaneously, typically over a short period of time.

Papules and nodules result from a focal or global overabundance of product and most commonly stem from suboptimal product reconstitution or placement. All products should be well hydrated prior to use (no shaking immediately after reconstitution because this deposits dry product on the walls of the vial that will not hydrate). Be aware that the product may precipitate out of suspension and should be evenly suspended in the syringe immediately prior to injection. Injection should be in the subcutaneous or supraperiosteal plane. Superficial injection into the dermis should be avoided because this can lead to visible neocollagenesis seen as lumps and

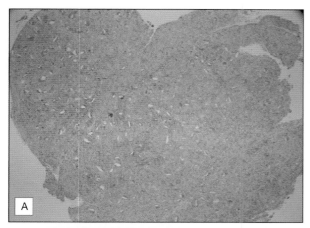

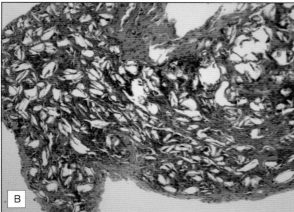

**Figure 8.8** Nodule versus granuloma/low-power histopathology: **(A)** nodule with an overabundance of product trapped in skeletal muscle; **(B)** true granuloma showing an overabundance of host reaction to a small amount of product. *Reproduced with permission from Fitzgerald R, Vleggaar D. Facial volume restoration of the aging face with poly-L-lactic acid. Dermatol Ther. 2011;24:2–27.*

bumps. Placement in or through areas of dynamic muscle, particularly around the eyes or lips, should also be avoided because this can lead to clumping of particles trapped in muscle fibers, as seen in Fig. 8.8A. Histopathology of papules or nodules will show an overabundance of product with a few foreign body giant cells. The presence of these few foreign body giant cells may lead to a histopathologic diagnosis of "granuloma," although these lesions are not true clinical granulomas. True clinical granulomas are a systemic inflammatory response showing an overabundance of host reaction (i.e., foreign body giant cells) to a relatively small amount of product, as seen in Fig. 8.8B. Because this is a systemic response, true clinical granulomas occur in all treated sites simultaneously, in contrast with papules and nodules that occur in a limited area. Because true clinical granulomas represent an overabundance of proliferating foreign body giant cells, they

respond well to treatment with antimetabolites like intralesional corticosteroids or 5-fluorouracil (5-FU) (0.1 mL of 40 mg/mL Kenalog mixed with 0.9 mL 5-FU 50 mg/mL; no more than 2 mL at one session. This can be injected once per week for 2 weeks, then weekly until resolution. Resolution is usually seen in 2 to 3 weeks). True clinical granulomas have been reported with all currently available commercial fillers and are fortunately rare (0.01% to 0.1%). In contrast, as papules and nodules represent product, not proliferating cells, they do not respond to treatment with antimetabolites, such as intralesional steroids or 5-FU. Indeed, intralesional steroids may make the problem even more visible by causing atrophy around the "bump." This was a common mishap in the early days with this product that is now disappearing due to evolution of our methodology and a wider understanding of the difference between true clinical granulomas and papules and nodules. Excision is an option but results in a permanent scar. Reassuring the patient that this is a transient process that will resolve spontaneously over time may suffice. Hyaluronic acid filler to camouflage the nodule until it resorbs is a good option. Late-onset (14 to 24 months) inflammatory nodules have also been described and may represent end-stage degradation of the PLLA product. This can also be treated with injections of steroids or 5-FU but may resolve spontaneously over time.

Vascular complications may occur when the product is injected into a blood vessel. This can cause ischemia and skin necrosis or more rarely blindness secondary to retrograde embolization of product into the ocular vessels. A reflux maneuver should be carried out prior to each injection to avoid intravascular injection. Injections should be performed slowly without using excessive pressure. Chapter 28 reviews prevention and management of vascular occlusion in more detail.

## Conclusion

PLLA is a safe and effective treatment for cosmetic enhancement. By stimulating new collagen, PLLA can restructure the face and gradually restore volume. Optimizing outcomes and minimizing adverse events requires awareness and attention to the technical details outlined above. Careful patient selection and thoughtful facial analysis of changes in all structural tissues will enhance site-specific augmentation and maximize satisfaction.

## Further reading

Alessio R, Rzany B, Eve L, et al. European expert recommendations on the use of injectable poly-L-lactic acid for facial rejuvenation. *J Drugs Dermatol.* 2014;13(9):1057–1066.

Bartus C, Hanke W, Daro-Kaftan E. A decade of experience with injectable poly-L-lactic acid: a focus on safety. *Dermatol Surg.* 2013;39:698–705.

Beer K. A single-center, open label study on the use of injectable poly-L-lactic acid for the treatment of moderate to severe scarring from acne or varicella. *Dermatol Surg.* 2007;33:s159–s167.

Butterwick K, Lowe NJ. Injectable poly-L-lactic acid for cosmetic enhancement: learning from the European experience. *J Am Acad Dermatol.* 2009;61:281–293.

Fitzgerald R, Vleggaar D. Facial volume restoration of the aging face with poly-L-lactic acid. *Dermatol Ther.* 2011;24:2–27.

Geirloff M, Stohring C, Buder T, Gassling V, Acil Y, Wiltfang J. Aging changes of the midfacial fat compartments: a computed tomographic study. *Plast Reconstr Surg.* 2012;129(1):263–273.

Goldberg D, Guana A, Volk A, Daro-Kaftan E. Single-arm study for the characterization of human tissue response to injectable poly-L-lactic acid. *Dermatol Surg.* 2013;39:915–922.

Lambros V. Observations on periorbital and midfacial aging. *Plast Reconstr Surg.* 2007;120:1367–1376.

Lemperle G, Gauthier-Hazan N. Foreign body granulomas after all injectable dermal fillers. Part 2. Treatment options. *Plast Reconstr Surg.* 2009;123(6):1864–1873.

Levy RM, Redbord KP, Hanke CW. Treatment of HIV lipoatrophy and lipoatrophy of aging with poly-L-lactic acid: a prospective 3-year follow-up study. *J Am Acad Dermatol.* 2008;59(6):923–933.

Lorenc ZP. Techniques for the optimization of facial and nonfacial volumization with injectable poly-L-lactic acid. *Aesthet Plast Surg.* 2012;36:1222–1229.

Narins RS, Baumann L, Brandt FS, et al. A randomized study of the efficacy and safety of injectable poly-L-lactic acid versus human-based collagen implant in the treatment of nasolabial fold wrinkles. *J Am Acad Dermatol.* 2010;62(3):448–462.

Palm M, Goldman M. Patient satisfaction and the duration of effect with PLLA: a review of the literature. *J Drugs Dermatol.* 2009;10:S15–S20.

Rohrich R, Pessa J. Discussion: aging of the facial skeleton: aesthetic implications and rejuvenation strategies. *Plast Reconstr Surg.* 2010;127(1):discussion 384–385.

Rohrich RJ, Pessa JE, Ristow B. The youthful cheek and the deep medial fat compartment. *Plast Reconstr Surg.* 2008;121(6):2107–2112.

Shaw R, Katzel E, Koltz P, et al. Aging of the facial skeleton: aesthetic implications and rejuvenation strategies. *Plast Reconstr Surg.* 2011;127:374.

Stuzin J. Restoring facial shape in face lifting: the role of skeletal support in facial analysis. *Plast Reconstr Surg.* 2007;119(1):362–376.

Vanaman M, Fabi SG. Décolletage: regional approaches with injectable fillers. *Plast Reconstr Surg.* 2015;136(5 suppl): 276s–281s.

Vleggaar D, Fitzgerald R, Lorenc ZP, et al. Consensus recommendations on the use of injectable poly-L-lactic acid for facial and nonfacial volumization. *J Drugs Dermatol.* 2014;13(4 Suppl):s29–s51.

# 9

# Emervel family

## Gary D. Monheit, Berthold Rzany

### Summary and Key Features

- The Emervel family comes in several products with and without lidocaine.
- The Emervel family is one of the few hyaluronic acid families with good clinical data behind their products.
- The products have been on the market for several years now in Europe and appear to be efficacious and safe.
- From 2016 on, the Emervel family is going to be subsummarized under the name of the Restylane family. The Emervel family can be still identified by the blue color of the boxes and mostly strange appearing names with an 'e' at the end. The previous name appears as small text on the box.

## Introduction

Soft tissue filling with hyaluronic acid (HA) began with single-purpose fillers designed and tested for nasolabial folds but subsequently used for multiple facial areas. This began in 2004 with the use and approval of Restylane and was followed rapidly with other HA fillers with similar physical characteristics and rheology. The need for HA filling material that is designed for more than the nasolabial folds coincided with the global approach to treating multiple areas of the face to achieve a natural yet more youthful look sought by our patients. Filling material that will restructure deep facial defects and others that are designed for more superficial defects with a natural appearance stimulates the need for customized filling material for each area. The Emervel family of HA fillers has evolved with specific products designed to treat variable facial indications, including nasolabial folds, marionette lines, perioral lines, cheek folds, tear troughs, and fine dermal wrinkles. Each has specific physical properties and flow characteristics to solve these specific facial problems of aging skin and soft tissue.

## Physical properties of the Emervel family

Emervel (Galderma, Lausanne, Switzerland) is a family of five fillers with a range of physical properties designed to accommodate all levels of facial correction. The variables that determine the nature of each product include the following:

1. HA concentration (20 mg/mL)
2. Cross-linking (by 1,4-butanediol diglycidyl ether [BDDE])
3. Calibration (this is the preferred term of the company) or particle size

Because all of the Emervel products maintain the same concentration (20 mg/mL), they vary the degree and type of cross-linking, as well as the three levels of calibration or particle size. This approach to customized filling nature is referred to as "optimal balance technology" (Table 9.1). From 2016 on, the Emervel family will be subsummarized under the Restylane brand. For this, several new names were created, making the Emervel brand still distinguishable from the old Restylane brand (Table 9.2).

Calibration is a unique term that is used for this group of fillers and describes the process of processing bulk cross-linked HA into smaller particle sizes to produce optimal size for the area to be treated. This is produced through a "sieving" process for optimal homogenicity. The products with a low cross-linking and with small calibration are designed for superficial injection (e.g., Emervel Touch) as the products with high cross-linking and larger calibration are designed for deeper and more volumetric injections (e.g., Emervel Volume). Except for Emervel Touch, they are available with and without lidocaine.

## Clinical studies

### European and South American clinical studies on Emervel

In contrast to the United States, in Europe generally no clinical trials are required to place an HA filler on the market. Therefore it is quite unique that the Emervel family entered the market with several concomitant trials. Two trials were comparative using Restylane products as the benchmark (Table 9.3).

Both trials showed a comparability of the tested products. However, Emervel Deep did show a better efficacy compared with Restylane Perlane.[1]

Three other trials, all case series, focused on real-life scenarios (e.g., treating patients with different members of the Emervel-family) (Table 9.4). Results from one trial (the Fresh study trial Rzany et al.[3,4]) have appeared in several subpublications (e.g., Cartier et al.[5], Kestemont et al.[6], and Rzany et al.[3,4]). These studies do not focus on comparability but more on effectiveness (how is the product working when its use is less restricted) and how safe is the product (usually the numbers of included patients are quite high, which allows also statements on less frequent adverse effects). However, one large trial did only follow up the patients for a couple of weeks.[8]

In addition, two smaller comparative trials have been presented at European meetings, comparing Emervel Lips versus Juvéderm Ultrasmile and Juvéderm Volbella, respectively.[9,10] Both trials comprised approximately 50 patients, mostly women. Interestingly the efficacy between the products compared was quite similar (Table 9.5).

## US clinical study

The Emervel US study was a multicenter, randomized, evaluator-blinded, intraindividual right–left comparing effectiveness and safety of Emervel Classic and Emervel Deep to Juvéderm Ultra and Juvéderm Ultra Plus to correct contralateral nasolabial folds.

This was a study for effectiveness: noninferiority versus a comparator. A blinded evaluation assessed safety, and adverse events were assessed by patient and evaluator. The Emervel Classic wrinkle scale was used with a baseline of three (moderate) to four (severe) nasolabial folds. An initial touchup was allowed, if needed, and injected volumes of both filler were the same.

The results at 6 months showed that the mean change in wrinkle severity score at 24 weeks were effective equally. This was true for both studies: Emervel Classic versus Juvéderm Ultra and Emervel Deep versus Juvéderm Ultra Plus. The adverse event profiles were also similar, as well as patient satisfaction (Table 9.6). This pivotal trial will be submitted to the US Food and Drug Administration (FDA) for final approval.

## Emervel in clinical practice—use of the different types in different areas (i.e., nasolabial folds, lips, volume filling)

The Emervel family is quite large, ranging from Emervel Touch for very superficial lines to Emervel Volume for deep augmentations. In contrast to the rest of the family

**Table 9.1** Properties of the Emervel family and their clinical impact

|  | Calibration | Cross-linking | Concentration |
|---|---|---|---|
| Benefit | Lifting effect | Firmness | Filler longevity |
| Adversity | Too big Uneven flow | Implant perceptible with inflammation | Hardness |

**Table 9.2** New and old names for the Emervel family*

| Indication | Old name | New name |
|---|---|---|
| For very superficial indications, such as fine periocular wrinkles | Emervel Touch | Restylane Fynesse |
| For medium-sized lines and folds, infraorbital hollow | Emervel Classic | Restylane Refyne |
| For deeper lines and folds as well as volume deficits | Emervel Deep | Restylane Defyne |
| For volume substitution, such as cheeks, chin, etc. | Emervel Volume | Restylane Volume |
| For lip volume augmentation | Emervel Lip | Restylane Kysse |

*The Emervel family is now subsummarized under the name of Restylane. The boxes differ from the Restylane boxes by the blue color and for non-Scandinavians mostly a bit strange appearing names ending with an 'e.' The previous names appear as a small text at the box.

**Table 9.3** Comparative European trials with Emervel

| Reference | Products | Randomized/ blinded | Area assessed | Duration of study | No. of patients | Objective outcome criteria | Comments |
|---|---|---|---|---|---|---|---|
| Ascher et al.[1] | Emervel Deep vs. Restylane Perlane | Y/Y | NLF | 6 months | 60 | 5-points WSRS | Emervel Deep provides better efficacy and similar tolerability compared with Restylane Perlane |
| Rzany et al.[2] | Emervel Classic vs. Restylane | Y/Y | NLF | 18 months | 52 | 5-points WSRS* | Emervel Classic provides similar efficacy and better overall tolerability compared with Restylane |

*Wrinkle Severity Rating Scale.

**Table 9.4** Case series with the Emervel family

| Reference | Products | Randomized/blinded | Area assessed | Duration of study | No. of patients | Objective outcome criteria | Comments |
|---|---|---|---|---|---|---|---|
| Rzany et al.[3,4] | Emervel Touch, Classic, Deep, Volume and Lips | Case series, multicenter study (58 physicians), collected between September 2010 and July 2011 | At least three of the eight indications (periorbital lines, tear troughs, cheek folds, nasolabial folds, upper lip lines and marionette lines; cheek and lip enhancement) | 6 months | 77 | Lemperle Rating scale (6 points) and Lip Fullness Scale, overall aesthetic improvement | At 6 months, 79.7% of participants were satisfied or very satisfied with the durability of the results* |
| Talarico et al.[7] | Emervel Volume | Case series, multicenter study | At least two indications among chin, temporal areas, cheeks, cheekbones, jawline, nasolabial fold | 18 months | 60 subjects | Volume loss scale (4 points), as well as Lemperle Rating scale (6 points), GAIS, Vectra 3D | At 18 months still one-point improvement in 68.3% of patients, 6 patients with nodule formation, mostly mild |
| Fahri et al. [8] | Emervel Classic, Deep, Volume and Lips | Consecutive case series, multicenter | Nasolabial folds and marionette lines by score— other areas only for treatment (cheek, lips, supramental crease, tear trough) | 2–4 weeks | 1822 | 5-point score for nasolabial folds and marionette lines | No long-term data on efficacy and safety are given |

*Several subpublications came out of this trial, all published in a supplement of the Journal of Drugs in Dermatology (e.g., Cartier et al.[5], Kestemont et al.[6], Rzany et al.,[3,4]).

**Table 9.5** Comparative lip volume trials with Emervel Lips

| Reference | Products | Randomized/blinded | Area assessed | Duration of study | No. of patients | Objective outcome criteria | Comments |
|---|---|---|---|---|---|---|---|
| Hilton[9] (presented at AWMC 2015) | Emervel Lips versus Juvéderm Ultrasmile | Randomized, evaluator-blinded, single-center study | Upper and lower lip | 6 months (24 weeks) | 40 all females | GAIS, subject satisfaction | GAIS and subject satisfaction results were similar, more swelling with Juvéderm Ultrasmile |
| Hilton et al.[10] (presented at IMCAS 2016) | Emervel Lips versus Juvéderm Volbella | Randomized comparative multicenter study | Thin to moderately thick lips | 12 months | 60 (58 females) | LFGS (5 points) | The improvement in the LFGS was similar. More treatment-associated adverse events occurred in the Juvéderm Volbella group |

up to now, Emervel Touch comes only without lidocaine. It is a beautifully smooth product; however, without lidocaine it makes the superficial injections more painful (up to now it is not clear why the company does not offer this product also with lidocaine). Very unique is Emervel Lips. It is a very good product for augmenting the lip red (Fig. 9.1A and B). However, in contrast to other products, it is quite firm, so that patients might feel the filler for a couple of weeks after the injection—which some patients do not like so much. Some colleagues use Emervel Lips also for evening the infraorbital hollows (Fahri et al.[8]).

| The EMERVEL® range | EMERVEL® TOUCH | EMERVEL® CLASSIC | EMERVEL® LIPS | EMERVEL® DEEP | EMERVEL® VOLUME |
|---|---|---|---|---|---|
| Gel texture | | | | | |
| Rheological characteristics Optimal Balance Technology™ | | | | | |
| Cross-linking | 1 out of 4 | 2 out of 4 | 3 out of 4 | 4 out of 4 | 3 out of 4 |
| Calibration | 1 out of 3 | 1 out of 3 | 1 out of 3 | 2 out of 3 | 3 out of 3 |
| Viscosity | Soft, subtle | Intermediate firmness | Firm | High firmness | Firm |
| Lifting capacity | Moderate volume effect | Moderate volume effect | Moderate volume effect | High volume effect | Very high volume effect |
| Depth of injection | Superficial Dermis | Dermis | Vermilion lip/Vermilion border | Deep dermis/Subcutaneous | Subcutaneous/Supraperiostic |
| Size of Ultra Thin Wall needle | 30 G 1/2 | 30 G 1/2 | 30 G 1/2 | 27 G 1/2 | 23 G 1 |
| Indications | Perioral lines / Periorbital lines | Nasolabial folds / Marionette lines | Lip enhancement / Lip contour | Deep nasolabial folds / Deep marionette lines | Cheekbones Cheeks / Chin Facial oval |
| Comfort | Without lidocaine | With* or without lidocaine | With* or without lidocaine | With* or without lidocaine | With* or without lidocaine |
| Blister packaging | 1 x 1 mL | 1 x 1 mL | 1 x 1 mL | 1 x 1 mL | 1 x 2 mL |

* 0.3 % of lidocaine

CE 0459 · EMERVEL is a medical device. Injectable solution for wrinkles filling. EMERVEL is a trademark owned by Galderma S.A

**Table 9.6** Comparative US trials with Emervel*

| Products | Randomized/blinded | Area assessed | Duration of study | No. of patients | Objective outcome criteria | Comments |
|---|---|---|---|---|---|---|
| Emervel Classic Lidocain versus Juvéderm Ultra | Y/Y | NLF | 6 months | 171 | 5-points WSRS[†] | Similar efficacy and safety |
| Emervel Deep Lidocain versus Juvéderm Ultra Plus | Y/Y | NLF | 6 months | 162 | 5-points WSRS[†] | Similar efficacy and safety |

*Study data have not been published so far (basic information comes from www.clinicaltrials.gov)
[†]Wrinkle Severity Rating Scale.

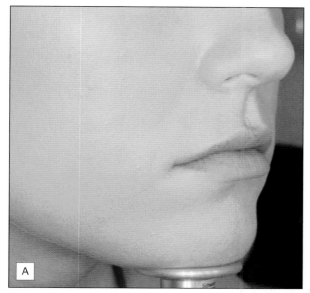
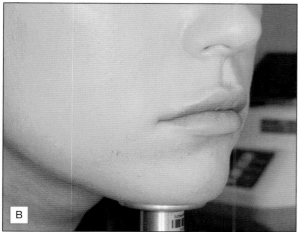

**Figure 9.1 A and B,** Lips before and 1 week after augmentation with 1 mL Emervel Lips in a 23-year-old patient.

## How does it compare with other HA fillers in different areas?

There are not a lot of comparative trials between different HA products. Based on the comparative trial of Emervel Deep and Classic it shows not much difference than Restylane Perlane and Restylane. In two further non-published studies between Emervel Lips and Juvéderm Ultrasmile, and Emervel Lips and Juvéderm Volbella from Hilton[9] and Hilton et al.[10] no clinical difference could be noted at least for the 6-month data when looking at efficacy. However, there were more adverse events with Juvéderm Volbella, reflecting similar data from Israel.[11] Concerning other Emervel products our guess would be that there are no clinically relevant differences when comparing Emervel Touch to say Restylane Vital (except for the pain because Emervel Touch so far is not available with lidocaine).

## Summary

In summary, the Emervel family of customized fillers present five unique HA products designed for facial rejuvenation in various locations of the face and at variable depths. The science, product analysis, and clinical validation all indicate this to be a useful product for the cosmetic physician.

## References

1. Ascher B, Bayerl C, Brun P, et al. Efficacy and safety of a new hyaluronic acid dermal filler in the treatment of severe nasolabial lines—6-month interim results of a randomized, evaluator-blinded, intra-individual comparison study. *J Cosmet Dermatol.* 2011;10:94–98.
2. Rzany B, Bayerl C, Bodokh I, et al. Efficacy and safety of a new hyaluronic acid dermal filler in the treatment of moderate nasolabial folds: 6-month interim results of a randomized, evaluator-blinded, intra-individual comparison study. *J Cosmet Laser Ther.* 2011;13:107–112.
3. Rzany B, Cartier H, Kestemont P, et al. Full-face rejuvenation using a range of hyaluronic acid fillers: efficacy, safety, and patient satisfaction over 6 months. *Dermatol Surg.* 2012; 38(7 Pt 2):1153–1161.

4. Rzany B, Cartier H, Kestermont P, et al. Correction of tear troughs and periorbital lines with a range of customized hyaluronic acid fillers. *J Drugs Dermatol.* 2012;11(suppl 1):s27–s34.

5. Cartier H, Trevidic P, Rzany B, Sattler G, Kerrouche N, Dhuin JC. Perioral rejuvenation with a range of customized hyaluronic acid fillers: efficacy and safety over six months with a specific focus on the lips. *J Drugs Dermatol.* 2012;11(suppl 1):s17–s26.

6. Kestemont P, Cartier H, Trevidic P, et al. Sustained efficacy and high patient satisfaction after cheek enhancement with a new hyaluronic acid dermal filler. *J Drugs Dermatol.* 2012;11(suppl 1):s9–s16.

7. Talarico S, Meski AP, Buratini L, et al. High patient satisfaction of a hyaluronic acid filler producing enduring full-facial volume restoration: an 18-month open multicenter study. *Dermatol Surg.* 2015;41(12):1361–1369.

8. Farhi D, Trevidic P, Kestemont P, et al. The Emervel French survey: a prospective real-practice descriptive study of 1,822 patients treated for facial rejuvenation with a new hyaluronic acid filler. *J Drugs Dermatol.* 2013;12(5):e88–e93.

9. Hilton S. A randomized evaluator blinded parallel group study on the safety of lip injections with Emervel Lips and Juvederm Ultra Smile. *Abstract and Poster at Aesthetic & Anti-aging Medicine World Congress Monaco;* 2015.

10. Hilton S, Sattler G, Samuelson U. A randomised comparative study of the safety and efficacy of lip injections with Emervel Lips and Juvéderm Volbella. *Abstract and Poster at International Master Course on Aging Science Paris;* 2016.

11. Artzi O, Loizides C, Verner I, Landau M. Resistant and recurrent late reaction to hyaluronic acid-based gel. *Dermatol Surg.* 2016;42(1):31–37.

# 10

# Safe fat transplantation

## Kyle M. Coleman, William P. Coleman III

Summary and Key Features

- Fat transplantation is a great tool for facial volumization.
- Fat transplantation can produce long-lasting results.
- Good harvesting and injection technique is paramount in achieving great results.
- Using safe and common sense techniques can minimize the risk of surgical sequelae, especially vascular occlusive events.

Fat transplantation has traditionally been the most efficient technique to restore facial volume to create more youthful features. This technique has also proved effective in filling soft tissue defects all over the body. With the advent of commercially available soft tissue fillers, facial volumization has become more commonly performed. Facial volumization with soft tissue fillers can be an excellent solution to the aging face; however, the use of these commercially available fillers for volume restoration is limited by several factors, especially cost and longevity. In contrast, fat transplantation can be performed on almost any area of the face and can provide long-lasting results in often a more cost-effective way. In addition, it provides appealing contouring of the donor site. With repeated injections, patients can often enjoy results that last for several years.[1] In the age of commercially available fillers, fat transplantation remains an important technique in the armamentarium of aesthetic medicine.

## Fat biology

### Patient selection and preoperative considerations

As with any aesthetic procedure, the most important factor in achieving excellent results is appropriate patient selection. It is important to discuss reasonable expectations and expected timelines for results. Appropriate candidates should be evaluated for the amount of volume loss, skin quality, sufficient fat volume source, and previous trauma or surgical procedures. Patients with larger degrees of volume loss generally need larger volumes injected per treatment and more treatments. Patients

also need to be prepared for potential social downtime resulting from edema and ecchymosis. It is important to make sure patients are in good general health prior to the procedure; laboratory values, such as blood chemistry, blood counts, and clotting factors, may be drawn preoperatively. It is recommended to avoid any potential blood thinning agents for at least a week prior to the procedure. In many cases a short course of broad-spectrum antibiotics is used in conjunction with the procedure to prevent potential infections.

## Harvesting

Selection of the most appropriate area for harvesting is based upon physician preference and viable store of fat volume. Some authors have suggested that certain areas of the body lead to more viable fat for transplantation.[2] However, other reviews have failed to show a difference in adipocyte survival based upon harvest site.[3] Liposuction of fibrous or areas of previous surgery tends to lead to a more bloody or fractured aspirate which could affect the viability of grafts. Cannula choice has also been an area of debate. Some authors have suggested that larger-bore cannulas are less traumatic to the fat grafts, whereas other research has shown that there appear to be no differences in fat graft retention related to cannula size.[4-6] In general, it is recommended to harvest under low pressure so as not to traumatize potential grafts.[6,7] Harvesting can be accomplished via negative pressure with a syringe or with vacuum assistance with sterile collection.[7,8] There are a multitude of collection systems that are commercially available that claim to assist in infranate separation or concentration of adipocytes. Currently, for small-volume fat transplantation (<100 cc harvested), we recommend the use of a negative-pressure syringe for harvesting (Fig. 10.1). For larger-volume transplantations, we use vacuum-assisted (<20 mm Hg) harvesting with a sterile collection canister.

## Preparation

Preparation of adipocytes for grafting has been an area of great debate. Many authors have advocated centrifugation of adipocytes after harvesting to concentrate adipocytes and remove potentially unwanted substrates that could impair graft survival.[8,9] However, some authors contend that centrifugation may lead to unnecessary adipocyte trauma and advocate for gravity separation of infranate.[3,10]

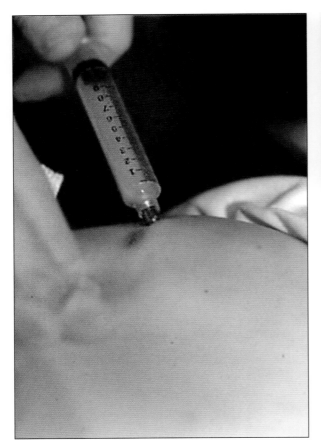

**Figure 10.1** Harvesting of fat with negative pressure via sterile syringe. *(Copyright William P. Coleman III, MD.)*

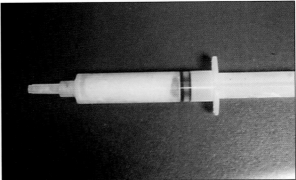

**Figure 10.2** Sterile syringe with cryopreserved fat to be prepared for transplantation. *(Copyright William P. Coleman III, MD.)*

storage medium (usually a syringe) and its container (Fig. 10.2). If cryopreserved fat is to be used, the fat should be brought to room temperature slowly using a warm water bath (water should not make direct contact with the syringe to maintain sterility).

## Injection technique

Prior to the procedure, patients are marked in an upright position. Anesthesia in both the donor and recipient sites can be achieved with tumescent anesthesia alone or in combination with oral analgesics; the tumescent anesthesia provides additive benefits of vasoconstriction and tissue cushioning through tissue separation with fluid. Some physicians perform the procedure under intravenous (IV) sedation, but with adequate tumescent anesthesia, this is not necessary. Preapplication of cold compresses can be helpful in providing additional anesthesia and in reduction of the potential for ecchymosis.

Like all surgical procedures, it is important to maintain a degree of sterility to minimize the potential for infection. Fat, being a larger molecule, must be harvested and injected through a larger-bore device than soft tissue fillers. In general, 12- to 16-gauge blunt cannulas are used for harvesting; 18- to 22-gauge blunt cannulas are used for injection because these are atraumatic and less likely to lead to intravascular injection. Entry points are planned at appropriate locations to provide access to the areas needing volumization. In almost all cases these heal without a visible scar. The authors recommend the use of an 18-gauge needle to create an entry point for the cannula. Care should be taken to not traumatize the cannula entry point to avoid any scarring.

Fat survival is improved by injecting very small aliquots (microdroplets) over multiple passes to enable contact between a large portion of the transplanted fat surface area with the surrounding vasculature (Fig. 10.3). Fat grafts should be injected via small syringes (i.e., 1 cc) and smaller cannulas to confer a greater degree of control and prevent large bolus injections. Determining the end

We typically allow the fat to separate in 10 cc harvesting syringes for several minutes and then withdraw the infranate. During the past decade there has been a fair amount of discussion about adding stem cell solutions or platelet-rich plasma preparation to increase adipocyte viability.[11,12] Although there have been data showing increased graft volume and survival with the addition of adipocyte stem cell preparations, the US Food and Drug Administration (FDA) has warned specific clinics that the use of adipose-derived stem cells or excessively manipulated adipose tissue could be considered a drug.[13]

There has also been some controversy on the use of cryopreserved fat for transplantation. Some authors contend that freshly harvested fat is more viable and will thus lead to increased transplant survival. It has been shown that fat that has been frozen at −15 to 20°C does not retain viability;[14] however, studies have shown that previously frozen fat can create an equivalent volumetric response to freshly harvested fat.[15,16] It is important to fully remove any infranate from the fat before it is cryopreserved. For patient safety, any cryopreserved fat should be labeled with patient demographics both on the

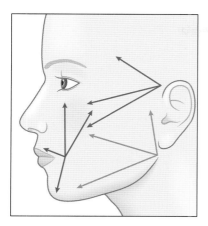

**Figure 10.3** Common locations for cannula insertion for transplantation.

point for correction comes with experience. Overcorrection is generally preferred because reabsorption rates vary from 40% to 60%. Relatively fixed areas, such as the cheek, generally have a higher degree of success than highly mobile areas, such as the lips and chin.[10,17] With repeated treatments to full correction, patients can expect long-lasting results; with many patients, results can remain for several years.[1] Some physicians prefer very large augmentations at one time instead of a series of smaller ones. In our experience, this leads to massive edema and long recoveries.

## Postoperative care

Postoperative care varies from physician to physician. Cold compresses or ice packs are recommended to decrease edema and the potential for ecchymosis. Patients are advised to sleep elevated to facilitate lymphatic drainage, especially around the eyes. Patients are advised to avoid strenuous activity and leaning over for the first few post-operative days to lower the risk of ecchymosis and possibly decrease the amount of fat reabsorption. Follow-up varies from physician to physician, but generally it is a good idea to have contact with the patient during the first 24 hours after surgery, preferably in person. Repeat treatments are generally performed at 1 to 2 months after the first procedure. It is important to explain to patients that the results that they perceive in the first week are deceiving because swelling is still a factor in their contours.

The donor site is covered with a light dressing, and elastic garments should be worn for several days to maximize contour improvement and decrease bruising and swelling.

## Complications and sequelae
### Surgical sequelae

As a minimally invasive procedure, there are higher rates of procedural sequelae and complications from fat transfer than from commercially available soft tissue volumization. Some degree of the risk is related to the size of the cannula used. In general, postoperatively patients experience edema, tenderness, and ecchymosis to varying degrees; however, the use of tumescent anesthesia tends to decrease the risk of edema and ecchymosis. Lymphedema can occur from overvolumization; this tends to resolve as reabsorption occurs. Hematoma and seromas, although rare, can occur; again, the risk of this is reduced from the use of tumescent anesthesia. Infection is also a potential complication because this is a surgical procedure; however, with good sterility and antibiotic coverage this is very rare.

### Nodules and calcification

Nodule formation is an uncommon complication of fat transplantation that results most likely from fat necrosis. Fat necrosis occurs as a result of incomplete vascular supply of the center of an area of transplanted fat. Inflammation as a result of the necrosis leads to nodule formation. These nodules occasionally self-resolve, but interventions, such as intralesional steroid injections, are often necessary to reduce these nodules. Calcification and ossification of transplanted fat is thought to be the end stage of fat necrosis. Nodules that are calcified or ossified most likely will need to be surgically excised. Avoid large volume and bolus injections of fat because these can potentially lead to fat necrosis.

### Vascular occlusion and blindness

Any time a substance is injected into the skin, there is a risk of intravascular injection or compression of vascular structures. As a result of vascular occlusion or compression, vascular compromise can lead to partial-thickness (ending in vesiculation) or full-thickness (ending in necrosis) injuries. Injection of substances into the ophthalmic circulation (most likely through supratrochlear, supraorbital, or dorsal nasal branches) can lead to retinal artery occlusion and blindness.[18,19] Fat is no exception; indeed, a review of the literature of retinal vascular occlusion showed that fat was the most common culprit in injectable-related retinal artery occlusion (47.9% of reported cases).[20] Most cases have occurred in the Asian literature; however, there have been three reported cases in the United States.[20] It is possible that the incidence is underreported in the United States; however, the fewer amount of cases may represent better training or differing aesthetic concerns between the United States and Asian countries. The most common locations associated with retinal artery occlusion are, in order, the glabella, nose, nasolabial fold, and forehead.

When it comes to vascular compromise, prevention is key. The use of small blunt cannulas, small volume injection, and epinephrine in anesthetic agents can decrease the risk of intravascular injection (Table 10.1). The authors believe the use of 1 cc syringes with microdroplet techniques for transplantation is extremely important to avoid

**Table 10.1** Techniques for decreasing the risk of vascular compromise

| Considerations for safe fat transplantation |
| --- |
| Injection via blunt cannula (18–22 gauge) |
| Injection of small aliquots (microdroplet) |
| Slow injection technique |
| Low-pressure injections |
| Use of small-volume syringes to inject (1 cc) |
| Use of tumescent anesthesia with epinephrine |
| Caution in high-risk areas (especially nasal dorsum and glabella) |

placement of large volumes of fat that could potentially compress or occlude a vessel. Injections should be performed only with low pressure and slowly, to avoid bolus injections to prevent potential retrograde flow if a vessel is accidentally canulized. Needles should be avoided, and only blunt-tipped cannulas should be used to avoid possible intravascular injection. Entry points should be placed at the periphery of the face and distant from vascular watershed areas to avoid canulization of a vessel. We also believe that the use of tumescent anesthesia with epinephrine can decrease the incidence of vascular compromise by causing vasoconstriction and plane separation with the tumescent fluid.

If vascular compromise is suspected, vasodilation through heat, vigorous massage, β-blockers, and topically applied nitrates can help to attempt to revascularize an impaired area. Anticoagulation with aspirin may also be helpful in reducing the impact of vascular occlusion. Unfortunately, retinal artery occlusion is not reversible if not reperfused within 90 minutes. Avoidance of injections into the at-risk areas, especially with needles, is paramount because treatment of retinal artery occlusion does not seem to be effective; 80.9% of the reported ocular complications from fat transplantation to the face have led to complete vision loss.[20]

## Conclusion

Fat transplantation remains an appealing option for facial rejuvenation and volumization. Aptly available supply, cost-effectiveness, and longevity may make fat transplantation a more viable option than treatment with commercially available soft tissue fillers in some patients. As a surgical procedure, fat transplantation requires additional training and consideration of potential sequelae and attention to safe techniques.

## References

1. Coleman S. Structural fat grafting: more than a permanent filler. *Plast Reconstr Surg.* 2006;118(suppl 3):108–120.
2. Hudson D, Lambert E, Bloch C. Site selection for fat autotransplantation: some observations. *Aesthetic Plast Surg.* 1990;14:195–197.
3. Rohrich R, Sorokin E, Brown S. In search of improved fat transfer viability: a quantitative analysis of the role of centrifugation and harvest site. *Plast Reconstr Surg.* 2004;113:391–395.
4. Ozsoy Z, Kul Z, Bilir A. The role of cannula diameter in improved adipocyte viability: a quantitative analysis. *Aesthet Surg J.* 2006;26:287–289.
5. Shiffman M, Mirrafati S. Fat transfer techniques: the effect of harvest and transfer methods on adipocyte viability and review of the literature. *Dermatol Surg.* 2001;27:819–826.
6. Nguyen PS, Desouches C, Gay AM, Hautier A, Magalon G. Development of micro-injection as an innovative autologous fat graft technique: the use of adipose tissue as dermal filler. *J Plast Reconstr Aesthet Surg.* 2012;65:1692–1699.
7. Leong DT, Hutmacher DW, Chew FT, Lim TC. Viability and adipogenic potential of human adipose tissue processed cell population obtained from pump-assisted and syringe-assisted liposuction. *J Dermatol Sci.* 2005;37:169–176.
8. Ozkaya O, Egemen O, Barutça SA, Akan M. Long-term clinical outcomes of fat grafting by low-pressure aspiration and slow centrifugation (Lopasce technique) for different indications. *J Plast Surg Hand Surg.* 2013;47:394–398.
9. Butterwick K. Lipoaugmentation for aging hands: a comparison of the longevity and aesthetic results of centrifuged versus noncentrifuged fat. *Dermatol Surg.* 2002;28:987–991.
10. Strong AL, Cederna PS, Rubin JP, Coleman SR, Levi B. The current state of fat grafting: a review of harvesting, processing, and injection techniques. *Plast Reconstr Surg.* 2015;136:897–912.
11. Bae YC, Song JS, Bae SH, Kim JH. Effects of human adipose-derived stem cells and stromal vascular fraction on cryopreserved fat transfer. *Dermatol Surg.* 2015;41:605–614.
12. Li F, Guo W, Li K, et al. Improved fat graft survival by different volume fractions of platelet-rich plasma and adipose-derived stem cells. *Aesthet Surg J.* 2015;35:319–333.
13. <http://www.fda.gov/ICECI/EnforcementActions/WarningLetters/2015/ucm479837.htm>. Accessed 10.13.16.
14. Moscatello DK, Dougherty M, Narins RS, Lawrence N. Cryopreservation of human fat for soft tissue augmentation: viability requires use of cryoprotectant and controlled freezing and storage. *Dermatol Surg.* 2005;31:1506–1510.
15. Erol O, Agaoglu G. Facial rejuvenation with staged injections of cryopreserved fat and tissue cocktail: clinical outcomes in the past 10 years. *Aesthet Surg J.* 2013;33:639–653.
16. Butterwick K, Bevin A, Iyer S. Fat transplantation using fresh versus frozen fat: a side-by-side two-hand comparison pilot study. *Dermatol Surg.* 2006;32:640–644.
17. Mojallal A, Shipkov C, Braye F, et al. Influence of the recipient site on the outcomes of fat grafting in facial reconstructive surgery. *Plast Reconstr Surg.* 2009;124:471–483.
18. Dreizen N, Framm L. Sudden unilateral visual loss after autologous fat injection into the glabellar area. *Am J Ophthalmol.* 1989;107:85–87.
19. Danesh-Meyer HV, Savino PJ, Sergott RC. Case reports and small case series: ocular and cerebral ischemia following facial injection of autologous fat. *Arch Ophthalmol.* 2001;119:777–778.
20. Beleznay K, Carruthers JD, Humphrey S, Jones D. Avoiding and treating blindness from fillers: a review of the world literature. *Dermatol Surg.* 2015;41:1097–1117. Coleman, W. Commentary, p. 1118.

# 11

# Introduction to permanent fillers: pros and cons

## Shilpi Khetarpal, Jeffrey S. Dover

### Summary and Key Features

- Permanent fillers are materials composed of nonabsorbable or permanent materials.
- These agents can provide long-lasting results but carry more potential risk.
- Polymethylmethacrylate and liquid injectable silicone are the only currently available permanent fillers available in the United States.
- Nonbiodegradable fillers can achieve full and long-lasting correction but carry the risk of permanent adverse effects.

## Introduction

In the past 15 years, with the approval of hyaluronic acid (HA) fillers, there has been a dramatic change in the rejuvenation of the aging face with injectable facial fillers. With more than 2.2 million soft tissue filler procedures performed in 2013, there has been increasing interests in research and development of both temporary and permanent agents.[1] There is no universally accepted classification for soft tissue fillers; however, they can be classified by their origin—natural animal, synthetic, or natural synthetic. They can be further classified by their longevity: temporary, semipermanent, or permanent.[1] An ideal soft tissue filler is one that is effective, easy, and painless to inject, feels natural, is nontoxic, nonreactive, noncarcinogenic, nonimmunologic, has a low incidence of adverse events, and is long-lasting.[2] The US Food and Drug Administration (FDA) defines permanent fillers as materials that are composed of nonabsorbable or permanent materials. These agents can provide excellent, long-term results but carry more potential risk and require a higher level of injector skill given that complications are more common compared with temporary agents and can be more difficult to resolve. In the United States the currently available permanent fillers are polymethylmethacrylate (PMMA) and liquid injectable silicone (LIS). Several other agents are available for use outside the United States or are currently being developed (Table 11.1).

## Polymethylmethacrylate

Bellafill (Suneva Medical, San Diego, CA) is a third-generation PMMA and collagen filler that is an updated version of its predecessor created more than 20 years ago. The original form was never commercially available in the United States (Arteplast/Artecoll); however, a refined version called Artefill was used in the United States.[3] Although these agents were effective, they had a high incidence of foreign body granuloma formation at 2.5%, due to the small PMMA microsphere size (<20 µm) that provoked a foreign body response due to macrophages digesting these small particles.[4] The latest generation, Bellafill, has 20% larger PMMA microspheres (30 to 50 µm) suspended in a water-based gel containing 3.5% bovine collagen and 0.3% lidocaine. The larger particle size decreases digestion by macrophages and overall immunogenicity. Due to the bovine collagen component, the FDA recommends a skin test at least 28 days prior to use because of a 3% rate of collagen hypersensitivity.[2] The collagen component is absorbed 1 to 3 months after injection, and the PMMA microspheres act as a scaffold for the development of autologous collagen.[4] Fibroblasts encapsulate each PMMA microsphere then the bovine collagen is replaced by the patient's own connective tissue over a period of several months, with eventual formation of new collagen. A series of multiple injections are necessary to achieve the best outcome. Results can take several months to more than a year after injection.[5] It is essential for the practitioner to take a conservative approach and wait months between injections. Although complications with Bellafill are less than with its predecessors, they can still occur. If injections are placed too superficially, nodules, beading, and scarring can occur. The new generation of PMMA has a lower incidence of delayed granuloma formation due to the more uniform and larger size and shape of microspheres. PMMA microsphere size is critical to avoid phagocytosis, and particles less than 20 µm in size cause a foreign body response.[3] The original generation of PMMA agents had granuloma rates of 2.5% at 5 years compared with 1.7% with the latest-generation product.[5] In 2006 Bellafill received FDA approval for nasolabial folds and in late 2014 for moderate-to-severe, atrophic, distensible facial acne scars on the cheeks.[5] The product has strict manufacturing requirements and unique formulation characteristics that make it superior when

**Table 11.1** Permanent fillers by category and composition

| Category | Branded product | Composition |
|---|---|---|
| Liquid injectable silicone | Silikon-1000 | Purified polydimethylsiloxane polymer |
| | Adatosil-5000 | Purified polydimethylsiloxane polymer |
| Other "silicones" | Adulterated and unknown products | Variable and often unknown |
| Polyalkylimide gels (hydrophilic) | Bio-Alcamid | 3% or 4% polyalkylimide gel in 97% or 96% sterile water |
| Polyacrylamide gels (hydrophilic) | Amazingel | Polyacrylamide gel in sterile water |
| | Aquamid | 2.5% polyacrylamide gel in 97.5% sterile water |
| Polymethylmethacrylate (hydrophobic) | Arteplast/Artecoll/Artefill | <20 μm PMMA microspheres in a bovine collagen carrier |
| | Bellafill | 30–50 μm PMMA microspheres in a bovine collagen carrier |
| Acrylic hydrogel (hydroxyethylmethacrylate/ethylmethacrylate) (hydrophobic) | Dermalive | 45–65 μm polygonal fragments acrylic hydrogel (40%) in HA (60%) |
| | Dermadeep | 80–110 μm polygonal fragments acrylic hydrogel (40%) in HA (60%) |

*HA*, Hyaluronic acid; *PMMA*, polymethylmetacrylate.
Modified from 3rd edition of Soft Tissue Augmentation, Complications of Permanent Fillers.

compared with prior PMMA products.[6] Bellafill is the only PMMA filler manufactured in the United States and uses a more refined collagen carrier matrix derived from bovine collagen sources that come from a restricted herd. The differences in manufacturing and quality in PMMA formulations play a large role in the product safety and effectiveness. The new class of PMMA-based fillers have longevity greater than 5 years and if injected properly can be safe for its approved indications in the appropriate patient type—one who desires long-lasting correction.[7]

## Liquid injectable silicone

LIS is one of the oldest and longest-lasting injectable fillers. It received FDA approval in 1959 for intraocular use as retinal stabilizing agents, for retinal tamponade during vitreous surgery. It is used off-label for cosmetic therapy, including for human immunodeficiency virus (HIV) lipoatrophy, acne scarring, and facial volume enhancement. Its use as a filler is controversial due to potential long-term complications.[6] Similar to PMMA, LIS induces new collagen production in addition to producing a direct volume-filling effect. Complications vary from minor and temporary to serious and permanent. Minor complications include erythema, ecchymoses, and edema at injection sites, which can occur with any soft tissue filler.[8] More serious complications include infection, silicone granuloma formation (weeks to years after placement), ulceration, inflammatory nodules, vascular occlusion, and migration.[6] Many of these complications occur when using contaminated industrial-grade products or improper injection technique. It is recommended that one of the FDA-approved, medical-grade silicone oils be used—Silikon 1000 (Alcon, Fort Worth, TX) or Adato Sil-ol-5000 (Bausch & Lomb, Rochester, NY)—with the microdroplet technique.[6] With this technique, droplets of 0.01-mL aliquots are injected in the subcutaneous fat or deep dermis in the desired locations. Silicone oil is available from manufacturers in Mexico and South America; however, these formulations can be contaminated and impure, resulting in a high rate of complications.[1] Before the microdroplet technique was developed, LIS was injected in large boluses in a single session, resulting in high rates of migration of the product.[9] Despite potential complications, LIS has many "ideal" qualities for soft tissue filling. It is colorless, odorless, nonvolatile, noncarcinogenic, thermally stable for heat sterilization, chemically stable at room temperature (allowing for storage for long periods of time), does not have to be reconstituted prior to use, and when injected properly looks very natural.[10] If used for the correct indications in the hands of a skilled injector, medical-grade silicone oil is a safe, economic, permanent dermal filler with minimal complications that has been used for more than half a century under the practice of "off-label use of an approved medical device."[1]

## Other permanent fillers

Synthetic facial implants serve a similar purpose to permanent fillers. Most are composed of either silicone or poly-tetraflurothene (Gore-tex).[11] Downsides of these implants are that they are often visible through the skin (especially with movement), they can become visible as facial anatomy changes, and they also may compress nearby structures.

There are other categories of injectable products that are available outside the United States or are currently in development. Polyacrylamide hydrogel—Aquamid (Polymekon, Milan, Italy)— is a biocompatible, nonabsorbable hydrogel containing water and cross-linked polyacrylamide.[12] Aquamid is available and approved in several European, Middle Eastern, and Asian countries for the treatment of rhytides, facial contouring, and HIV lipoatrophy. Although the studies conducted with Aquamid demonstrate high rates of patient satisfaction, the complication rates are high when compared with the temporary hyaluronic acid (HA) fillers. Side effects include unevenness, nodule formation, and displacement of the gel.[12] Delayed immune-mediated events have been reported approximately 10 months after the product had been injected; these include inflamed nodules and pseudoabscesses.[12]

Bio-Alcamid is a 97% hydrophilic polyalkylimide gel that was a permanent filler previously approved for use in Canada for facial contouring and the treatment of HIV-related lipoatrophy. After injection, an inflammatory reaction occurs within 45 to 60 days and leads to a thin fibrous capsule forming around the injected material.[13] It was most commonly used in the malar and lower midface region, and success has also been reported with its use for chin augmentation. Overall patients reported a high success rate with the product when small amounts were used with each injection session (10 to 30 cm$^3$ per side).[13] There have been no reports of foreign body granulomas. Unfortunately, the product becomes mobile after approximately 4 years and tracks around the face giving unsightly lumps (Fig. 11.1A and B). Removal can be achieved through tumescent analgesia with puncture and drainage with manual compression over several sessions. In a study with 2000 injections, 12 patients had infections (0.06%), which were all caused by *Staphylococcus* and treated successfully with oral antibiotics and needle aspiration.[14]

## Pros of permanent fillers

The use of medical-grade LIS and PMMA is now supported by a wide array of scientific evidence that shows these permanent fillers can be used safely and effectively by a skilled injector. After correction with these agents there is no need for maintenance injections, which contribute to additional discomfort, cost, and inconvenience.[6] Bellafill is the only dermal filler FDA-approved to treat acne scarring. It is also the only nonreabsorbable filler approved by the FDA for the correction of nasolabial folds.

## Cons of permanent fillers

Unlike permanent fillers, the HA group of injectable agents has a unique characteristic which is their reversibility with enzymatic digestion with hyaluronidase.[15] Their lack of permanence and ease of correction, with the ability to be dissolved, makes the HA group of fillers attractive to physicians and patients alike. A concern for the use of permanent, synthetic dermal fillers is the safety profile of these long-lasting agents.[16] Many clinicians avoid these

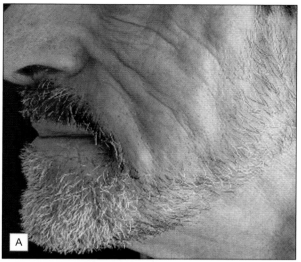

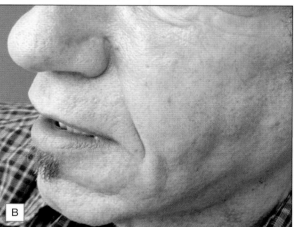

**Figure 11.1 A and B,** Four years after injection with Bio-Alcamid, both patients present with unsightly lumps on the cheeks. *(Photos courtesy of Drs. Jean Carruthers and Alastair Carruthers.)*

agents because of this fear that after the agent has been injected, it cannot be easily removed. Although all fillers have potential side effects, the side effects associated with permanent agents tend to be longer-lasting due to continued presence of product. The other concern of permanent fillers is their irreversibility as facial shape changes with age. Nonbiodegradable fillers can achieve full and long-lasting correction but carry the risk of permanent adverse effects.

## References

1. Wilson Y, Ellis D. Permanent soft tissue fillers. *Facial Plast Surg.* 2011;27(6):540–546.
2. Nettar K, Maas C. Facial filler and neurotoxin complications. *Facial Plast Surg.* 2012;28(3)288–293.
3. Attenello NH, Maas CS. Injectable fillers: review of material and properties. *Facial Plast Surg.* 2015;31:29–34.

4. Lemperle G, Knapp TR, Sadick NS, Lemperle SM. ArteFill permanent injectable for soft tissue augmentation: I. Mechanism of action and injection techniques. *Aesthetic Plast Surg.* 2010;34(3):264–272.

5. Joseph JH, Eaton LL, Cohen BR. Current concepts in the use of bellafill. *Plast Reconstr Surg.* 2015;136(5S):171–179.

6. Narins RS, Cohen SR. Novel polymethylmethacrylate soft tissue filler for the correction of nasolabial folds: interim results of a 5-year long-term safety and patient satisfaction study. *Dermatol Surg.* 2010;36:766–774.

7. Mills DC, Camp S, Mosser S, Sayeg A, Hurwitz D, Ronel D. Malar augmentation with a polymethylmethacrylate-enhanced filler: assessment of a 12-month open-label pilot study. *Aesthetic Surg J.* 2013;33(3):421–430.

8. Fulton J, Caperton C. The optimal filler: immediate and long-term results with emulsified silicone with cross-linked hyaluronic acid. *J Drugs Dermatol.* 2012:11(11):1336–1341.

9. Duffy D. The silicone conundrum: a battle of anecdotes. *Dermatol Surg.* 2002;28(7):590–595.

10. Ellis L, Cojen J, High W. Granulomatous reaction to silicone injection. *J Clin Aesthet Dermatol.* 2012;5(7):44–47.

11. Conrad K, Togerson CS, Gillman GS. Applications of GORE-TEX implants in rhinoplasty reexamined after 17 years. *Arch Facial Plast Surg.* 2008;10(4):224–231.

12. Yamauchi PS. Emerging permanent filler technologies: focus on aquamid. *Clin Cosmet Investig Dermatol.* 2014:7;261–266.

13. Ellis DAF, Segall L. Review of non-FDA approved fillers. *Facial Plast Surg Clin N Am.* 2007;15(2):239–246.

14. Pacini S, Ruggiero M, Morucci G, Cammarota N, Protopapa C, Gulisano M. Bio-Alcamid: A novelty for reconstructive and cosmetic surgery. *Ital J Anat Embryol.* 2002;107:209–214.

15. Carruthers J, Carruthers A, Humphrey S. Introduction to fillers. *Plast Reconst Surg.* 2015;136(5S):120–131.

16. Joseph JJ. The case for synthetic injectables. *Facial Plast Surg Clin N Am.* 2015;23:433–445.

# 12

# Liquid injectable silicone

## Derek H. Jones, Jeanette M. Black, Harold J. Brody

### Summary and Key Features

- Two forms of highly purified injectable liquid silicone (Silikon-1000 and Adatosil-5000) are US Food and Drug Administration (FDA)-approved for intraocular tamponade of retinal detachment.
- Both products may be legally injected off-label for skin augmentation, according to the 1997 FDA Modernization Act.
- Industrial liquid silicone, including "medical-grade" industrial liquid silicone, may contain contaminants that cause granulomatous reactions.
- Industrial-grade liquid silicone should never be injected into the human body.
- Three rules should always be followed when using liquid injectable silicone (LIS) for skin augmentation, as follows:
- Rule 1: Inject only FDA-approved highly purified liquid silicone.
- Rule 2: Use only microdroplet technique.
- Rule 3: Inject limited amounts of volume at monthly intervals or longer.
- There is much evidence supporting the safety and efficacy of LIS for human immunodeficient virus-associated lipoatrophy.
- With proper protocol, serious adverse events are rare and are usually treatable.

## Introduction

Physicians and patients continue to strive for the "ideal filler," which would offer consistent, sustained results that remain natural and free of complications over time and that would be biocompatible, safe, cost-effective, and versatile. When injected properly, highly purified liquid injectable silicone (HPLIS) meets the majority of these criteria. Although use of injectable silicone has historically been met with controversy, when modern HPLIS is properly injected in small amounts using the microdroplet technique with repeat treatments spaced at least a

month apart, the physician may routinely achieve optimal and enduring correction of scars, rhytides, and facial atrophy.

HPLIS may be much less forgiving than temporary fillers and is a potential liability when it is injected incorrectly, results in undesired augmentation, or serves as a nidus for inflammation and infection. Therefore to achieve good outcomes, experience and precise technique are imperative. Physicians should use HPLIS only after extensive training in proper technique and patient selection. Candidates for treatment should have clear treatment objectives and understand that multiple treatment sessions may be required to achieve optimal correction. Patients who desire immediate correction or are uncertain of their treatment goals are better treated with temporary fillers rather than HPLIS.

## Basic science

*Silicon* (Si) is a relatively inert element that is essential to humans in small amounts and is second only to oxygen as the most abundant element of the Earth's crust. "Silicone" describes a group of synthetic polymers containing elemental silicon. Polymers in the silicone family may exist in solid, liquid, and gel states, with various chemical, physical, and thermal properties. Silicone polymers also vary with regard to purity, sterility, and biocompatibility. Although various silicone polymers are used for medical use, *polydimethylsiloxane* is the liquid injectable silicone (LIS) used for soft tissue augmentation. The molecular structure of this colorless, odorless, nonvolatile oil consists of repeating dimethylsiloxane units with terminal trimethylsiloxane ends.

The viscosity of a given liquid silicone product is dependent upon the mean number and chain length of the dimethylsiloxane subunits within the polymer, with longer chain molecules conferring a higher viscosity. Viscosity is measured in centistokes (cs), where 1 cs equals the viscosity of water. Current HPLIS is either 1000 cs (similar to the viscosity of honey) or 5000 cs.

Silicones have not been found to be carcinogenic and have demonstrated "an enviable record of safety," according to a 1998 National Science Panel investigating silicone implants, reported by Diamond et al. HPLIS is not altered in vivo, although small amounts may be phagocytized and enter the reticuloendothelial system.

## Mechanism of action

HPLIS first creates immediate volume enhancement by a direct space-filling effect. Additional filling occurs by the deposition of new collagen via fibroplasia. After injection, a localized inflammatory reaction ensues, consisting of neutrophil migration and some degree of macrophage phagocytic activity, with fibroblasts depositing a thin-walled collagen capsule around the silicone microdroplet. This capsule effectively anchors the microdroplet in place and prevents migration.

Several filler products, both temporary and permanent, were reported by Jones in 2009 to induce collagen fibroplasia as a partial mechanism of action for aesthetic improvement.

Rather than attempting to reach optimal correction in one session, fibroplastic fillers require that smaller amounts of product be injected over several sessions spaced 1 to 2 months apart or longer. This avoids overcorrection by allowing the fibroplastic process adequate time to occur prior to subsequent treatment sessions.

## Controversy

The past several decades have witnessed notable debate regarding the safety of LIS, with both critics and advocates arguing their positions based largely on anecdotal data rather than rigorous trials. The true number of patients treated with liquid silicone available prior to 1990 who have historically experienced treatment success versus significant complications is simply unknown.

A further difficulty in historically analyzing the safety of "silicone" as an augmenting agent is that, apart from the modern, FDA-approved products available since the 1990s, an unknown number of products claiming to be silicone have likely been adulterated, impure, or non-silicone substances altogether. Although highly purified 1000 and 5000 cs products intended for injection into the human body were FDA-approved for human use in the 1990s, various substances masquerading as silicone have been injected for the past 60 years, at times with significant complications, as reported by Delage et al., Baselga and Pujol, and Rapaport et al. Even products labeled as "medical-grade" silicone have not historically been regulated or authenticated. A 1989 analysis by Parel of six "medical-grade" silicone oils commonly used for injection revealed six different products of variable viscosity, each with significant amounts of elemental impurities and low-molecular-weight adulterants that can produce inflammatory and granulomatous reactions.

Critics argue that liquid silicone is an inherently unpredictable implant, fraught with potential complications. Several anecdotal reports of complications, such as cellulitis, nodules, granulomatous reactions, and migration, have been described by the groups previously discussed, although variables, such as product purity, volume, and injection technique, could not be established with certainty. Furthermore, complications were reported by Rapaport et al. to occur as long as 36 years after treatment. Migration of product to other areas of the body may occur when large boluses of liquid silicone are injected, but this has never been reported when using the microdroplet technique, as in the studies by Duffy in 2005 and Price et al. in 2006.

Advocates posit that HPLIS is extremely safe and beneficial when three rules of injection are strictly followed: (1) use only FDA-approved products intended for injection into the human body, (2) exclusively use the microdroplet technique, and (3) strictly follow a protocol using limited volumes injected over multiple sessions spaced monthly or longer.

Several authors have published excellent safety records of longer-term follow-up on patients treated with liquid silicone. Wallace et al. reported long-term follow-up over 41 years using liquid silicone as a soft tissue substitute for plantar fat loss in more than 1500 patients, with 25,000 recorded silicone injections; they found that the host response to injections consisted of a "banal and stable fibrous tissue formation." Other authors, including Jones et al., Chen et al., Orentreich and Leone, and Hevia, have published multiple reports of their extensive and successful experience with liquid silicone and reiterate that the three principles of product purity, appropriate technique, and proper protocol are imperative for success. Duffy, who has written extensively on the subject, gathers that LIS has been used for soft tissue augmentation worldwide for at least 40 years and hypothetically in at least 200,000 patients in the United States. He cautions that, although pure liquid silicone may be a superior filler for the permanent correction of certain defects, physicians who use it must realize that its misuse, or the use of other materials masquerading as pure silicone, have created "a pervasive climate of distrust and a veritable minefield of extraordinarily unpleasant medico-legal possibilities." Such perceptions reiterate the importance of ongoing trials because they replace anecdotal reports with more rigorously obtained data. Despite 60 years of use, only within the past 12 years have well-designed trials begun with the newer generation of standardized, highly purified products injected according to strict protocol. These studies have so far demonstrated an excellent profile of safety and efficacy. Collection of ongoing objective data and longer-term follow-up are necessary to provide clarity into the true risks and benefits of soft tissue augmentation with modern HPLIS.

## Indications and patient selection

Although there are currently no FDA-approved cosmetic indications for HPLIS, it may be legally injected off-label for the augmentation of human immunodeficiency virus (HIV)-associated facial lipoatrophy, nasolabial folds, labiomental folds, mid-malar depressions, lip atrophy, hemifacial atrophy, acne scarring, other atrophic scarring, age-related atrophy of the hands, corns and calluses of the feet, and healed diabetic neuropathic foot ulcers (see the studies by Orentreich and Jones, Balkin, and Fulton et al.) (Figs. 12.1 to 12.4). HPLIS is specifically contraindicated for injection into the breast, eyelids, or bound-down scars or injection into an actively inflamed site. Its safety has not been studied in pregnant or breast-feeding women. It should not be injected into patients with chronic bacterial sinusitis, dental caries, or other active bacterial infection or in those who may be predisposed to trauma in the treated area. In addition, HPLIS is not a substitute for surgical lifting, chemical or laser resurfacing, dermabrasion, or treatment of dynamic rhytides with botulinum toxin. The ideal patient is one with appropriate insight into the permanent and off-label nature of LIS, a realistic attitude regarding achievable results, in good physical health, and compliant with recommendations. Patients seeking immediate correction or temporary augmentation should be treated with temporary fillers. Serious consideration by both the patient and physician must be given to the longevity of results obtained with HPLIS. Although permanent fillers may be preferred to temporary fillers owing to their longevity, one must consider the possibility that personal and societal aesthetic goals may change over time. Furthermore, an undesirable result will be unlikely to diminish with time and may be difficult to correct.

The previously mentioned indications for HPLIS are also well served by modern, temporary fillers, such as hyaluronic acid, calcium hydroxylapatite, and poly-L-lactic acid. However, in the authors' opinion, HPLIS is the most practical and has been demonstrated as an excellent choice for the correction of more severe HIV-related facial lipoatrophy (HIV FLA), in which large volumes and a durable correction are required. Those affected may be stigmatized, leading to psychologic distress, social and career impediments, and impaired compliance with HIV medications. Temporary treatment options are limited by excessive cost and necessity of frequent treatments. An open-label pilot trial by Jones et al. published in 2004 evaluated the safety and efficacy of highly purified 1000 cs silicone oil injected by microdroplet technique for the treatment of HIV FLA. Data on 77 patients with a complete correction were analyzed, and it was determined that the volume of silicone, number of treatments, and time required to reach optimal correction were directly related to initial severity of lipoatrophy ($p < 0.0001$). Supple, even facial contours were routinely restored, with all patients tolerating treatments well. Approximately 3-monthly treatments using 2 mL of HPLIS were required for each stage of severity on the James/Carruthers lipoatrophy severity rating scale. No initial adverse events were noted. In this pilot trial it was demonstrated that highly purified 1000 cs silicone oil is a safe and effective treatment option for HIV FLA.

Jones reported in 2010 on safety outcomes in 135 patients with 5-year and beyond follow-up after treatment with HPLIS for HIV FLA. At 5-year follow-up, 4

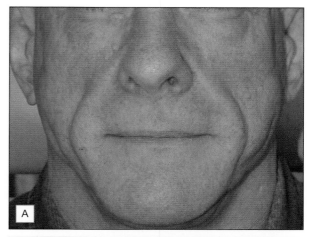

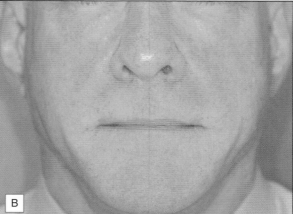

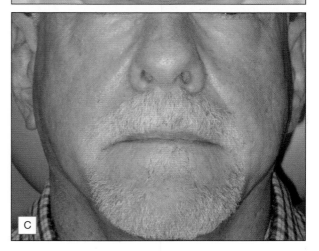

**Figure 12.1 A,** Human immunodeficiency virus (HIV) facial lipoatrophy. **B,** After correction with a series of monthly injections with Silikon-1000. **C,** Ten-year follow up.

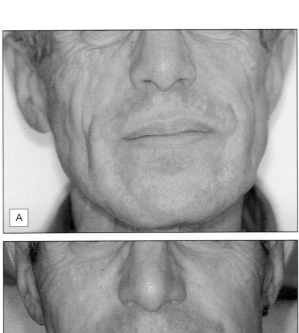

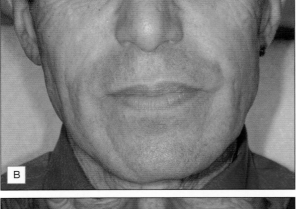

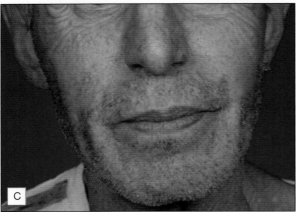

**Figure 12.2 A,** Human immunodeficiency virus (HIV) facial lipoatrophy after Gore-tex thread implants. Note the uneven facial contour. **B,** After a series of monthly injections with Silikon-1000 to restore volume and even contour. **C,** Ten-year follow-up.

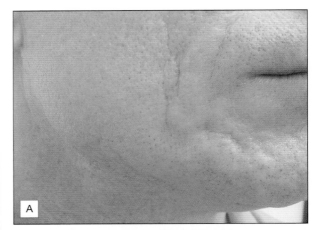

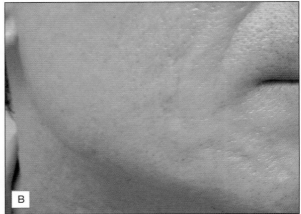

**Figure 12.3 A,** Acne scarring. **B,** After a series of injections with Silikon-1000.

of the 135 patients experienced a palpable subcutaneous nodule or firmness at the injection site. All events responded completely to intralesional triamcinolone and oral minocycline, and none were considered serious. The specific histories of each patient support a bacterial and/or immunologic basis for such reactions. In 2016, Black and Jones presented a report on the safety outcomes in 113 patients with 10-year and beyond follow-up after treatment with HPLIS for HIV FLA. Of the 113 patients, 10 experienced mild and treatable adverse events resulting from either excessive fibroplasia manifesting as mild subcutaneous firmness and/or nodules or acute inflammatory events manifesting as tenderness and swelling. All adverse events were treatable and none were considered serious. Jones currently prefers to treat these adverse events of excessive fibroplasia with intralesional subcutaneous injections of injectable liquid 50 mg/mL 5-flourouracil, admixed with 40 mg/mL triamcinolone. Usually 0.1 mL of 40 mg/mL triamcinolone is added to 1 mL of 50 mg/mL 5-flourouracil. This is injected monthly until satisfactory improvement is achieved.

Using the microdroplet, multiple-injection technique, Barnett and Barnett have had success with injections of LIS for acne scars lasting over a 10-, 15-, and 30-year follow-up period (as reported by Jones in 2010).

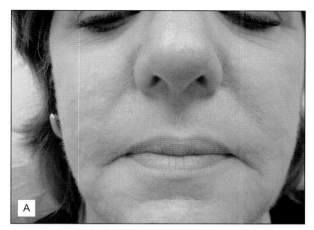

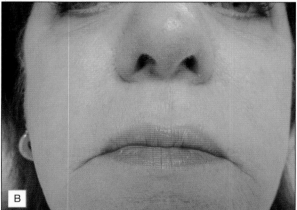

**Figure 12.4 A,** Acne scarring. **B,** After a series of injections with Silikon-1000.

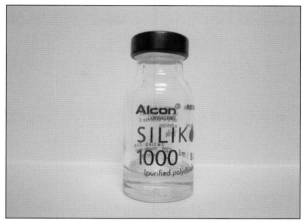

**Figure 12.5** Silikon-1000, which is specifically US Food and Drug Administration (FDA)-approved for ophthalmic use but may be legally used off-label for skin augmentation.

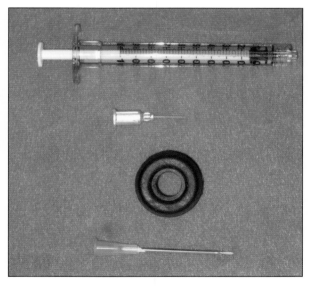

**Figure 12.6** Instrumentation; from top to bottom, 1 mL BD syringe, 27-gauge ½ inch needle, autoclaved electrical bushing, 16-gauge needle.

## Materials

The most appropriate HPLIS for off-label soft tissue augmentation is Silikon-1000 (Alcon, Fort Worth, TX) (Fig. 12.5); 5000 cs Adatosil (Bausch & Lomb, Rochester, NY) may also be used off-label but is too viscous to inject through small-gauge needles. Using a 16-gauge Nokor needle, 0.5 mL of LIS is drawn into a 1 mL Becton Dickinson (BD) Luer-Lock syringe (Fig. 12.6), using sterile technique. As molecules from the rubber stopper of the syringe could theoretically contaminate the HPLIS after a long exposure period, it should be drawn into the injecting syringe immediately prior to treatment and should never be stored in the syringe. HPLIS is most easily injected through a 27-gauge 0.5-inch (6 mm) Kendall Monoject aluminum-hubbed needle. Plastic-hubbed needles tend to pop off with the higher injection pressures needed for injection through smaller-gauge needles. To increase injector comfort, 0.5-inch inner diameter rubber electrical bushings purchased from a hardware store may be autoclaved and placed over the barrel of the syringe to cushion the physician's second and third fingers during injection.

### Pearl 1

Of the two FDA-approved liquid silicones, Adatosil-5000 and Silikon-1000, Silikon-1000 is more suitable for injection through small-gauge needles, and hence for skin augmentation, due to its lower viscosity.

## Patient preparation

As with all fillers, patients should avoid blood thinners, such as aspirin, nonsteroidal antiinflammatory preparations, and anticoagulants for 7 to 10 days prior to injection. It is mandatory to discuss with the patient the risks, benefits, and alternative treatments to HPLIS and document this prior to injection. Patients must understand that HPLIS is a permanent filler and must understand that it is being used off-label. Written informed consent must be obtained.

Furthermore, high-quality pretreatment photographs should be taken. Makeup is removed, and the skin is washed with an antibacterial cleanser and prepared with a povidone–iodine antiseptic or other surgical preparatory solution. Areas to be injected are outlined under good lighting, with the patient in a sitting position, using a fine-tip marking pen. Target areas for volume restoration should be marked in both the smiling and resting position, as these often change remarkably with facial activity. When treating HIV facial lipoatrophy, mid-malar depressions often become slightly elevated on smiling, and overcorrection of this area may result in a "chipmunk" appearance.

## Injection technique

Although temporary fillers may be injected with varied techniques, HPLIS should be injected only by the microdroplet technique originally described in 2000 by Orentreich. Other injection techniques risk undesirable consequences, including pooling or beading of silicone macrodroplets in the injection tract and possible migration via escape from the anchoring fibroplastic capsules. A microdroplet is defined as 0.005 to 0.01 mL of product, an amount that possesses a very large surface area to volume ratio. A larger surface area to volume ratio effectively allows the microdroplet to be anchored into place by the ensuing fibroplasia around the periphery. With larger macrodroplets, defined as greater than 0.01 mL, encapsulation may not be sufficient to prevent product migration. A given volume of HPLIS dispersed into many microdroplets provides for a greater total surface area than would be provided by fewer, larger droplets. Maximizing the total surface area of injected product effectively maximizes the degree of augmentation.

Injections are made into the immediate subdermal plane or deeper. Often, as the needle enters the subdermal plane, there is a slight give in the tissue resistance to the needle. Intradermal injection should be diligently avoided, as it may result in dermal erythema and ridging. Attention should be given to make sure that the needle is in the subdermal plane prior to depressing the plunger. Furthermore, the injector's thumb should be removed from the plunger prior to removing the needle. Injections should be placed at 2- to 5-mm intervals along the skin surface at the optimal angle for penetration and deposition into the subdermal plane. The optimal angle varies with the intended depth of LIS placement. For areas where deeper placement is desired, a more oblique (approaching perpendicular to the skin surface) angle of insertion is best, whereas a more acute (approaching parallel to the skin surface) angle of insertion works best for more superficial deposition.

As a rule, multiple passes over the same treatment area in a single session should be avoided, although experienced injectors may sometimes make a second pass at a different subcutaneous level and use a tunneling technique to inject microdroplets in different subdermal areas. Importantly, greater correction should be accomplished over a longer period of time rather than with a larger per-session volume. Per-session treatment volumes should be limited to 0.5 mL for smaller surface areas, such as the nasolabial fold, and no more than 2.0 mL for larger surface areas, such as facial lipoatrophy. Such per-session volumes allow approximately 100 to 200 individual microdroplet deposits at 2- to 5-mm intervals, allowing a large treatment area to be covered in a single session if necessary.

Injection sessions should be spaced at least 1 month or more apart to allow for a limited fibrous tissue reaction to occur around each silicone microdroplet. Overcorrection should be avoided. As optimal correction approaches, treatment intervals should be extended to allow complete deposition of fibrous tissue prior to the next injection.

## Side effects and managing complications

The immediate injection-related side effects commonly seen with all fillers also occur with HPLIS. Needle-associated pain is usually well controlled with pretreatment topical lidocaine anesthetics. Pretreatment with oral analgesics (e.g., 0.5 mg alprazolam and two tablets of hydrocodone/acetaminophen 5/300 mg) 1 hour prior to treatment may occasionally be necessary in the pain-intolerant patient. Mild postinjection edema and erythema are common and resolve within a few days. The transient edema may even be representative of what optimal correction may look like after several treatments. Purpura, when it rarely occurs, usually resolves within a few days and may be treated with a pulsed dye laser to hasten resolution.

When injected with the appropriate technique, LIS is remarkably similar in texture and sensation to natural soft tissue. However, when larger cumulative volumes are injected, as in HIV FLA, the treated area may occasionally feel slightly rubbery and firmer than natural soft tissue. Migration of injected liquid silicone is an often-mentioned and undesired adverse event. Using small volumes over multiple treatment sessions with the microdroplet technique avoids this problem because microdroplets of silicone are anchored to the surrounding soft tissue by fibroplasia. However, LIS may track along tissue planes in the path of least resistance when injected in large boluses all at once.

Skin dyschromia is a rare side effect of LIS, occurring most often when too much liquid silicone is inadvertently injected into the dermis. When the inflammatory response to LIS extends into the dermis then postinflammatory erythema, postinflammatory hyperpigmentation, and telangiectasia may occur. Dermal ridging often occurs in conjunction with the dyschromia. Erythema and telangiectasia may be treated with a pulsed dye laser or intense pulsed light device. Hyperpigmentation may be treated with hydroquinone and sun protection. Dermal ridging may improve with intralesional steroid injection, but the response is often incomplete and the problem persistent.

A more concerning potential adverse event to LIS is excessive fibrosis or acute inflammation presenting as a palpable subcutaneous nodule or firmness. Such reactions were described in 2009 by Jones with liquid silicone, as well as a variety of other permanent or longer-lasting fillers, such as polymethylmethacrylate and polylactic acid. They are thought to be immune-mediated, although the basis of the immune mechanism remains unclear. It has been postulated that granulomatous reactions may be a result of infection at a distant site because granulomatous reactions to liquid silicone have been noted to appear with the development of acute bacterial dental abscesses or sinusitis and to resolve upon treatment of the infection. Another theory, proposed by Christensen, is that bacterial biofilm formation around the LIS microdroplet may create a low-grade, chronic infection resulting in an inflammatory host response. Biofilms may occur if bacterial organisms are introduced upon filler injection, or seed the filler later during bacteremic episodes. Once present, they may remain dormant for months or years on foreign body surfaces, such as injected liquid silicone. Biofilms may serve as a target of a delayed immune response by the patient when organisms convert back to a planktonic state, explaining the potential for granuloma formation years after injection. Should granulomatous reactions develop, they may be treated with high concentrations of intralesional triamcinolone (20 to 40 mg/mL) at 2- to 4-week intervals. It should be noted that HIV infection or ritonavir (Norvir) might predispose individuals to adrenal suppression with higher doses of cortisone. In these cases injectable 5-fluorouracil may be beneficial. Based on the biofilm hypothesis, institution of a full-dose, broad-spectrum antibiotic, such as minocycline, once or twice daily should also occur. Isotretinoin and etanercept have also been used successfully to treat LIS granulomas, in studies by Desai et al., Lloret et al., and Pasternack et al. However, granulomas that fail to resolve may ultimately require surgical removal.

### Pearl 7

HIV-infection or ritonavir (Norvir) may predispose individuals to develop adrenal suppression when higher doses of cortisone are used. In cases where higher doses may be needed to treat rare granulomatous reactions, injectable 5-FU may be useful.

## Conclusion

HPLIS is a safe, effective filler when appropriately used by experienced injectors using the microdroplet technique. Currently its greatest application is for the permanent correction of HIV FLA, although it is effective for the correction of a variety of facial atrophies and deformities. Injectable liquid silicone has generated controversy in decades past. However, modern, highly purified silicone oils studied in controlled clinical settings have so far been demonstrated to be safe agents that warrant distinction. As with any procedure, complications may still occur and may be more difficult to treat, owing to the permanent nature of the product. For this reason, physicians must use proper injection method and inject only in appropriate patients who have had full disclosure as to the off-label nature of its use and adequate informed consent. Continued studies are ongoing to further examine both long-term safety and efficacy.

## Further reading

Balkin SW. Injectable silicone and the foot: a 41-year clinical and histologic history. *Dermatol Surg.* 2005;31(11 pt 2): 1555–1559.

Barnett JG, Barnett CR. Treatment of acne scars with liquid silicone injections: 30-year perspective. *Dermatol Surg.* 2005;31(11 pt 2):1542–1549.

Baselga E, Pujol R. Indurated plaques and persistent ulcers in an HIV-1 seropositive man. *Archives Dermatol.* 1994;130(6):785–789.

Benedetto AV, Lewis AT. Injecting 1000 centistoke liquid silicone with ease and precision. *Dermatol Surg.* 2003;29(3):211–214.

Black JM, Jones DH. A report of 113 patients with 10-year and beyond follow up after treatment with highly purified liquid injectable silicone for HIV associated facial lipoatrophy. Poster abstract. American Society for Dermatologic Surgery Annual Meeting, New Orleans, LA; 2016.

Chen F, Carruthers A, Humphrey S, Carruthers J. HIV-associated lipoatrophy treated with injectable silicone oil: a pilot study. *Dermatol Surg.* 2013;69(3):431–437.

Christensen L. Normal and pathologic tissue reactions to soft tissue gel fillers. *Dermatol Surg.* 2007;33:s168–s175.

Delage C, Shane JJ, Johnson FB. Mammary silicone granuloma: migration of silicone fluid to abdominal wall and inguinal region. *Arch Dermatol.* 1973;108(1):105–107.

Desai AM, Browning J, Rosen T. Etanercept therapy for silicone granuloma. *J Drugs Dermatol.* 2006;5(9):894–896.

Diamond B, Hulka B, Kerkvliet N, et al. *Summary of report of National Science Panel: silicone breast implants in relation to connective tissue diseases and immunologic dysfunction.* Online. <http://www.fjc.gov/BREIMLIT/SCIENCE/summary.htm>; 1998. Accessed 31.01.09.

Duffy DM. Tissue injectable liquid silicone: new perspectives. In: Klein AW, ed. *Augmentation in Clinical Practice: Procedures and Techniques.* New York: Marcel Dekker; 1998:237–263.

Duffy DM. The silicone conundrum: a battle of anecdotes. *Dermatol Surg.* 2002;28:590.

Duffy DM. Liquid silicone for soft tissue augmentation. *Dermatol Surg.* 2005;31(11 pt 2):1530–1541.

Duffy DM. Liquid silicone for soft tissue augmentation: histological, clinical, and molecular perspectives. In: Klein A, ed. *Tissue Augmentation in Clinical Practice*, 2nd ed. New York: Taylor & Francis; 2006:141–237.

Fulton JE Jr, Porumb S, Caruso JC, et al. Lip augmentation with liquid silicone. *Dermatol Surg.* 2005;31(11 pt 2):1577–1586

Hevia O. Six-year experience using 1,000-centistoke silicone oil in 916 patients for soft-tissue augmentation in a private practice setting. *Dermatol Surg.* 2009;35:1646–1652.

Jones D. HIV facial lipoatrophy: causes and treatment options. *Dermatol Surg.* 2005;31(11 pt 2):1519–1529.

Jones D. Semi-permanent and permanent injectable fillers. *Dermatol Clin.* 2009;27(4):433–444.

Jones D. *A report of 135 patients with 5 year and beyond follow up after treatment with highly purified liquid injectable silicone (LIS) for HIV associated facial lipoatrophy (HIV FLA).* American Society for Dermatologic Surgery Annual Meeting, Chicago, IL; 2010.

Jones D. Treatment of delayed reactions to dermal fillers. *Dermatol Surg.* 2014;40(11):1180.

Jones DH, Carruthers A, Orentreich D, et al. Highly purified 1000-cSt silicone oil for treatment of human immunodeficiency virus-associated facial lipoatrophy: an open pilot trial. *Dermatol Surg.* 2004;30:1279–1286.

Jones DH. Injectable silicone for facial lipoatrophy. *Cosmet Dermatol.* 2002;15:13–15.

Lloret P, Espana A, Leache A, et al. Successful treatment of granulomatous reactions secondary to injection of esthetic implants. *Dermatol Surg.* 2005;31(4):486–490.

Orentreich D, Leone AS. A case of HIV-associated facial lipoatrophy treated with 1000-cs liquid injectable silicone. *Dermatol Surg.* 2004;30:548–551.

Orentreich DS, Jones DH. Liquid injectable silicone. In: Carruthers J, Carruthers A, eds. *Soft Tissue Augmentation.* New York: Elsevier; 2006:77–91.

Orentreich DS. Liquid injectable silicone: techniques for soft tissue augmentation. *Clin Plast Surg.* 2000;27:595–612.

Parel JM. Silicone oils: physiochemical properties. In: Glaser BM, Michels RG, eds. *Retina*, vol 3. St Louis: Mosby; 1989:261–277.

Pasternack FR, Fox LP, Engler DE. Silicone granulomas treated with etanercept. *Arch Dermatol.* 2005;141(1):13–15.

Price EA, Schueler H, Perper JA. Massive systemic silicone embolism: a case report and review of literature. *Am J Forensic Med Pathol.* 2006;27(2):97–102.

Rapaport MJ, Vinnik C, Zarem H. Injectable silicone: cause of facial nodules, cellulitis, ulceration, and migration. *Aesthetic Plast Surg.* 1996;20:267–276.

Rapaport MR. Silicone injections revisited. *Dermatol Surg.* 2002;28:594–595.

Selmanowitz VJ, Orentreich N. Medical grade fluid silicone: a monographic review. *J Dermatol Surg Oncol.* 1977;3:597–611.

Spanoudis S, Koski G. *Sci.polymers.* Online. <http://www.plasnet.com.au/index.php?option=com_content&view=article&id=89:polymer-faq&catid=118:FAQ&Itemid=258>; 2009. Accessed 31.01.09.

Turekian KK, Wedepohl KH. Distribution of the elements in some major units of the earth's crust. *Bull Geol Soc Am.* 1961;72(2):175–192.

Wallace WD, Balkin SW, Kaplan L, et al. The histological host response of liquid silicone injections for prevention of pressure-related ulcers of the foot: a 38-year study. *J Am Podiatr Med Assoc.* 2004;94:550–557.

# 13

# Bellafill

## Neil S. Sadick

### Summary and Key Features

- Bellafill is currently the only US Food and Drug Administration (FDA)-approved permanent filler indicated for the correction of the nasolabial folds and atrophic acne scars.
- The latest generation of Bellafill is composed of smooth and round microspheres of nonresorbable polymethylmethacrylate (PMMA), which are 30 to 50 µm (20% by volume) suspended in a water-based gel containing 3.5% bovine collagen gel (80% by volume) and 0.3% lidocaine.
- Because the PMMA microspheres stimulate the production of the patient's collagen, there is both immediate and lasting improvement, with studies showing no decrease in visible results after 5 years and a favorable safety profile.
- Bellafill is the filler of choice for people who want long-lasting, natural-looking results and who do not want to have to return regularly for maintenance treatments.
- Bellafill is currently the only permanent dermal filler currently approved by the FDA for nasolabial fold correction and atrophic acne scars.
- Five-year safety data show a stellar safety profile and longevity of clinical results.
- Success in Bellafill depends on using only the latest third-generation formulation and intimate knowledge of injection techniques.

## Introduction

Soft tissue fillers have become one of the most popular minimally invasive aesthetic procedures in the past several decades. Most available fillers, to ensure a safe and biocompatible profile, consist of biologic materials that are reabsorbed, thus significantly reducing their longevity and clinical efficacy. Polymethylmethacrylate (PMMA), currently branded as Bellafill, is the only US Food and Drug Administration (FDA)-approved permanent filler for injection in the nasolabial folds and atrophic acne scars. PMMA has long been used in medicine, particularly in the fields of orthopedics and dentistry, before its application in the field of aesthetics was evaluated. Early formulations of PMMA had an unfavorable safety profile, thus the product underwent considerable development and refinements to meet safety and clinical standards (Fig. 13.1). The first-generation product, called Arteplast (Arteplast, George Lemperle), was developed in the 1980s in Europe. It consisted of PMMA that was suspended in gelatin, which allowed the microspheres to clump together.[1] The microspheres varied in size and had rough surfaces, leading to macrophage infiltration, particle phagocytosis, and subsequent inflammation. In the second-generation product, Artecoll (Artecoll, Rofil Medical), developed in Europe, gelatin was replaced with bovine collagen, which allowed a more even distribution of the microspheres.[2,3] The addition of a wet sieving process eliminated some electrostatic charges that helped to minimize clumping, and microspheres were more refined but still varied in size with some rough surfaces. Bellafill, the third and latest generation of PMMA, previously called Artefill (Artefill, Artes Medical), is the result of 25 years of continuous scientific development and refinement specifically developed to have a superior efficacy and safety profile. In Bellafill the microspheres are rigorously controlled to be within 30 to 50 µm with even smoother surfaces. They undergo seven wet sieving filters to remove negatively charged particles and an ultrasound bath to remove any irregular particles. This process results in producing the most biocompatible PMMA filler for dermal injection.[4,5]

## Product overview and mechanism of action

Bellafill (Artefill) is a nonbiodegradable PMMA injectable filler composed of 30 to 50 µm smooth and round PMMA microspheres (20% by volume) suspended in a water-based gel containing 3.5% bovine collagen gel (80% by volume) and 0.3% lidocaine.[6] Bellafill has an immediate and delayed mechanism of action (Fig. 13.2). The collagen volume that constitutes 80% of the syringe volume provides an immediate lift and volumizing effect. Over time, collagen is reabsorbed and the PMMA microspheres, which make up 20% of the volume in the syringe, act as

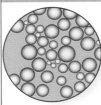

Generation 1
Arteplast
Introduced in 1989

- Bovine collagen suspension
- Single wet sieving process introduced to eliminate negative charges on microspheres to minimize clumping
- More evenly sized microspheres but some less that 20 microns still present

Generation 2
Artecoll
Introduced in 1994*

- High-bloom gelatin suspension
- Dry sieving process
- Non-uniform size of microspheres and rough surface
- Small microspheres (0.5–20 microns) may be phagocytosed by skin cells

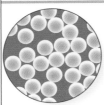

Generation 3
Bellafill
Introduced in 2007

- Bovine collagen from a US closed herd and US manufacturing plant
- Additional wet sieving steps limit microsphere size to 30–50 microns and further reducing clumping
- PMMA particles in this range are not ingested by cells tested, nor do they stimulate TNFα production
- Smoother beads

Figure 13.1 Overview of three generations of PMMA. *PMMA*, Polymethylmethacrylate.

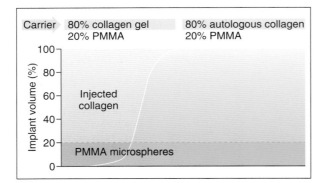

Figure 13.2 Bellafill mechanism of action. *PMMA*, Polymethylmethacrylate.

a matrix to biostimulate collagen production. Histologic analysis has shown that within days of injection monocytes infiltrate the injection sites, differentiate into fibroblasts, and produce a fibrous capsule around the microspheres. Dermal remodeling and angiogenesis are seen as early as 3 weeks post treatment, as capillaries and connective tissue develop and collagen fibers are detected. Over the next weeks to months, collagen fibers increase in density and volume, and by a period of 4 months, the process is complete.[7,8]

## Technical considerations

Each box of Bellafill contains 0.8- and 0.4-mL syringes that may be equipped with a double stopper for use in a metered dose delivery (MDD) device that delivers precise and consistent microdroplets. The carrier collagen of PMMA contains the local anesthetic lidocaine (0.3%) for injection comfort. To maximize comfort, local anesthetics, such as a topical anesthetic spray, 5% lidocaine cream, or others products like EMLA (Akorn Medical), Betacaine, may be used 30 minutes before the procedure.[9] Bellafill product shelf life is 12 months, and refrigeration is recommended. The product must be discarded if phase separation between the collagen and microspheres is detected.

Before use, allergy testing is required 4 weeks prior to planned treatment to minimize the risk of hypersensitivity reactions by intradermal collagen test injection in the volar forearm. Currently, acne scars and the nasolabial folds are the only FDA-approved clinical indications for Bellafill. Injection in lips is contraindicated, and off-label use in the periocular area and tear troughs must be performed judiciously to avoid vascular occlusion of major vessels in the area; globe injury can lead to irreversible blindness.

## Acne scars injection technique

The first decision point for use of Bellafill in acne is whether the scar is distensible or not because distensible scars respond the best when treated with Bellafill. After marking of the scars and application of anesthetic, the Bellafill syringe should be inserted with the bevel up at a 30- to 40-degree angle relative to the surface of the skin (Fig. 13.3). The entry point should be outside of the actual scar area. The needle is advanced underneath the scar to the far edge of the scar into the deep dermis. In cases of very deep acne scars, the needle may be inserted closer to the subcutaneous junction. After the needle is inserted to the far side of the scar, the angle of the needle is reoriented parallel to the skin and moved repeatedly at 90 degrees until a pocket is created for Bellafill to be placed. Bellafill is then injected as the needle is withdrawn, and pressure may be applied to ensure even distribution. A variety of injection techniques may be used to fill in the area underneath the scar, such as serial puncture, or linear threading. Undercorrection is recommended and, in cases of successive treatments, the new Bellafill should be placed above the previous implant, thus building a scaffold.

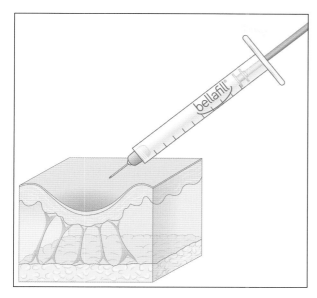

**Figure 13.3** Injection technique for acne scars.

## Nasolabial fold injection technique

Ideal candidates for Bellafill treatment in the nasolabial folds are patients with well-defined wrinkle lines and furrows and little excess skin. Patients with sebaceous skin and large pores but few deep folds are preferred to patients with extremely thin and loose skin because Bellafill implants may be palpable, show through with tension on the skin, or even be visible. Nasolabial folds are best supported by two to three bands of Bellafill injections done parallel to each other and medial to the fold. Because the filler is viscous during the first 3 days after implantation and may be moved laterally by facial muscle movement, it should not be placed too superficially. Strict injection of Bellafill along the dermal–subdermal junction is essential, and a second implantation is often necessary, especially in the lower third of the nasolabial crease adjacent to the corner of the mouth. Undercorrection is recommended, and the filler should not be injected as a large bolus but as small aliquots.

## Pivotal clinical studies

Despite the publication of several clinical studies using PMMA for aesthetic indications, results using the latest generation branded as Bellafill have only been demonstrated in the two pivotal clinical studies conducted for Bellafill FDA approval in the treatment of acne scars and nasolabial folds, respectively.

The Bellafill US Acne Scar pivotal study was a prospective, randomized, placebo-controlled, double-blinded, multicenter (10 centers) clinical trial of 147 subjects older than 18 years who desired correction of moderate-to-severe, atrophic, distensible facial acne scarring.[10] The primary effectiveness end point was the success rate at 6 months, based on the blinded evaluating investigator's (EI's) assessment using the validated four-point Acne Scar Rating Scale (ASRS) with success defined as at least a two-point improvement on the ASRS for at least 50% of treated scars. The average initial injection volume of Bellafill in randomized subjects was 0.11 mL per scar, and the average initial volume injected per subject was 0.93 mL. Touch-ups were conducted as needed at follow-up visits at weeks 2, 4, 6, and 8 and months 3, 6, 9, and 12. Results from the study showed that the primary effectiveness end point was achieved with 64.4% responders in the Bellafill group and 32.6% responders in the control group ($p$ = 0.0005) at 6 months. Subject satisfaction was assessed using the six-point SASC scale. Greater than 83% of Bellafill subjects judged themselves to be at least somewhat to very satisfied with the appearance of their treated scars at all time points. There were no treatment-related severe adverse effects. Unblinded evaluation out to 12 months confirmed a consistent level of effectiveness. Based on these results, acne scar treatment with Bellafill was shown to occur relatively quickly, was sustained, and was effective in all races, genders, and adults of all ages.

A large-scale 5-year postapproval study of Bellafill was required by the FDA to obtain full approval for the use of Bellafill for nasolabial folds with the aim of documenting the incidence of granuloma formation and satisfaction of long-term treatment.[11] Thus a prospective, multicenter, open-label postapproval study was conducted at 23 centers across the United States, and 1008 subjects were enrolled. Compliance with follow-up was outstanding, with an 87% completion rate (871/1008) at 5 years. Subjects received treatment with Bellafill in the nasolabial folds, and safety follow-up visits were conducted at 3 months and 60 months. Result of the study demonstrated an overall granuloma incidence rate of 1.7%, the majority of which were mild to moderate in severity. This 5-year study that represents the largest and longest follow-up study of a US-approved dermal filler product to date substantiated the safety and efficacy of Bellafill for use in nasolabial folds.

Other notable studies using third-generation PMMA, branded as Artefill, include a single-center, open-label, pilot study of 14 qualified subjects treated for atrophic acne scars.[12] Investigator ratings after 8 months post procedure indicated that 96% of the atrophic acne scars showed some degree of improvement, with the majority of patients reporting a moderate correction. No adverse events or side effects were noted. In another prospective, multisite, open-label study including 24 patients with age-related lipoatrophy, Artefill was injected in the supraperiosteal layer of the malar region, at a maximum volume of 6 mL (3 mL/side). Touch-up injections were performed at weeks 4 and 6, up to a maximum total volume of 8.8 mL. Based on both the patient- and physician-rated evaluation, 95.8% of study participants were reported as being "improved" or "very much improved." The change in malar lipoatrophy grade was significantly improved from baseline to 1 year by $0.96 \pm 0.98$ ($p < 0.0003$). Patients also reported high levels of satisfaction, with 87.5% being "satisfied" or "very satisfied." There were no reported adverse safety events in the study.[13]

## Complications and management

As with any foreign entity injected into the body, there is risk of complications.[14–16] Bellafill has been demonstrated to have a stellar safety product profile, and key to minimizing potential complications lies in the hands of the injection technique.[7,8,17]

- In the case of potential technique-dependent adversities, such as uneven filler distribution that appears in the form of a string of pearls, a second implantation into the gaps may alleviate the problem.
- Deep placement of the filler in the subcutaneous fat, together with muscle movements, may result in inadequate treatment, in which case a successive implant is required.
- On the other hand, superficial treatment may lead to itching and erythema that can be treated with corticosteroid cream or intradermal corticosteroid injections. Irregularities or filler nodules that are palpable due to superficial injection can be removed by dermabrasion or shaving.
- Filler dislodgement or migration may be treated with intralesional corticosteroid injections or, if palpable intraorally, excision. Excision should be performed thoroughly and completely because residual Bellafill

may potentially cause secondary hypertrophic scarring, especially in patients prone to keloid formation (Asians and African Americans).

- Patients with thin skin overlying the implant may experience visible dilated capillaries that can be treated and resolved by laser or intense pulsed-light (IPL) therapy.
- Granulomas are the most serious potential complications that occur with soft-tissue fillers, and the concern was more pronounced in the case of Bellafill due to the earlier product formulations and the filler being nonreabsorbable.[18] The etiology of granulomas in dermal implants is multifactorial and potential factors include an excessive immunologic response, bacterial seeding of the implant acquired around the time of implantation, late contamination of the implant site with organisms presumptively spread hematogenously, and biofilms produced by seeded microorganisms.[17,19,20] The safety results from the 5-year study of Bellafill demonstrated that the overall granuloma rate was only 1.7%, with all confirmed cases being mild to moderate and treated was intralesional corticosteroid injections with and without 5-fluorouracil. Granuloma treatment is effectively resolved with intralesional corticosteroid (Kenalog) injections. A 1 : 1 mixture of lidocaine and triamcinolone = fluorprednisolone ((Kenalog or Volon-A)up to 20 mg/mL, or betamethasone (Diprosone) up to 5 mg/mL), can be injected safely through a 1-mL syringe with a Luer-Lock and a 30-gauge needle. The steroid must be injected strictly into the nodule while guiding the needle tip back and forth.[19]

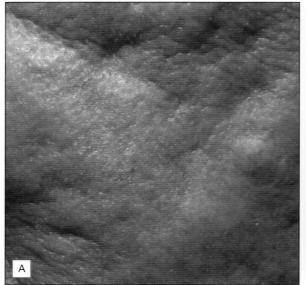 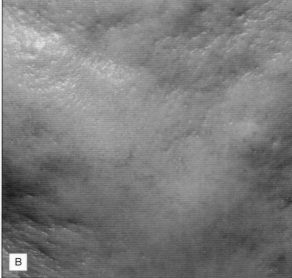

**Figure 13.4** Thirty-five-year-old patient before (A) and after (B) 12 months of two treatments of Bellafill for acne.

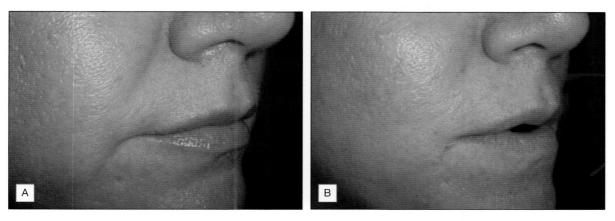

**Figure 13.5** Fifty-year-old patient before (A) and after (B) 3 years of four treatments of Bellafill for acne.

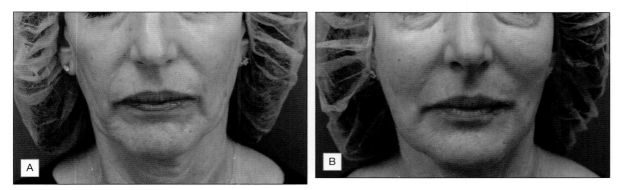

**Figure 13.6** Sixty-five-year-old patient before (A) and after (B) 12 months of two treatments of Bellafill for panfacial volumization.

## Conclusion

The latest generation of PMMA Bellafill has proven an important addition to the armamentarium of soft tissue fillers available for aesthetic applications. Based on sound data supporting its safety and efficacy, Bellafill is currently cleared for use in nasolabial folds and atrophic acne scars (Fig. 13.4). In the author's experience, off-label use for Bellafill for panfacial augmentation and other indications has favorable results, especially in older patients who seek a permanent solution and need considerable structural facial support (Fig. 13.5). Bellafill may also serve as an adjunct to other treatments, such as energy-based devices within a whole-body rejuvenation regimen. Ultimately, it is the practitioner's responsibility to engage in judicious training, commitment to staying up-to-date with research and treatment protocols to capitalize the benefits and minimize risk when treating patients with multifaceted goals and needs in facial reconstruction with Bellafill (Fig. 13.6).

## References

1. Haneke E. Polymethyl methacrylate microspheres in collagen. *Semin Cutan Med Surg*. 2004;23(4):227–232.
2. Solomon P, Sklar M, Zener R. Facial soft tissue augmentation with Artecoll(®): a review of eight years of clinical experience in 153 patients. *Can J Plast Surg*. 2012;20(1):28–32.
3. Bagal A, Dahiya R, Tsai V, Adamson PA. Clinical experience with polymethylmethacrylate microspheres (Artecoll) for soft-tissue augmentation: a retrospective review. *Arch Facial Plast Surg*. 2007;9(4):275–280.
4. Lemperle G, de Fazio S, Nicolau P. ArteFill: a third-generation permanent dermal filler and tissue stimulator. *Clin Plast Surg*. 2006;33(4):551–565.
5. Broder KW, Cohen SR. ArteFill: a permanent skin filler. *Expert Rev Med Devices*. 2006;3(3):281–289.
6. Joseph JH, Eaton LL, Cohen SR. Current concepts in the use of Bellafill. *Plast Reconstr Surg*. 2015;136(5 suppl): 171s–179s.
7. Lemperle G, Sadick NS, Knapp TR, Lemperle SM. ArteFill permanent injectable for soft tissue augmentation: II. Indications and applications. *Aesthetic Plast Surg*. 2010;34(3):273–286.

8. Sadick N. The manufacturer of the FDA approved non-resorbable aesthetic dermal filler Artefill. *J Drugs Dermatol.* 2010;9(7):751, author reply 751.

9. Smith KC, Melnychuk M. Five percent lidocaine cream applied simultaneously to the skin and mucosa of the lips creates excellent anesthesia for filler injections. *Dermatol Surg.* 2005;31(11 pt 2):1635–1637.

10. Karnik J, Baumann L, Bruce S, et al. A double-blind, randomized, multicenter, controlled trial of suspended polymethylmethacrylate microspheres for the correction of atrophic facial acne scars. *J Am Acad Dermatol.* 2014;71(1):77–83.

11. Cohen S, Dover J, Monheit G, et al. Five-year safety and satisfaction study of PMMA-collagen in the correction of nasolabial folds. *Dermatol Surg.* 2015;41(suppl 1):s302–s313.

12. Epstein RE, Spencer JM. Correction of atrophic scars with artefill: an open-label pilot study. *J Drugs Dermatol.* 2010;9(9):1062–1064.

13. Mills DC, Camp S, Mosser S, Sayeg A, Hurwitz D, Ronel D. Malar augmentation with a polymethylmethacrylate-enhanced filler: assessment of a 12-month open-label pilot study. *Aesthet Surg J.* 2013;33(3):421–430.

14. Lee SC, Kim JB, Chin BR, Kim JW, Kwon TG. Inflammatory granuloma caused by injectable soft tissue filler (Artecoll). *J Korean Assoc Oral Maxillofac Surg.* 2013;39(4):193–196.

15. Kadouch JA, Kadouch DJ, Fortuin S, van Rozelaar L, Karim RB, Hoekzema R. Delayed-onset complications of facial soft tissue augmentation with permanent fillers in 85 patients. *Dermatol Surg.* 2013;39(10):1474–1485.

16. Park TH, Seo SW, Kim JK, Chang CH. Clinical experience with polymethylmethacrylate microsphere filler complications. *Aesthetic Plast Surg.* 2012;36(2):421–426.

17. Lemperle G, Rullan PP, Gauthier-Hazan N. Avoiding and treating dermal filler complications. *Plast Reconstr Surg.* 2006;118(3 suppl):92s–107s.

18. Conejo-Mir JS, Sanz Guirado S, Angel Munoz M. Adverse granulomatous reaction to Artecoll treated by intralesional 5-fluorouracil and triamcinolone injections. *Dermatol Surg.* 2006;32(8):1079–1081, discussion 1082.

19. Lemperle G, Gauthier-Hazan N. Foreign body granulomas after all injectable dermal fillers: part 2. Treatment options. *Plast Reconstr Surg.* 2009;123(6):1864–1873.

20. Honma T, Hamasaki T. Ultrastructure of multinucleated giant cell apoptosis in foreign-body granuloma. *Virchows Arch.* 1996;428(3):165–176.

# 14

# Forehead reflation

Kavita Mariwalla, Marguerite Germain

## Summary and Key Features

- Rejuvenation of the upper face relies on toxins, but for some patients with etched-in lines, true correction requires replacement of volume in the forehead concavity and filling of lines at the superficial dermal level. Although multiple fillers are available to correct the upper third of the face, we recommend calcium hydroxylapatite for deep volumization and hyaluronic acid fillers for fine lines specifically.

- Forehead correction is achieved by placing a bolus of material into the inferior frontal eminence. Fine-line correction is achieved by placing hyaluronic acid fillers directly into the lines themselves, although occasionally a bolus to add support to the forehead concavity can be done simultaneously.

- Postoperative edema is a common side effect that resolves spontaneously by 72 hours.

- Relative ptosis of the eyebrows is also a temporary side effect and is a result of lidocaine and edema, typically resolving within 24 hours.

## Introduction

Although fillers are typically used for restoring volume loss to create a youthful appearance, an additional role of fillers is often overlooked—facial recontouring. The recontouring process not only corrects for defects but also aims to restore facial proportion that may or may not have been present naturally in the patient who presents for correction.

One of the prime areas amenable to restructuring through fillers is the forehead area. With time, the upper third of the face elongates as the hairline moves upward and the brow moves downward. Both intrinsic and extrinsic factors play a role. Gender, age, family history, and styling practices can influence hairline position, while gravity, smoking, and sun exposure can cause keratinocytic dysplasia, which manifests as coarse wrinkles and a rough skin surface.

Initially, changes associated with aging, such as rhytides, can be corrected through neurotoxin use. Over time, skin laxity and relative muscle atrophy create temporal wasting and some brow ptosis, leading to decreased efficacy of neurotoxin for this area. Even in patients who are neurotoxin naïve, brow descent can occur through repetitive contractions of forehead depressor muscles and loss of elastic fibers. Although many physicians focus on brow elevation, it is important to consider complementary filler placement in the forehead to optimize a younger appearance. (Coincidentally, brow elevation is on occasion noted in patients treated for forehead recontouring.)

In this chapter, we review a simple technique to replenish volume loss in the forehead, improve skin laxity, and reposition facial structures to correct for descent using calcium hydroxylapatite (CaHA; Radiesse or Radiesse Plus [Merz Aesthetics, San Mateo, CA]) and hyaluronic acid (HA) fillers. Though we primarily use CaHA and HA, autologous fat and poly-L-lactic acid (PLLA; Sculptra [Sanofi-Aventis US, Bridgewater, NJ]) are also options and will be reviewed briefly.

## Patient evaluation

Changes in the forehead region in terms of texture are typically sun-related, whereas age-related changes cause volume loss, descent of brow position, and muscle atrophy, along with a seeming permanence of horizontal lines. For horizontal lines that are etched into the skin surface, it is important to use neurotoxin first to assess the degree of amelioration through that route, and evaluation for fillers in this region should only occur after the full effect of the neurotoxins has taken place. Questions regarding malignancy, human immunodeficiency virus (HIV) status, diabetes, and thyroid dysfunction should be asked because these are all medical conditions that can contribute to lipoatrophy. In addition, it is important to be aware if the patient is allergic to lidocaine or if he or she has had an adverse reaction to fillers in the past. This is especially important when using PLLA, which can cause granulomas. Informed consent should always be obtained in addition to preoperative photographs. Baseline facial asymmetry is also important to assess. Prior to injection, these authors recommend prepping the skin with alcohol or with chlorhexidine gluconate. Because additional diluted anesthetic is added to the product (CaHA is now available with lidocaine added to it), it is not necessary to anesthetize the patient topically prior to the procedure.

## Anatomy

### Forehead

The skin of the forehead is typically thick compared with other areas on the face, is richly vascularized, and abundant in sebaceous and sweat glands. Though the forehead appears to be a convex structure, there is a concavity that becomes more prominent with age in the suprabrow region. It is located between the frontal eminence of the forehead and the superciliary arches. The superciliary ridges are prominences of the frontal bone above the orbital margins that meet in the midline in the glabella and are typically more visible in men.

The forehead constitutes the upper third of the face and is superiorly bordered by the hairline and inferiorly by the glabella and the eyebrows. For multiple reasons, the hairline is not a reliable landmark among individuals, and depending on the hairline, rhytids can extend almost into the lower hairline area. Remember that the frontal branch of the facial nerve passes through the temple and forehead, placing this nerve at risk of injury during filler use. For this reason, fanning is not encouraged because it can cause nerve injury. The frontal branch of the facial nerve supplies motor innervation to the muscles of facial expression of the eyebrows and forehead. The usual trajectory of the nerve is from a point 5 mm below the tragus to a point 15 mm above the lateral extremity of the brow. The most common method of finding this "danger zone" is to draw a line from the ear lobe to the lateral eyebrow and then from the tragus to the superior-most forehead rhytid. The result will be a zone that corresponds to the usual trajectory path of the frontal branch. Transection with a needle can result in brow ptosis.

Injury to the supraorbital nerve is of concern when treating the forehead. The nerve exits the supraorbital notch, which lies along the orbital rim medially. Although we often teach palpation along the superior orbital rim to find this notch, notches are present bilaterally in only 49% of skulls. A compression injury to the nerve can be avoided by injecting laterally and at least 1 cm lateral to the supraorbital foramen. Adjacent to the supraorbital nerve is the supraorbital artery. Retrograde injection can decrease the risk of vascular embolization, as can the use of blunt-tipped cannulas.

The tissue layers of the forehead are as follows: skin, subcutaneous fat, galea aponeurotica, loose areolar tissue, and periosteum. In the region of the eyebrow, galea gives way to the muscles of facial expression. The preferred injection plane is posterior to the frontalis muscle.

Transverse fibrous septa from the frontalis muscle to the dermis in the forehead are partially responsible for the deep, horizontal forehead creases. The subcutaneous prefrontalis muscle level has been used for PLLA injections. More cohesive fillers, such as CaHA, may not spread as easily and may require multiple injections, thus causing more tissue trauma. Cases of blindness have been reported when injecting near the glabella, making it critical to understand the anatomy of this area before injecting. For this reason we will often use HA fillers in patients with noticeable atrophy due to its pliability and ability to be dissolved.

## Selecting the right filler

There are many fillers to choose from when rejuvenating the upper third of the face. Autologous fat transfer can provide long-lasting results, although multiple treatment sessions are required and significant swelling and edema are postoperative consequences. Autologous fat is also less amenable in patients with HIV-associated lipoatrophy because the fat cells are more difficult to harvest and the fat graft tends to be less successful.

PLLA is another choice for filling, but again multiple treatment sessions spaced 4 to 6 weeks apart are required for optimal results. In these authors' experience the ideal dilution for PLLA is 8 mL of sterile water and 1 mL of 1% or 2% lidocaine. The product can be premixed days in advance, despite package instructions to mix 2 hours prior to injection with the final 1 mL of lidocaine added just prior to patient injection. Injection with $1\frac{1}{4}$ -inch

(35 mm), 25-gauge needles attached to 3 mL syringes allows for even injecting and controlled dispersion of the product. It is critical that the patient massage the area post procedure using the "rule of fives" (5 times a day for 5 days for 5 minutes each time).

HA fillers are viable in this area. For concavity filling, the more viscous products, such as Restylane Lyft (Galderma Laboratories LP, Fort Worth, TX) and Juvéderm Ultra Plus (Allergan, Irvine, CA), are preferable, whereas for individual creases, Restylane Silk (Galderma Laboratories LP, Fort Worth, TX) and Belotero Balance (Merz Aesthetics, San Mateo, CA) are optimal. Some practitioners "thin" Juvéderm Ultra (Allergan, Irvine, CA) by adding 0.5 mL of lidocaine to a 1-mL syringe and injecting this into the mid-dermis in a small depot fashion along the horizontal forehead creases. Placement of these products can occur high in the dermis without Tyndall effect, making it an ideal choice for softening of lines in patients who have become toxin-immune or who require frontalis action to raise the brow and thus cannot tolerate toxin injection (especially the lateral frontalis). Placement of Restylane Silk or Belotero Balance directly into the lines will still allow for muscle movement though it will create a relative softening.

The HA family of fillers is ideal when a reversible correction is desired. Adding 0.5 mL of 1% lidocaine per HA syringe and injecting the retrofrontalis muscle facilitates an even correction.

Again, assessments of the degree of frontal atrophy and skin thickness are necessary before choosing which product is best. For HA fillers the duration of action is typically 4 to 6 months.

In our clinical practices we use both HA and CaHA for these specific applications. The CaHA, especially mixed with lidocaine, lends itself to reliable placement without migration and provides longevity, whereas the HAs have a unique role in the correction of deep, etched in lines. Injection with CaHA and HA is described in detail in the following sections.

## Materials, injection sites, and injection techniques

### Materials

CaHA is a filler with relatively high viscosity. Meland, et al. (J Drugs Dermatol. 2016;15:1107-1110) in addition to original Sundaram, et al. reference for Radiesse viscosity (Dermatol Surg 2010; 36 Suppl 3:1859-65). Alterations in the viscosity can be implemented without compromising long-term efficacy. Consequently, prior to administration of CaHA into the forehead, the product should be homogeneously mixed with lidocaine. In our clinical practice the 1.5-mL syringe of CaHA is combined with 1.0 mL of 1% lidocaine/normal saline diluent mixture for the forehead. If using CaHA that already contains 2% lidocaine, then constitute with 1.0 mL of 1% lidocaine/normal saline diluent only. This mixing enhances the ease of distributing the product throughout the treatment area.

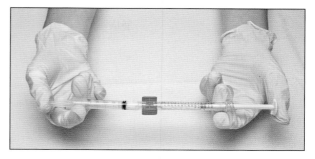

**Figure 14.1** A Luer-Lock connector is used to mix the 1.5-mL calcium hydroxylapatite (CaHA) syringe with the 3.0-mL syringe containing either lidocaine or lidocaine/normal saline diluent. *Courtesy of Merz North America, Inc., Raleigh, NC*

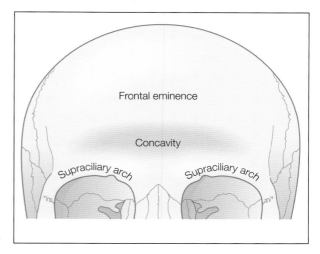

**Figure 14.2** The suprabrow concavity extends inferiorly to the frontal bone supraciliary ridge and superiorly to the frontal eminence.

An ordinary 3.0-mL syringe containing the diluent can be connected to the 1.5-mL syringe, using a female-to-female Luer-Lock adapter (Fig. 14.1). Typically 10 to 15 passes of the CaHA and the diluent back and forth from syringe to syringe is sufficient for homogeneous distribution of both diluent and dermal filler. When using an HA, addition of diluent is typically not needed unless filling lines specifically—in this case, if a more viscous product is used (other than Restylane Silk or Belotero Balance), 0.5 mL of 1% lidocaine should be similarly added to the syringe. Voluma, Restylane Lyft, and Juvéderm Ultra Plus are not recommended for this area.

### Injection site for the forehead

The target in the suprabrow area is the suprabrow concavity. Specifically, this area extends inferiorly to the frontal bone supraciliary ridge and superiorly to the frontal eminence, approximately 3 cm away from the supraciliary arches. Laterally, the space to be injected is marked by extension into the temporal compartment below the temporal cheek fat (Fig. 14.2). The floor of the target

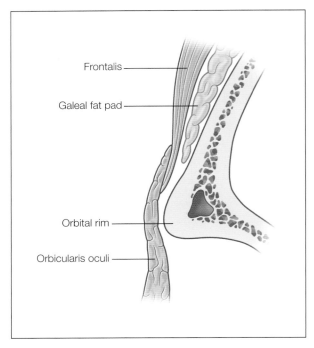

**Figure 14.3** Injections should be executed at the subcutaneous level, with dermal filler placed at the supraperiosteal level behind the galeal fat pad. *Reproduced from Busso M. Forehead contouring with calcium hydroxylapatite.* Dermatol Surg. *2010;36(s3):s1910–s1913.*

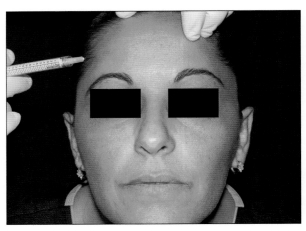

**Figure 14.4** A threading bolus is used to place calcium hydroxylapatite (CaHA) in the inferior frontal eminence. *Reproduced from Busso M. Forehead contouring with calcium hydroxylapatite.* Dermatol Surg. *2010;36(s3):s1910–s1913.*

---

**Pearl 4**

Patients taking blood thinners are susceptible to bruising. When reflating the forehead, bruising can be expected, and in patients on some of the newer blood-thinning agents that do not require routine blood monitoring, the bleeding risk is significant and can leave hemosiderin deposition, especially at the temples. For this reason, patients on blood thinners other than aspirin are asked to have an INR check the day prior to the cosmetic appointment. For those on blood thinners that do not require monitoring, we extensively discuss bleeding and bruising risk and in our experience have found the most bleeding from skin procedures occurs in patients on a combination of clopidogrel and aspirin or on prasugrel. Other thinners that cause extensive bruising include apixaban, dabigatran, edoxaban, and rivaroxaban.

---

injection area is the frontal supraperiosteum, and the ceiling is the frontalis muscle.

When addressing the medial aspects of the area, injections should extend lateral to the projection of the supraorbital nerve. This projection is located >1 cm from the supraorbital notch or foramen. Injections should be executed at the subcutaneous level, with dermal filler placed at the supraperiosteal level behind the galeal fat pad (Fig. 14.3).

When correcting superficial lines that cannot be corrected with neurotoxin alone, place the needle of the HA filler (30 gauge) into the line itself in the dermal place with bevel up. Inject using a retrograde, threading technique, and massage the area immediately afterwards. Keep in mind that overcorrection is not necessary with HA fillers and that swelling is common and should be expected for 24 hours after filler placement.

### Injection technique for forehead recontouring

A 27-gauge, 1¼-inch (35-mm) needle is used to introduce the CaHA–lidocaine solution into the forehead. A threading bolus is used to place the product in the inferior frontal eminence (Fig. 14.4). The amount of product varies with each patient, but the stated objective is reconstitution of the suprabrow arch. When sufficient product has been deposited using retrograde injection for introduction of

the bolus, the area is then massaged so that the product is evenly distributed throughout the borders described in the section above. Volumes may range from 1.5 mL to 3.0 mL of CaHA, in addition to the volumes of diluent necessary for mixing.

In some cases a brow lift has also been a fortunate consequence of forehead recontouring. This has occurred without any placement of product directly behind the brow. However, even in the absence of a brow lift, the filler placement of the patients in a "horseshoe" pattern has resulted in cosmetic benefits, including projection of the lateral eyebrow and reduction of transitions between the suprabrow, temporal, and cheek regions.

When filling individual lines, use a 30-gauge ½ inch needle attached to the HA syringe. Be prepared to replace the needle frequently because 30-gauge needles can burr quickly after multiple injections into thick forehead skin. Inject in a retrograde motion with the bevel of the needle pointed up. Do not inject with the patient lying down because this will give a false sense of improvement. For comfort, the patient should be at a 45-degree angle because patients who are sitting upright can sometimes develop vasovagal syncope due to the number of injections placed into individual lines.

---

**Pearl 5**

Using a bolus technique is preferable to fanning in the forehead region. A 1¼-inch (35 mm) needle facilitates placement.

---

*Note*: After injection, the treated area will likely become edematous. This condition is self-limiting and will resolve in as little as 24 hours in some cases but as long as 10 days in others. An initial temporary brow droop, as opposed to brow lift, is the likely consequence of the diffusion of the lidocaine in the injected solution. The droop is quite short-lived, resolving within several hours.

## Safety considerations and adverse events

The anatomy of the forehead can pose a challenge to experienced and inexperienced physicians alike. The superficial temporal artery and the frontal branch of the facial nerve, both closely associated with the superficial temporal fascia, are to be avoided. Tenting the forehead may be difficult because of the relatively low skin laxity, but tenting the temporal area can separate the subcutaneous layer from the fascia and help to identify the area where the filler is to be injected. Retrograde injection and the use of blunt cannulas can decrease vascular complications, although reliance on a cannula itself is not advised to avoid this complication.

Even with the most careful injection technique into the forehead, edema is likely. This edema is short-lived and usually resolves without any need for ice, cool presses, or analgesic at home. However, our patients are always instructed to contact us when edema lasts beyond 72 hours. Delayed bruising is also possible with ecchymosis, appearing up to 48 hours after injection. To avoid excessive or long-lasting edema, upper face recontouring can be staged, limiting the total volume of CaHA to 1.5 mL per visit. Short-lived brow ptosis has also been observed in some patients, lasting only a few hours post injection of filler.

## Conclusion and discussion

As the 21st century opened, aesthetic physicians were accustomed to seeing the application of dermal fillers as an endeavor that involved chasing lines and wrinkles. Indeed, even the indications for CaHA and other fillers address remediation of fine lines and wrinkles. However, within

10 years, a sea change has occurred in the profession of dermatology in its approach to the use of fillers. Dermatologists now see fillers as tools to volumize the mid- and lower face. We believe that the upper face can also profit from volumizing, in particular by restoring the original contours of the forehead and softening creases that are resistant to neurotoxin use alone. Although PLLA and perhaps even fat transfer may have utility in upper face recontouring, at present we have found that CaHA and HAs offer us the best treatment option for the forehead and temples.

---

**CASE STUDY 1**

Sara is a 55-year-old female patient who consulted us to learn about nonsurgical options for facial rejuvenation. On examination, it was established that periorbital volume reconstitution should be part of the antiaging regimen. CaHA was injected at the retrofrontalis level. Soon after the injection was started, a treelike blanching with the base at the orbital rim was observed, most likely caused by vascular occlusion or compression of a supraorbital artery branch. Subsequent steps included immediate cessation of injection of filler and commencement of vigorous massage. No further changes were observed in subsequent days. Had a HA filler been injected, a hyaluronidase would have been administered.

It is important to watch for any skin color changes while injecting any filler. Injecting lateral to the supraorbital vessels with a blunt cannula, in small amounts, diluted with anesthetic, will help to avoid this complication.

---

## Further reading

Busso M. Vectoring approach to midfacial contouring using calcium hydroxylapatite and hyaluronic acid. *Cosmet Dermatol*. 2009;22(10):522–528.

Busso M. Commentary on extrinsic addition of lidocaine to calcium hydroxylapatite. *Dermatol Surg*. 2010;36(11):1795.

Jones D. Semi-permanent and permanent injectable fillers. *Dermatol Clin*. 2009;27(4):433–444.

Knize DM. An anatomically based study of the mechanism of eyebrow ptosis. *Plast Reconstr Surg*. 1996;97(7):1321–1333.

Knize DM. Anatomic concepts for brow lift procedures. *Plast Reconstr Surg*. 2009;124(6):2118–2126.

Le Louarn C, Buthiau D, Buis J. The face recurve concept: medical and surgical applications. *Aesthet Plast Surg*. 2007;31(3):219–231; discussion 232.

Patel B, Gupta R. *Forehead Anatomy*. <emedicine.medscape.com/article/834862>. Accessed 28.06.16.

Rohrich RJ, Pessa JE. The fat compartments of the face: anatomy and clinical implications for cosmetic surgery. *Plast Reconstr Surg*. 2007;119(7):2219–2227.

Sundaram H, Voigts R, Beer K, Meland M. Comparison of the rheological properties of viscosity and elasticity in two categories of soft tissue fillers: calcium hydroxylapatite and hyaluronic acid. *Dermatol Surg*. 2010;36(S3):1859–1865.

Sullivan PK, Salomon JA, Woo AS, Freeman MB. The importance of the retaining ligamentous attachments of the forehead for selective eyebrow reshaping and forehead rejuvenation. *Plast Reconstr Surg*. 2006;117(1):95–104.

# 15

# Temple reflation

## Derek Jones, Bhushan Hardas, Diane K. Murphy

### Summary and Key Features

- Lipoatrophy of the temporal region can result from the aging process, low body fat, certain genetic disorders, treatment with antiretroviral therapy, or physical trauma.
- Effective reflation of the temporal region with soft tissue fillers can produce gratifying results for both the patient and the physician.
- Administration of hyaluronic acid dermal fillers to reflate the temple has gained significant popularity because of their ease of use and predictable treatment outcomes.
- To avoid the risk of severe complications associated with vascular occlusion, superior knowledge of temporal anatomy and injection technique is essential to achieve safe and effective reflation of the temple.

## Introduction

The appearance of soft tissue fullness in the face results from the multifaceted interplay of all facial tissues, including bone, fat, muscle, and skin.[1,2] Age-related lipoatrophy, the slow, symmetrical loss of subdermal adipose tissue, can result in loss of fullness in many facial areas.[2,3] Lipoatrophy is not only related to aging but can also result from low body fat, certain genetic disorders, treatment with antiretroviral therapy, or physical trauma at any age.[1,3,4] Disease-related lipoatrophy is often more rapid and asymmetric and may be associated with psychologic issues (e.g., body image distortions, social anxiety/withdrawal).[3]

One of the earliest and frequently unaddressed signs of aging is lipoatrophy of the temples (i.e., temple hollowing).[1] With age, the temporal bone progressively becomes more concave, and the overlying temporalis muscle reduces in volume.[5,6] Deflation of the temple causes the tail of the eyebrow to appear shorter, results in the loss of smooth arcs of light around the temporal orbit, and emphasizes the lateral orbital rim.[1,6] Importantly, hollow temples may also be a hallmark of thin individuals and not related to aging.[1] Regardless, individuals who experience lipoatrophy of the temples lose the convexity and fullness of the temporal region that is associated with a

youthful appearance. Individuals with substantial volume loss, especially thinner patients, can have a skeletonized appearance. Successful treatment and correction of the temporal region can produce satisfying results for both the patient and the physician.[1]

### Pearl 1

The temporal fossa is a large, concave area located on the lateral surface of the skull that extends almost to the end of the parietal bone and is bordered by the superior temporal line, zygomatic arch, and zygoma. The anterior region near the hairline is the focus of cosmetic augmentation procedures.

## Aesthetic procedures used for temple reflation

Numerous aesthetic techniques have been used to revolumize or augment hollowed temples, including surgical alloplasty, autologous fat transfer, or soft tissue filler injections.[5,6] Alloplastic implants need to be customized for each patient, often during the surgical procedure. Undercorrection or overcorrection is a limitation of this technique, with implant malpositioning and migration as possible outcomes.[7,8] Limitations of autologous fat transfer include nonstandardization of fat harvesting and fat processing techniques, unpredictability of fat graft retention, and potential for fat necrosis.[9,10] Poly-L-lactic acid (PLLA; Sculptra Aesthetic; Sanofi-Aventis) is a biostimulatory injectable that can deliver natural-appearing temple reflation for up to 2 years. However, numerous injections are required over several months to achieve the desired effect, and the effectiveness is dependent on the strength of the patient's immune system response. As such, treatment can be unpredictable and in some cases result in nodule formation. Calcium hydroxylapatite (CaHA; Radiesse; Merz Aesthetics) is considered "combined filler" because it provides gradual revolumization for 10 to 14 months and has an immediate effect due to the aqueous vehicle; however, treatment can be painful due to deep placement of injection.[6]

Use of hyaluronic acid (HA) dermal fillers to reflate the temple has substantially increased in popularity because of ease of use, consistent, predictable outcomes, and physician and patient satisfaction.[1,11] The immediate aesthetic effects of HA fillers can last up to 1 year; however, these

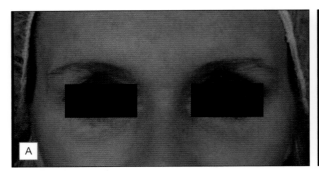
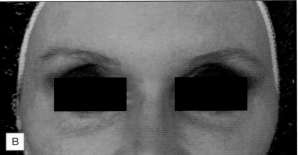

**Figure 15.1** Patient before (**A**) and after (**B**) Juvéderm Voluma XC treatment (2 mL injected) for temple hollows. *Photographs courtesy of Jean Carruthers.*

agents have the unique quality of being reversible (i.e., dissolvable) with hyaluronidase should vascular occlusion occur.[6] As shown in **Fig. 15.1**, satisfactory reflation of the temple with the HA filler Juvéderm Voluma XC (Allergan plc, Dublin, Ireland) can restore a convex shape, provide an upward lift of the face and brow, and result in considerable enhancement in the appearance of the upper face. Based on these outcomes, temple reflation with HA dermal fillers may be part of a comprehensive approach to facial aesthetic treatment.[1,5,12,13]

## Scales to assess temple hollows

Standardized, graded scales are critical to provide objective assessments of the severity of temple hollowing before and after treatment. Two scales are currently available to assess temple appearance. The Hollowness Severity Rating Scale (HSRS) is a four-point numeric scale that scores temple hollowness as absent (one), mild (two), moderate (three), or severe (four).[14] Although the HSRS has yet to be validated, physicians and patients can use this standardized grading system to objectively evaluate outcomes following treatment to augment or enhance the temporal region. The Allergan Temple Hollowing Scale is a validated 5-point photonumeric scale for physician assessment of temple volume deficit (**Fig. 15.2**) (Carruthers, 2016 submitted to *Derm Surg*) and has demonstrated almost perfect interrater and intrarater agreement, suggesting the substantial reliability of numerous assessments for the same individual across different raters. The scale has also shown sufficient sensitivity for detecting clinically significant improvements in volume deficit in the temple area. Scale components include an assessment guide, verbal descriptors, morphed images, and real-world patient images representing both genders and several skin types. Because it was validated in live subjects and included both morphed and unaltered images, the Allergan Temple Hollowing Scale provides standardized ratings that can be applied in day-to-day clinical practice and in clinical trials of individuals seeking temple enhancement.

## Injection technique for placement of hyaluronic acid dermal fillers in the temple

Exceptional knowledge of temporal anatomy is critical to safely achieving optimal temple reflation.[1,11,15] The complexity of the network of blood vessels and nerves in the temporal region increases the risk of vascular compromise and severe complications. Thus it is paramount for the individual injecting the dermal filler to know the exact location of these specific neurovascular structures to avoid injury to the patient. For example, the location of the middle temporal vein (MTV) deep to the superficial layer of the deep temporal fascia presents challenges in regard to avoiding this vein during injection.[16] Likewise the medial zygomaticotemporal vein (MZTV) is located within the same anatomic area and may also be prone to injection-related vascular damage.[15] Based on anatomic knowledge of the temporal fossa area, as well as clinical experience, it has been determined that planes for safe injection within the temple region include the immediate subcutaneous plane using a cannula only, or deep to the temporalis muscle on the periosteum using a needle.[1,11] Safe injection also depends on the type of filler being used.[11] The physician should consider specific attributes of the product because formulations with higher viscosity or elasticity can resist any downward pull of the mid or lower face. The lead author (DJ) recommends that the most effective option is to inject volumizing HA filler deep to the temporalis muscle into the avascular space directly on the periosteum, as described below. This specific placement achieves effective, long-lasting, and reversible reflation of temple.[1]

Prior to initiating the injection, the temporal region should be thoroughly cleaned with alcohol and chlorhexidine to prevent infection and formation of biofilm.[1] An HA dermal filler can be injected using a 27- or 30-gauge half-inch needle, and the injection should be initiated within the safe treatment window, which includes three facial landmarks that serve as safety boundaries. The temporal fusion line represents the superomedial boundary beginning at the tail of the eyebrow; all injections should

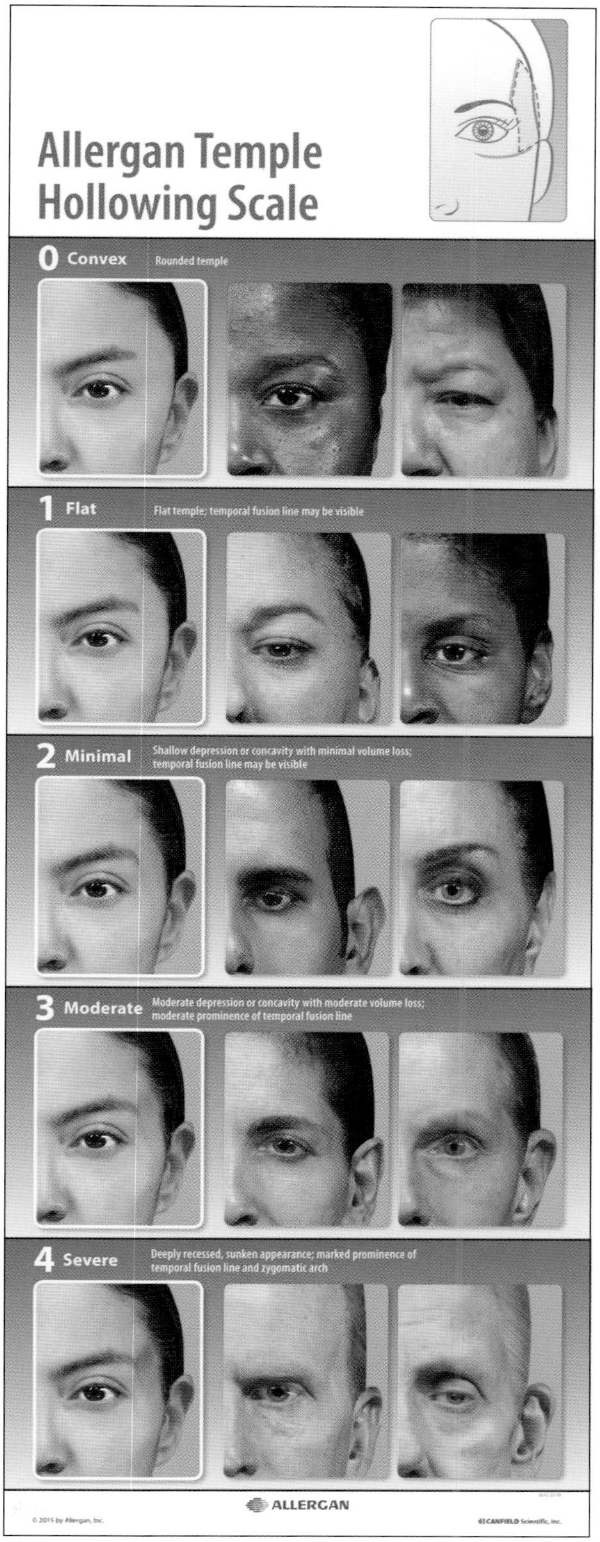

## Allergan Temple Hollowing Scale

**0 Convex** — Rounded temple

**1 Flat** — Flat temple; temporal fusion line may be visible

**2 Minimal** — Shallow depression or concavity with minimal volume loss; temporal fusion line may be visible

**3 Moderate** — Moderate depression or concavity with moderate volume loss; moderate prominence of temporal fusion line

**4 Severe** — Deeply recessed, sunken appearance; marked prominence of temporal fusion line and zygomatic arch

*© 2015 by Allergan, Inc.*　　　**ALLERGAN**　　　*©CANFIELD Scientific, Inc.*

**Figure 15.2** The Allergan Temple Hollowing Scale. The extent of temporal volume deficit (within area of diagram shown in upper right corner) is assigned a grade of 0 (convex) to 4 (severe). *Carruthers, 2016 submitted to Derm Surg.*

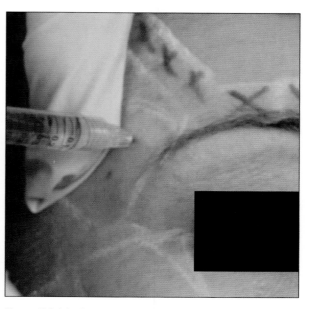

**Figure 15.3** Injection technique: position of needle and injection of product. It is critical that the needle is inserted within the safe injection window at an angle perpendicular to the skin and directed deep until it makes contact with bone. Once placed, the injector delivers a slow, steady depot of HA while placing a finger posteriorly to allow the filler to progress smoothly into the hollowed temple. *Reproduced with permission from Breithaupt AD, Jones DH, Braz A, Narins R, Weinkle S. Anatomical basis for safe and effective volumization of the temple. Dermatol Surg. 2015;41(suppl 1):s278–s283.*

be placed inferior and lateral to this point. All injections should occur 1.5 cm above the zygomatic arch to avoid contact with the MTV and should be placed anterior to the facial hairline because this area offers minimal results with regard to cosmetic enhancement.[1]

To successfully place the filler on the periosteum, the injector should insert the needle perpendicular to the skin and guide it deep until the needle makes contact with bone (**Fig. 15.3**).[1] The injector should then aspirate the syringe until air is visible; this will help to confirm that the needle was not placed intravascularly, although this is not always foolproof, especially with small-bore needles. A slow, steady injection of 0.5 to 1.0 mL of HA filler is recommended for each treatment per temple. The injector may choose to place a finger posteriorly to ease the flow of product into the temple and prevent diffusion to the hairline and massage the temporal area to ensure even distribution of product and achieve smooth, optimal contour (**Fig. 15.3**). An alternative but equally safe and effective method to that previously described involves vertical injection of HA dermal filler on bone at a single point 1 cm lateral to the temporal fusion line, approximately 1 cm superior to the brow.[11] Using this method, maintaining the needle tip in contact with bone is paramount to avoid intravascular injection. Overall, both injection techniques are considered reliable, safe, and effective for injection of HA dermal fillers into the hollow temple.

A cannula method can be used for products with less G′ or for situations that require superficial filling in the subdermal plane.[1,11] To successfully use the cannula technique, the injector should place an injection of lidocaine anterior to the hairline and 1.5 cm superior to the zygoma. Following injection of lidocaine, the injector should insert a 22-gauge needle and place a 27-gauge cannula in the subcutaneous plane of the entry point. Finally, the injector should slowly and steadily fan the cannula throughout the temporal region using a retrograde injection technique and massage the area to ensure even distribution of dermal filler. Importantly, cannula placement of filler in the periosteal plane should be avoided.[1]

> **Pearl 2**
>
> Thorough knowledge of temporal anatomy and appropriate injection technique are critical to achieving optimal temple reflation. One effective option is to inject volumizing HA filler deep to the temporalis muscle into the avascular space directly on the periosteum.

## Avoiding and treating complications of injecting hyaluronic acid dermal fillers

Potential complications associated with injection of HA dermal fillers can be minimized or prevented with sufficient knowledge of the product and the injection technique. The most common adverse events associated with dermal filler placement in the temples are often mild and transient (Fig. 15.4) and include lower eyelid bruising, prominence of superficial blood vessels, headache, injection site pain, and soreness or tenderness that worsens with chewing or eating.[1,12] The relatively mild adverse events of bruising and pain may be minimized by having patients avoid any medications that may increase the risk of bruising (aspirin, nonsteroidal antiinflammatory agents, fish oil, garlic, gingko). If prominent bleeding occurs upon needle withdrawal following injection, direct pressure should be applied to the injection site. To avoid pain while chewing or eating, patients should be instructed to eat soft foods until the pain resolves. Ice, pressure, and corticosteroids can be recommended for acute, intense swelling at the injection site.[1]

Severe complications associated with soft tissue reflation of the temple, using either biostimulatory agents or HA dermal fillers, are those related to vascular damage through puncture or pressure, or occlusion through direct intravascular injection. Although rare, these complications can include skin changes distant from the injection site, severe skin pain, visual acuity changes, ocular pain, or permanent blindness.[1,17] Occlusion of the MTV during HA filler placement may lead to ophthalmic complications in that this vein is connected to the cavernous sinus through the periorbital veins, potentially leading to cavernous sinus

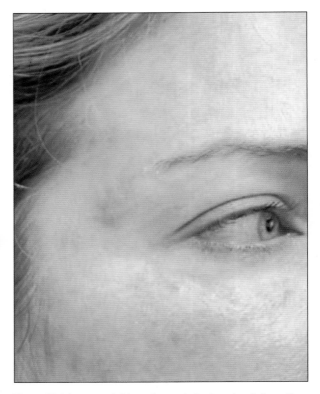

**Figure 15.4** Lumps and ridges observed after temple reflation with a hyaluronic acid filler (Perlane [Medicis, Inc, Scottsdale, Arizona]) injected into the superficial temporal fascia resolved within 1 month. *Reproduced with permission from Ross JJ, Malhotra R. Orbitofacial rejuvenation of temple hollowing with Perlane injectable filler. Aesthet Surg J. 2010;30:428–433.*

embolization.[16] The MZTV may also play a role in ocular complications given that this vein drains into the MTV.[15] Avoiding vascular compromise and occlusion is therefore critical, and the risk is substantially reduced with injection of the HA dermal filler in the avascular periosteal space. In addition, aspiration must be performed prior to injection, and it is absolutely required that the filler is placed slowly without force. If the needle becomes clogged, it should be removed and replaced before reinitiating the injection. If signs or symptoms of vascular occlusion become apparent, including skin changes, severe pain, change in vision, or ocular pain, the needle should be removed immediately, and the injection site should be thoroughly massaged using direct heat. In addition, to achieve optimal vasodilation, nitroglycerin paste can be massaged into the injection site. Hyaluronidase can be liberally injected to dissolve any product responsible for the vascular occlusion, including retrobulbar injection for blindness.[17] Other potentially beneficial treatments for vascular compromise include aspirin, sildenafil, and hyperbaric oxygen.[1]

## Pearl 3

Complications can be minimized by knowing the location of neurovascular structures to avoid injury to the patient. Planes for safe injection within the temple region include the immediate subcutaneous plane using a cannula only or deep to the temporalis muscle on the periosteum using a needle.

## Conclusions

Hollowing of the temples can be successfully corrected using HA dermal fillers. However, the complex anatomy of the temporal region increases the risk of potentially severe adverse effects and should not be overlooked. Safe, effective injections of HA dermal fillers to the temple can be achieved with superior knowledge of temporal anatomy and through use of appropriate injection techniques.

## References

1. Breithaupt AD, Jones DH, Braz A, Narins R, Weinkle S. Anatomical basis for safe and effective volumization of the temple. *Dermatol Surg.* 2015;41(suppl 1):s278–s283.
2. Coleman SR, Grover R. The anatomy of the aging face: volume loss and changes in 3-dimensional topography. *Aesthet Surg J.* 2006;26(suppl 1):s4–s9.
3. Szczerkowska-Dobosz A, Olszewska B, Lemanska M, Purzycka-Bohdan D, Nowicki R. Acquired facial lipoatrophy: pathogenesis and therapeutic options. *Postepy Dermatol Alergol.* 2015;32(2):127–133.
4. Pavicic T, Ruzicka T, Korting HC, Gauglitz G. Monophasic, cohesive-polydensified-matrix crosslinking-technology-based hyaluronic acid filler for the treatment of facial lipoatrophy in HIV-infected patients. *J Drugs Dermatol.* 2010;9(6):690–695.
5. Moradi A, Shirazi A, Perez V. A guide to temporal fossa augmentation with small gel particle hyaluronic acid dermal filler. *J Drugs Dermatol.* 2011;10(6):673–676.
6. Rose AE, Day D. Esthetic rejuvenation of the temple. *Clin Plast Surg.* 2013;40(1):77–89.
7. Cuzalina LA, Hlavacek MR. Complications of facial implants. *Oral Maxillofac Surg Clin North Am.* 2009;21(1):91–104, vi–vii.
8. Tantawi D, Eberlin S, Calvert J. Midface implants: surgical and nonsurgical alternatives. *Clin Plast Surg.* 2015;42(1):123–127.
9. Gause TM 2nd, Kling RE, Sivak WN, Marra KG, Rubin JP, Kokai LE. Particle size in fat graft retention: a review on the impact of harvesting technique in lipofilling surgical outcomes. *Adipocyte* 2014;3(4):273–279.
10. Rai S, Marsland AM, Madan V. Facial fat necrosis following autologous fat transfer and its management. *J Cutan Aesthet Surg.* 2014;7(3):173–175.
11. Sykes JM, Cotofana S, Trevidic P, et al. Upper face: clinical anatomy and regional approaches with injectable fillers. *Plast Reconstr Surg.* 2015;136(5 suppl):204s–218s.
12. Lambros V. A technique for filling the temples with highly diluted hyaluronic acid: the "dilution solution". *Aesthet Surg J.* 2011;31(1):89–94.
13. Ross JJ, Malhotra R. Orbitofacial rejuvenation of temple hollowing with Perlane injectable filler. *Aesthet Surg J.* 2010;30(3):428–433.
14. Moradi A, Shirazi A, Moradi J. A 12-month, prospective, evaluator-blinded study of small gel particle hyaluronic acid filler in the correction of temporal fossa volume loss. *J Drugs Dermatol.* 2013;12(4):470–477.
15. Yang HM, Jung W, Won SY, Youn KH, Hu KS, Kim HJ. Anatomical study of medial zygomaticotemporal vein and its clinical implication regarding the injectable treatments. *Surg Radiol Anat.* 2015;37(2):175–180.
16. Jung W, Youn KH, Won SY, Park JT, Hu KS, Kim HJ. Clinical implications of the middle temporal vein with regard to temporal fossa augmentation. *Derm Surg.* 2014;40(6):618–623.
17. Beleznay K, Carruthers JD, Humphrey S, Jones D. Avoiding and treating blindness from fillers: a review of the world literature. *Derm Surg.* 2015;41(10):1097–1117.

# 16

# Three-dimensional reflation of the glabella and adjacent forehead

Jean Carruthers, Alastair Carruthers

## Summary and Key Features

- Remodeling of cranial bone and fat is well described as part of the aging process, beginning earlier in women (25 years) than in men (45 years).
- The shallow hollows that are seen in the periglabellar area give a tired, careworn appearance.
- Filling the hollows in the underlying glide plane with diluted and thus malleable hyaluronic acid filler gives support which also helps to elevate the brows and to allow frontalis action to continue so that the subject can express interest and compassion.

## Introduction

Age-related loss of periocular bone and fat begins earlier in women (25 years) than in men (45 years).[1–4] The inevitable result is descent and flattening of the brows, furrowing of the glabella and forehead skin, hooding of the upper lids, and a tired discouraged expression. Both women and men wish to eliminate the disempowered appearance that results.

For many years the glabellar lines have been supported intradermally using hyaluronic acid (HA) fillers,[5] and the combination treatment with Botulinum Toxin A (BoNT-A) neuromodulators has been particularly successful. The problem comes with the descent of the brows seen with the aging process because neuromodulator treatment of the frontalis results often in further flattening and descent of the brows (brow ptosis) and a flat, uncaring, and rather wooden lack of forehead expression.

An acceptable alternative treatment is to reflate the glabella and forehead using diluted HA filler, which can be deposited in subgaleal vascular safe zones and then digitally massaged over the subgaleal glide plane. This can be performed at the same time as filler into intradermal glabellar folds, if needed.

The result is softening of the glabellar folds and horizontal frontalis rhytides, filling of the forehead concavities, elevation of the glabella and the brows, and restoration of a relaxed open expression. This treatment is often performed at the same time as temple reflation.

A detailed knowledge of the underlying neurovascular anatomy is essential to effective and safe treatment.

Informed consent must include discussion of the potential for both superficial and deep vascular occlusion and its management.[6]

## Vascular anatomy and forehead vascular safe zones

The forehead is supplied by both superficial and deep branches of the supratrochlear and supraorbital arteries, both of which are terminal branches of the ophthalmic artery. The supratrochlear vessels are found 18 to 22 mm lateral to the midline of the glabella, and the supraorbital vessels leave the orbit at the supraorbital notch or foramen approximately 1 cm lateral to the supratrochlear vessels. There are many variations in their branching patterns, but it is helpful to understand that there is a relative vasculature-free zone between the periosteum and the galea, also known as the forehead glide plane. A bolus of HA filler diluted and deposited as a depot in the glabella between the supratrochlear vascular arcades can be gently massaged to distribute the filler without further needle injections[5,7] (Figs. 16.1 and 16.2).

## Materials and methods

After discussion, photography, and full informed consent (including the discussion of the rare possibility of iatrogenic filler-induced blindness),[6,8] the authors mark the vessels to be avoided on the mid forehead—supratrochlear and supraorbital vessels.

Each subject is photographed before and after the injection session, and the digital photos are printed for the subject's chart and also shown to them before and after the injection treatment.

For pain relief, we apply topical 30% lidocaine in plasticized base to a clean face free of makeup, for 10 to 15 minutes prior to injection, and then continue after removal of the anesthetic gel with the use of the proprietary cold roller (Palomar). We prefer to use 100% diluted low-molecular-weight hyaluronic acid (HA-V) filler. Each 1-mL syringe of HA filler is first decanted into two polycarbonate syringes with ½ mL of HA-V in each syringe. Then 0.1 mL of 2% lidocaine with epinephrine 1:100,000 (20% by volume) is admixed with 20 back and forth movements through the double Luer Lock. A further 0.4 mL of preserved saline is added to each ½-mL syringe to bring the total volume in each syringe to 1 mL. This

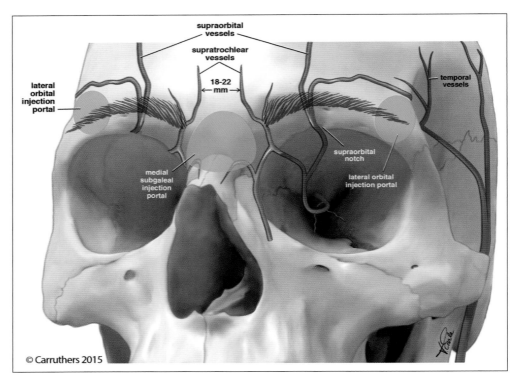

supraorbital vessels

supratrochlear vessels

18-22 ←mm→

lateral orbital injection portal

temporal vessels

supraorbital notch

medial subgaleal injection portal

lateral orbital injection portal

© Carruthers 2015

**Figure 16.1** Forehead depot injection zones. *(Copyright Jean Carruthers, MD, 2015. Previously published in Carruthers J, Carruthers A. Three-dimensional forehead reflation. Dermatol Surg. 2015;41(suppl 1):s321–s324.)*

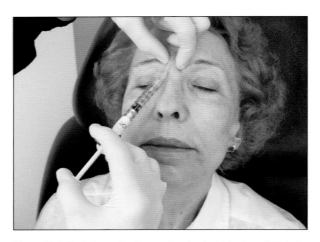

**Figure 16.2** Technique of anterograde subgaleal injection of diluted HA filler into the glide place between periosteum and galea. After the bolus of diluted filler is deposited, gentle upward digital massage distributed the product without further needle injections.

is also admixed with 20 back-and-forth movements using the double Luer Lock to ensure even mixing.

HA-V (Juvéderm Voluma) is injected below the procerus and frontalis muscles above the periosteum and in the subgaleal plane[7] using a 1-mL syringe with a 27/28-gauge Excel needle or 27-gauge cannula, using slow and gentle anterograde injection technique with radial fanning. After the tip of the injecting instrument is below the surface of the dermis, the plunger is withdrawn to see if any blood regurgitates into the hub. This has so far happened only on one occasion, and the video has been published.[9]

The product is distributed with gentle anterograde injection technique remaining in the correct plane deep to the frontalis and the galea and anterior to the periosteum (i.e., within the galeal glide plane). After a bolus of filler has been deposited, it is easy to spread the filler using digital pressure instead of using further punctures. The diluted HA-V is massaged gently in an upward direction to ensure that it is evenly distributed. Ice can be applied immediately following the procedure to reduce transient swelling and redness. It is important to explain to the subjects that for a period of 40 minutes to an hour the lidocaine in the HA-V will affect the function of the frontalis and the brows may transiently drop.

## Results

We began using Juvéderm Voluma in January 2009. To date we have volumized the glabella and forehead using radial fanning and the gentle anterograde injection technique from a subprocerus entry point in hundreds of

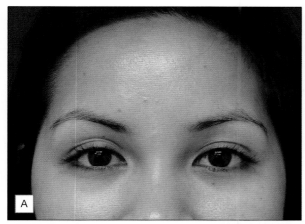

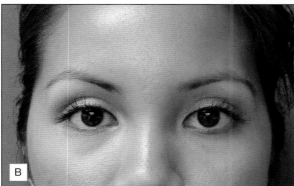

**Figure 16.3 A,** Before the three-dimensional glabellar reflation.
**B,** After three-dimensional brow reflation with HA-V and the
injection of 30 units of BoNT-A. *(Reprinted with permission from
Carruthers JDA, Carruthers JA. Volumizing the glabella and forehead.
Dermatologic Surg. 2010;36:1905–1909.)*

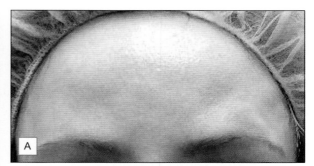

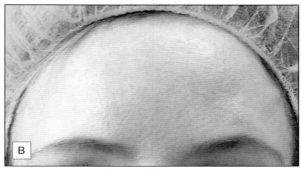

**Figure 16.4 A,** Paracentral forehead depressions before reflation
by massage from the central bolus. **B,** Forehead reflated after the
massage of the injected diluted bolus of HA-V.

injection sessions. The medial part of the eyebrow and
adjacent brow and the medial forehead are revolumized
and recontoured. The immediate medial brow lift is well
appreciated by the subjects, as is the more open appearance of their palpebral apertures and the softer, more
relaxed appearance to the periorbital region (Fig. 16.3).
When the immediate adjacent forehead is depressed, we
also reflate this area using massage of the injected bolus
(Fig. 16.4).

We have witnessed few side effects, except for the need
for further treatment after 2 to 3 weeks in approximately
30% of subjects to ensure ideal correction. Treatment
results typically last for at least 10 to 12 months, although
the associated brow depressor treatment with BoNT-A is
helpful in increasing longevity of response.

The subjects noted the immediate softening of their
horizontal frontalis rhytides without any dropping of their
brows or reduction in expressivity because they were still
able to lift their brows when expressing compassion,
sympathy, and interest. The improved mild convexity of

their forehead also married well with temple reflation
with filler, restoring the face that should be "five eyes
wide," as famously noted by Leonardo Da Vinci.

In addition they became aware of the new glow and
reflectivity of their forehead skin. We presume that the
HA and also BoNT-A injected was stimulating neocollagenesis from within the skin of the forehead.[10–12]

## Conclusions

Three-dimensional filling has reinvented the rejuvenation
of the upper face. It is particularly effective if used with
chemodenervation of the brow depressor musculature
and avoidance of chemodenervation of the only brow
elevator, the frontalis. The resulting brow elevation and
continued frontalis action give the subject back a rested
and interested and positive expression, most helpful in all
social interaction.

## References

1. Richard MJ, Morris C, Deen BF, Gray L, Woodward JA.
   Analysis of the anatomic changes of the aging facial skeleton
   using computer-assisted tomography. *Ophthal Plast Reconstr
   Surg.* 2009;25:382–386.
2. Wong C, Medelson B. Newer understanding of specific
   anatomic targets in the aging face as applied to injectables:
   aging changes in the craniofacial skeleton and facial ligaments.
   *Plast Reconstr Surg.* 2015;136:44s–48s.

3. Ramanadhan S, Rohrich R. Newer understanding of specific anatomic targets in the aging face as applied to injectables: superficial and deep fat compartments—an evolving target for site-specific facial augmentation. *Plast Reconstr Surg.* 2015;136:49s–55s.

4. Shaw RB Jr, Katzel EB, Koltz PF, et al. Aging of the facial skeleton: aesthetic implications and rejuvenation strategies. *Plast Reconstr Surg.* 2011;127(1):374–383.

5. Carruthers J, Carruthers A. A prospective, randomized, parallel group study analyzing the effect of BTX-A (Botox) and nonanimal sourced hyaluronic acid (NASHA, Restylane) in combination compared with NASHA (Restylane) alone in severe glabellar rhytides in adult female subjects: treatment of severe glabellar rhytides with a hyaluronic acid derivative compared with the derivative BTX-A. *Dermatol Surg.* 2003;29:802–809.

6. Carruthers JDA, Fagien S, Rohrich R, Weinkle S, Carruthers A. Blindness caused by cosmetic filler injection. *Plast Reconstr Surg.* 2014;134(6):1197–1201.

7. Carruthers JDA, Carruthers JA. Volumizing the glabella and forehead. *Dermatologic Surg.* 2010;36:1905–1909.

8. Beleznay K, Carruthers JDA, Humphrey S, Jones D. Avoiding and treating blindness from fillers: a review of the world literature. *Dermatol Surg.* 2015;41:1097–1117.

9. Sykes JM, Cotofana S, Trevidic P, et al. Upper face: clinical anatomy and regional approaches with injectable fillers. *Plast Reconstr Surg.* 2015;136(5 suppl):204s–218s [Video presentation of Carruthers forehead reflation technique included].

10. Wang F, Garza L, Kang S, et al. In vivo stimulation of de novo collagen production caused by cross linked HA dermal filler injections in photodamaged human skin. *Arch Dermatol.* 2007;143:155–163.

11. Quan. T, Wang F, Shao Y, et al. Enhancing structural support of dermal microenviroment activates fibroblasts, endothelial cells,and keratinocytes in aged human skin in vivo. *J Invest Dermatol.* 2013;133:658–667.

12. Oh S, Lee Y, Seo Y, et al. The potential effect of botulinum toxin type A on human dermal fibroblasts: an in vitro study. *Dermatol Surg.* 2012;38:1689–1694.

# 17

# Volumetric treatment of the brows

Val Lambros

## Summary and Key Features

- Orbits that are large, round, and hollow are associated with age, not youth.

- Young orbits are almond-shaped, the bone is not visible, and there may be considerable fullness of the upper lid.

- The same configurations that are seen in younger patients may be perceived as looking old in older ones.

- Communication is difficult in the periorbital area. Many patients want the eye "lifted" or skin and fat removed because that is what they have been told is done. Moreover, some patients like the hollow and defined look because it may look more dramatic and makeup can be used more liberally.

- The author prefers using a trial of local anesthetic in the upper lid to demonstrate the visual effect of filling in the upper lids and brow. If the patient likes the look, the injection is performed immediately; there is no need to wait. Local anesthetic provides a vasoconstricted environment. There is no better way of communicating the visual effect of the brow fill.

- Putting in the local anesthetic and avoiding overfills and fluid blobs in the upper lid are difficult to do well and easily; some practice is involved. The area is massaged and a few minutes should elapse to let the local anesthetic distribute before showing the patient.

- Underfill is better than overfill. This is not a method to fill in an abundance of skin, though the fill does inflate some skin. Nor is it a method to lift brows, though the brow can elevate in a few patients. Someone with full heavy lids is not a candidate for this procedure.

- The author favors hyaluronic acid (HA) products in the brow because they have more projection.

- One should expect at least 2 years' duration in this location with HA products.

- The injector should always be aware of the presence of the globe. Some upper orbits are very shallow, and the globe is immediately adjacent to the bone.

## Introduction

Thinning, deflation, and loss of subcutaneous volume are characteristic of periorbital aging. Though by no means universal, and seen largely in people who have not gained facial weight, this pattern of aging has been known through the ages and is frequently used as a caricature of the aging process. The term "nursing home eyes" provides an instant visual image of the problem.

Traditional treatments around the upper lid have been largely surgical, mainly because until recently the only tools available were excisional. "Extra" skin and fat around the upper lid were removed; for many eyes this proved to be an entirely satisfactory remedy. However, for some patients the apparent extra skin was secondary to a volume loss in the upper lid and brow, and removing further tissue had the dual effect of making the orbit look more defined but rounder and more hollow. Both of these have traditionally been considered beneficial. The perceived advantage of this look is that the orbit looks larger and dramatic in the vertical dimension and leaves more room for makeup. It is also the traditional look of upper lid "rejuvenation" and familiar. However, these are also characteristics of the nursing home eye, and in some people the overall appearance of the eye is clearly older, smaller, and more tired. With the advent of tools to reestablish volume in the face, alternatives have become available, which the patient (and clinician) should be aware of before making treatment decisions in the peri-orbital area.

There is nothing new in these observations. Volume fillers were used exactly as they are now in the 1890s, well before facelift surgery was developed. Unfortunately, all that was available at the time was paraffin and petroleum jelly (Vaseline); the complication rate was high, and these treatments fell into disfavor, as described by Kolle and by Goldwyn.

## The "local preview"

Patients usually have their own predetermined ideas about what looks good. If one has a choice of filling an area or defining it by removing tissue, the different potential effects must somehow be communicated to the patient. In other words, an adequate consultation should be able to explain the aesthetic alternatives to the patient. We have found no way in words to describe how the effects of filling the brow will improve the patient's overall look; this is entirely a visual concept. It is like trying to describe a dress and assuming that the customer will like it without trying it on.

What has proved extremely useful is the "local preview," as I have previously described (2009); 1 cc or two of 1/4% lidocaine with epinephrine is injected into the brow with the intention of visualizing the effect of filling the area and also to make it numb and vasoconstricted (Fig. 17.1). With the use of an ice cube for the initial injections, this is almost painless.

Filling the brow with local anesthetic in a realistic way is not easy, but is good practice for the final injection. The tendency for inexperienced injectors is to place the needle superficially and make individual lumps of fluid. This is convincing of nothing. The correct plane is around the orbicularis muscle or deeper, and the needle must be withdrawn on injection, leaving a horizontal and even flow of local anesthetic. This is performed across the brow,

trying to anticipate the final intended result. The area is massaged a little. After a few minutes the product has diffused enough to demonstrate the intended look.

We tell patients that what they see is approximately 80% accurate as to the final result. Most people, if correctly selected, like the look and say that it "opens their eyes." This is perceptually interesting because in reality the orbit is being narrowed. In addition to the demonstrative ability of the preview, the area is now vasoconstricted, making the possibility of an intravascular injection smaller. Strictly speaking, brow filling could be performed with topical anesthetic or none at all, but the communicative power of the preview is invaluable—patients determine whether they like the look before the clinician does anything definitive. The latter can also see whether he or she likes the effect. Because patients have seen the results of the injection and approved it before the product injection, no one in my experience has asked to have product removed. If they do not like the look of the preview, then nothing further is performed; no product has been injected, and other alternatives can be explored. Patients love the idea that they can see the results before a procedure is performed and embrace the concept enthusiastically.

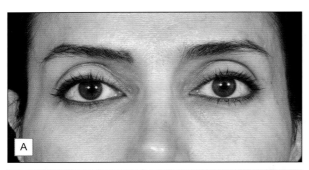

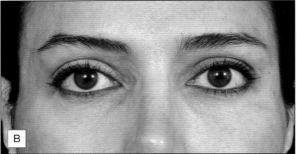

**Figure 17.1** The "local preview." It is difficult to communicate the visual effects of volume around the orbit without actually seeing it. An invaluable way of doing this is to inject the area with local anesthetic, which demonstrates the effect of fill and numbs and vasoconstricts the area at the same time. Patients approve or disapprove of the visual effect before any product is injected. It usually takes more fill—approximately 1/2 to 1 mL per side—than the actual product injection. The long-term result looks like the result at the end of the procedure and typically lasts 2 to 3 years. **A,** Before and **B,** after injection.

> ### Pearl 1
> There is a population of patients who have anxious-looking eyes with level brows. These patients do not have a well-developed medial upper lid crease, or it is absent. Restoring this crease makes the eyes look much more normal and less anxiety projecting.

> ### Pearl 2
> There are patients with small excesses of lid skin that get used up by increasing the volume of the brow down to the orbital rim.

> ### Pearl 3
> The anterior orbital rim can be pushed forward in some eyes, hiding the upper lid crease and making the eye look less bulgy.

## The injection

At the time of writing, hyaluronic acid (HA) products, calcium-based products, and poly-L-lactic acid are available. I use only HA fillers outside of the operating room, where I may use autologous fat. They are easy to use and can be removed with hyaluronidase if necessary. The duration of HA products in the brow and tear trough is 2 to 3 years, equal to or greater than other available products. To my mind there is no advantage to using products other than HAs in the periorbital region.

This is not an area for novice injectors. If the clinician has performed only lips and nasolabial folds and injects them with bolus injections and massage, the upper lid will be a source of disappointment and complications, some of them potentially catastrophic. Though not difficult for experienced injectors, technique in the upper lid is important. The goal is to create a pleasing shape across the brow, not just to fill a hollow. The depth of this injection should be around the level of the orbicularis muscle. There are very large immobile arteries at the periosteal level that one should avoid. Injection into the sulcus of the upper lid may result in ptosis, as described by Coleman. Keeping the plane of injection superficial to the bone also keeps the needle farther away from the globe as mentioned below.

I begin the injection at the conclusion of the local preview after the patient has approved the look. The area is now vasoconstricted and numb. The presence of the anesthetic in no way alters the ability to distribute the product evenly, which is performed partially visually and partially by feel. Though I cannot prove it, I believe that HAs distribute more evenly in a very wet environment.

As illustrated in Fig. 17.2, my preferred technique is to begin laterally and place three fanning longitudinal fills with a 30-g 1/2-inch (6-mm) needle: high, middle, and low. The process is repeated across the brow. Tiny amounts are placed with each pass. If the thumb moves perceptibly, then the volume is excessive. A small needle like the 30-g 1/2-inch one is protective in avoiding overfills. Palpation is an excellent way to determine the evenness of the injection. Typically the injection should not go inferior to the border of the orbital bone laterally and centrally. Unless one is confident of the intention and results, it is very easy to create irregularities or worse here. The expansion of the curve of the orbital bone suffices to improve the hollow of all but the most deep-set and hollow orbits. As one proceeds medially the injection might need to drop inferior to the level of the bone somewhat. Usually 1/2 mL per side is injected. For economic reasons this seems a good place to start, and indeed most brows and the expressive qualities of the face are improvable by even this small amount, even if undercorrected. I am always amazed by the ability of such a small amount of filler to create as much difference as it does. With experience, it is obvious where the product needs to be placed.

The injection should not be overdone. More is not better. The patient is given an ice pack to use later in the day. Bruising is occasional. There is not much swelling, although there is some. Usual complications are minor and are usually related to irregularities that can be dissolved

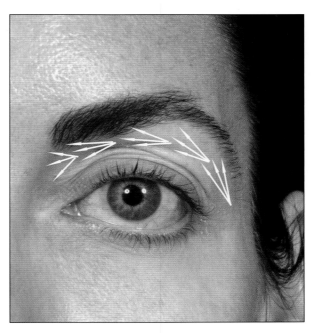

**Figure 17.2** Author's injection technique: after the area is numb and vasoconstricted, I use three passes from each injection site—high, medium, and low. The injection is repeated across the brow and repeated if necessary. The presence of local anesthetic in no way alters the ability of the injector to visualize the results.

or added to. In general, the appearance at the end of the injection is the final result.

## Intraarterial injection

Injections are by and large innocuous and low risk. However, the specter of intraarterial injection is ever present though fortunately uncommon. For this to occur, the needle tip must be in an artery and a bolus of sufficient size injected to cause upstream flow, as blindness from a periocular injection, or distal embolization, as in a lip or nasal necrosis from injection into the nasolabial fold, as described by Coleman. These are excellent arguments for not doing bolus injections. We favor threading injections, always keeping the tip of the needle moving with small low-pressure flows and vasoconstriction. We believe that this complication is largely technical and avoidable.

Some orbits are flat superiorly, without an upper lid sulcus. In orbits like these the globe is immediately adjacent to the orbital rim, and there is a distinct possibility of a direct needle injury. We have never seen this complication, but it is easy to see how it could happen. The clinician must focus on the position of the globe and needle tip. Keeping the tip of the needle away from the orbital bone will also keep it away from the globe. We are uncertain of the use of blunt cannulas here. Although they are blunt, they are also long and whippy and could easily track subcutaneously and wind up in unexpected places.

## Who is a candidate for brow volume treatments?

Unlike the lip or nasolabial fold, one cannot rely on formula or dogma to treat the brow. Though some brows may have

been fuller when younger, the look of the eye might be worse on restoring or amplifying the brow volume. There are configurations that lend themselves to this treatment and configurations that are made worse by adding volume. In general, except for some Asian eyelids, full upper lids are not made better by additional filling. Very hollow eyes are made only modestly better. As mentioned by Mancini et al., there is concern that injection into the actual sulcus may cause a space-occupying ptosis.

> **Pearl 7**
>
> This is not a technique that all eyes need. Experience will show which eyes improve.

Brows that have deflated evenly (Figs. 17.3 to 17.5) and brows in which the medial supraorbital crease peaks medially are excellent candidates. This latter group is interesting in that a medial peak of the supraorbital crease gives people a look of anxiety or worry. A very small amount of filler in this location alters the emotional projection of the face (Fig. 17.6). Though actual elevation of the brows of a millimeter or two is sometimes seen with

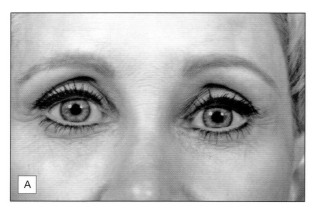

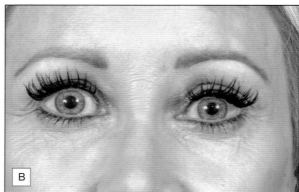

Figure 17.3 A 56-year-old patient seen in 2009, for whom 1/2 mL Restylane was injected into each brow. The patient returned in 2016 reporting no further surgery or injections into her brows, though she has had lip fillers. This is the most longevity I have seen with hyaluronic acid fillers in this location. Like the temples and tear troughs, 2 years is usual and 4 is common, but a 7-year duration is remarkable. The product could be palpated, as well as seen. Note the appearance of anxiety in the preinjection image, which is gone post injection. *(Photo courtesy of V. Lambros MD.)*

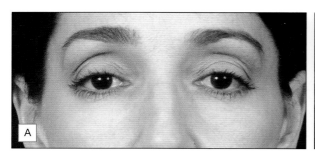

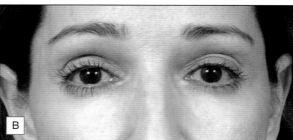

Figure 17.4 **A,** A 58-year-old patient with hollow superior orbit, **B,** seen 3 years after brow injection 1 mL/side. The temples were also filled 6 months previously.

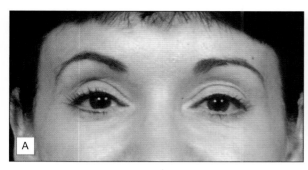
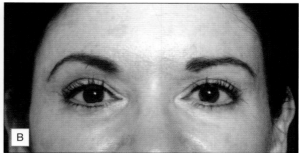

**Figure 17.5 A,** A 68-year-old patient with hollow brows, **B,** 3 years after 1 mL hyaluronic acid filler was placed in each brow.

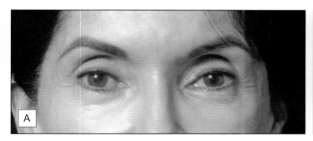
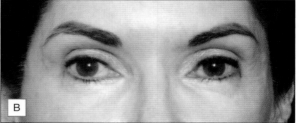

**Figure 17.6 A,** A 54-year-old patient with very hollow and anxious eyes, **B,** seen here 3 years after 1 mL HA filler per side and 10 months after a fill of her temples 2 mL per side with diluted HA fillers.

injection, we believe that the impression of elevation is largely illusory, based on greater light reflection from the now-filled and rounder brow. In any event, trying to lift brows with volume may provide a slight elevation at the cost of an unnaturally overfilled eye.

The point with these treatments is not necessarily to make the orbit fuller; rather it is to make the periorbital area look better, and if one does not have at least a rudimentary appreciation for what looks good on the face, one will have limited success in treating the area.

## Further reading

Coleman SR. Hyaluronic acid fillers. *Plast Reconstr Surg.* 2006;117(2):661–665.

Goldwyn RM. The paraffin story. *Plast Reconstr Surg.* 1980;65(4):517–524.

Kolle FS. Plastic and Cosmetic Surgery. New York: Appelton; 1911.

Lambros VS. Observations on periorbital and midface aging. *Plast Reconstr Surg.* 2007;120(5):1367–1376, discussion 1377.

Lambros V. Volumizing the brows with HA fillers. *Aesthet Surg J.* 2009;29:177–179.

Mancini R, Taban M, Lowinger A, et al. Use of hyaluronic acid gel in the management of paralytic lagophthalmos: the hyaluronic acid gel 'gold weight'. *Ophthal Plast Reconstr Surg.* 2009;25(1):23–26.

# 18

# Infraorbital hollow and nasojugal fold

## Shannon Humphrey, Steven Fagien

### Summary and Key Features

- The infraorbital hollow (IOH) refers to the U-shaped or curvilinear depression under the eyes and comprises the tear trough, nasojugal fold, and palpebromalar groove and has become a common presentation for those seeking cosmetic enhancement to the lower eyelid and mid-face.

- With thin skin overlying bone and little-to-no subcutaneous fat or muscle in this region, the IOH can be an unforgiving region and challenging to treat with injectable agents.

- Injections seem to work best in patients with thick and smooth skin and a well-defined tear trough, without excessively protruding eyelid fat or excess eyelid skin.

- Hyaluronic acid (HA) is currently the injectable agent treatment of choice for IOHs and lower eyelid and periorbital augmentation.

- Meticulous injection with small volumes, reduced volume speed, supraperiosteal placement, lower gauge needles and/or cannulas, and minimal number of injection sites will reduce the risk of complications.

- Some patients are not suited to fillers alone and require adjuvant therapy or surgery for further restoration of the IOH.

## Introduction

In youth the transition between the lower eyelid and cheek is imperceptible and smooth. The eyes are balanced and in harmony with the surrounding tissue and the face as a whole, with gentle sloping contours most often without distinct demarcations. Skin texture is consistent and smooth, and the surface is unblemished and uniform in color. Over the years, every aspect of youthful countenance changes through a cascade of events known simply as the aging process.

The infraorbital hollow (IOH) refers to the curvilinear or U-shaped depression under the eyes from the nasal bone to the outer corner of the eye and comprises three core elements: the "tear trough" and "nasojugal fold" medially and the palpebromalar groove laterally (Fig. 18.1). Although the terms tear trough and nasojugal fold have historically been used interchangeably, the former—which occurs mildly in all people across all ages—refers to the superior aspect of the latter. A sign of early aging, the deepening of the tear trough leads to a true indentation at the junction of the thin eyelid skin above and thicker skin of the cheek below. Later, the mid-cheek may descend, accentuating a flat or hollow crescent below the eye. The appearance of hollows and dark circles under the eye is the interplay of various factors. Genetics and habits and environmental exposures lead to dyschromias and pigmentation; soft tissue laxity, subcutaneous volume alterations, changes in bony landmarks, and redistribution of superficial fat all lead to shadowed contours and deepening folds. Periorbital volumetric shifting and loss is not an isolated event but part of a global shift in the contours of the aging face.

There is little to no superficial fat under the lower eyelid. The orbicularis oculi muscle has direct bony attachment for approximately one-third of the orbital rim length, from the nasal bone to the medial limbus. Laterally, orbicularis-retaining ligaments connect the deep surface of the skin to bone. Retaining ligaments weaken, facial bones recede, and volume decreases in the deep fat pads, causing the cheek to descend and superficial fat to accumulate under the eye, all of which combine with genetically predisposed discolorations and bony changes to produce the perception of hollowed and sometimes baggy eyes, deep and shadowed tear troughs, and an aged, fatigued appearance refractory to cosmetic attempts at concealment (see Fig. 18.1).

Treatment of the periorbital area with injectable agents allows little room for error and requires careful patient selection, careful choice of filling agent, and precise technique to avoid complications and ensure optimal outcome.

## Candidates for augmentation of the infraorbital hollow

Proper patient selection is critical and relies on careful ophthalmologic and medical history and physical assessment. Poor candidates are unlikely to obtain optimal results and may not be satisfied with results and are at higher risk of side effects, such as visibility and irregularity (Table 18.1). Patients with diseases or metabolic conditions

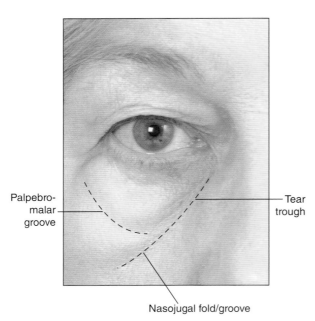

Palpebro-
malar
groove

Tear
trough

Nasojugal fold/groove

**Figure 18.1** Anatomy of the infraorbital hollow.

**Table 18.1** Identifying candidates for augmentation of the infraorbital hollow

| Best candidates | Poor candidates |
| --- | --- |
| Young patients with good skin elasticity | Elderly patients with poor skin elasticity |
| Thick smooth skin | Very thin skin |
| Good skin tone | Transparent or dyspigmented skin |
| Minimal laxity | Significant skin laxity |
| Mild-to-moderate tear troughs | Extremely deep tear troughs |

that predispose to lower eyelid irregularity or bleeding and infection should be excluded, and all manner of anticoagulant medications and supplements discontinued if medically safe for at least 2 weeks prior to treatment. Some patients have genetically determined pigmentation that may look like a tear trough but without an indentation that can be filled. Pigmented dark lower eyelid circles cannot be improved by fillers and can indeed be worsened by treatment. Older patients with thinner, crepelike, inelastic skin and individuals with preexisting malar edema—whether metabolic (thyroid disease) or otherwise (i.e., chronic sinus disease, prior surgery, etc.)—may not respond well and also have an increased risk for adverse events and dissatisfaction with these treatments. Patients with orbital fat herniation and significant skin laxity would

benefit first from lower lid blepharoplasty or other surgical procedures. Injection works best in patients with thicker and smooth skin and a well-defined tear trough or defined maxillary retrusion or hypoplasia (common in young Asian females), without excessively protruding eyelid fat or excess eyelid skin.

## Appropriate filling agents

Thin skin directly overlying bone, allowing any irregularity to be readily visible, propensity for discoloration, and vascularity make the IOH a challenging area to fill. The ideal filler is one with a low extrusion force or density to allow precise and delicate injection through lower-gauged needles, and one that is reversible or, at the very least, biodegradable. Because there is a tendency for anything injected into this area to form visible lumps, particularly on animation, permanent fillers should be considered only with great caution.

The use of autologous fat had gained popularity in recent years (also) as a replacement for surgery for the correction of contour defects and has been used for augmentation of the IOH, but results have been generally unpredictable and often associated with considerable side effects, such as lumpiness, long-lasting irregularities, volume distortion, and prolonged edema, as well as risks associated with any surgical procedure. More recently, hyaluronic acid (HA)—with its gel consistency, varying concentrations and the possibility of dilution with lidocaine or saline, favorable flow characteristics, fewer side effects, and nonpermanence—has emerged as the treatment of choice for augmentation of the lower periorbita by injection. Lumps or irregularities can be avoided with careful and precise injection techniques and can also be reversed through treatment with hyaluronidase, an important consideration when injecting in delicate areas requiring precise placement of filling agent. Surprisingly, HA in the periorbital region yields better than expected longevity. Lambros (and others) have described the persistence of effect, often in excess of 1 year (see Chapter 17). Donath et al. used three-dimensional imaging in 20 patients treated in the tear trough with HA and found an average 85% maintenance of effect at the final follow-up visit (average 14.4 months); the patient with the longest duration retained 73% volume augmentation at 23 months without any touch-ups. Side effects with HA can include visibility and nodules, a bluish tint (from the presumed Tyndall effect), along with injection-related bruising and swelling (see Complications).

Calcium hydroxylapatite (CaHA) has yielded positive outcomes in other areas of the face, and Hevia has detailed successful outcomes in the infraorbital region using CaHA diluted by 10% to 30% with 2% lidocaine. However, CaHA has a history of palpable (and sometimes visible) nodules, particularly in the lips, and Goldman has reported a case of superficial nodularity after injection of CaHA in the IOH. Its major drawback remains the lack of reversibility; despite its biodegradable nature, there is little to do but wait out the occurrence of adverse effects.

## Augmentation techniques

Techniques for augmentation under the eye vary. Replacing periorbital volume entails not only focusing on specific regions in the IOH requiring augmentation—the tear trough, the central and lateral aspect of the orbital rim, the palpebromalar groove—but other areas that influence the appearance of the lower eye. A deflated medial cheek, for example, will look unnatural without concurrent augmentation, particularly on animation. Correction of the cheek will sometimes improve the appearance of the IOH, necessitating smaller amounts of filling agent to achieve optimal results. However, Hill has demonstrated that treatment of the medial cheek alone does not significantly improve the tear trough deficit. Ideally, periorbital volume augmentation should be performed in conjunction with rejuvenation of the mid-face and sometimes to the entire face to preserve harmony and restore aesthetic proportion.

## Skin preparation, anesthetic, and syringes

Patients are treated sitting in an upright position. Photographs should be taken with controlled lighting, which can illuminate rather than disguise the appearance of rhytides, tear trough deformity, and lower lid fat prolapse. After all makeup has been removed and skin thoroughly cleaned with alcohol, the patient is asked to look upward to accentuate and delineate the borders of the tear trough, and all areas of injection can be marked using a fine-tipped marker, including adjacent areas requiring augmentation (Fig. 18.2).

The choice of anesthetic will depend on the area to be treated, needle size, number of injection sites, and patient tolerance. Usually a combination of topical anesthetic (or ice), the use of HA agents containing lidocaine, or dilution of filling agent with lidocaine with epinephrine provides adequate pain relief. Direct infiltration of local anesthetic can be used to numb the malar area and lateral orbit; infraorbital nerve block is administered with a small volume of 0.5% to 0.1% lidocaine with epinephrine. Only minimal volumes of the anesthetic solution are used so that the volume status of the mid-face and tear trough is not distorted. Sometimes topical anesthetic cream or gel applied to the area to be treated and left in place a minimum of 20 minutes may be all that is necessary for pain relief.

Type and size of syringe in the IOH range from a 30-gauge blunt-tipped cannula to 27- to 32-gauge needles, depending on injector preference, treatment area, and technique used. Blunt cannulas may eliminate the risk of inadvertent intravascular injection; however, some injectors believe needles allow more precise placement of filler material in the periorbital region and these adverse events can almost always be avoided with careful injection technique.

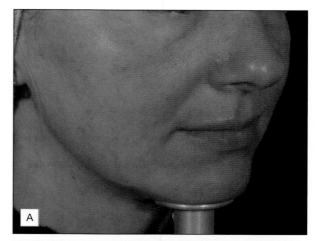

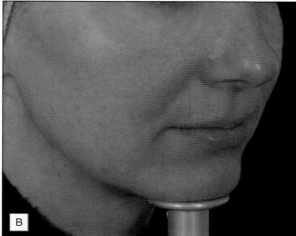

**Figure 18.2** Patient **(A)** before and **(B)** after treatment.

## General techniques

With thin skin overlying bone and little-to-no subcutaneous fat, the IOH is an unforgiving region and challenging to treat. Injections often produce discoloration or bruising, and any irregularity is readily visible. Anatomic areas of concern include the prominent infratrochlear vessels adjacent to the nasal bone and the infraorbital nerve, more often located approximately 14 mm below the bony orbital margin in the midpupillary line.

**Pearl 1**

Anatomic areas of concern in the IOH include the infratrochlear vessels and infraorbital nerve.

Small amounts of filler—generally no more than 1 mL in total for both sides—under low pressure will avoid complications, such as a "sausage roll" appearance under the eye and retrograde embolus into the periorbital vasculature as the filler inadvertently slips behind the orbital septum. If 0.2 to 0.4 mL of HA does not lead to a noticeable improvement, it is possible—or even likely—the filler has been misplaced. The attempt here is to place a confluent deposit of filler material along the orbital rim, beneath the apparent "hollow" without complete volume filling of the agent and allowing the additional physical properties of these filling agents (including hydrophilicity) to augment the overlying soft tissues to reduce the appearance of the "trough."

Injections are deep in the suborbicularis plane at or below the orbital rim at the supraperiosteal level except in the medial aspect of the orbicularis oculi, which attaches to bone and requires direct injection. Superficial injections in the periorbital region increase the risk of visibility and skin discoloration secondary to the Tyndall effect (see Complications), although some researchers (such as Hirmand) have described the occasional need for very superficial subdermal injection using a 32-gauge needle for spot application over a 1- to 2-mm surface area to "lift" the overlying skin.

Use of the smallest possible gauge but longer needles (i.e., a 1-inch [12-mm] 30-gauge needle) and reducing the number of injection sites can minimize postinjection bruising caused by trauma to blood vessels as the needle passes through the skin and the underlying orbicularis oculi muscle. When using multiple passes and layered techniques, it is best to withdraw the needle just enough to reposition it without exiting back through the muscle.

## Augmentation of the infraorbital hollow

Linear threading (the fanning technique) (Fig. 18.3) and serial puncture (Fig. 18.4) are the most commonly used techniques in the IOH. Goldberg and Fiaschetti describe deep injection using multiple needle passes to layer and feather the filler in a three-dimensional pattern in the IOH and cheek. Morley and Malhotra used the serial puncture technique with three to eight injections along the inferior IOH, depositing small aliquots of filling agent. Hirsch et al. detail the use of 1-inch needles and two or three injection sites just above the periosteum to augment the lateral to medial IOH, using the push-ahead technique, in which the submuscular layer is dissected by the forward movement of the filling agent rather than the tip of the needle. Small aliquots of 0.1 to 0.2 mL are deposited along the length of the groove, using digital manipulation instead of frank injection in the medial portion to avoid inadvertent injection of the infratrochlear vessels and infraorbital nerve. Hirmand describes a similar technique of discontinuous deposition using a blunt cannula, three to five injections of 0.01 to 0.5 mL deep in the supraperiosteal plane in the medial aspect of the tear trough, with gentle digital massage to disperse the filler into the intended location. The vertical supraperiosteal depot technique, pioneered by Sattler (see Chapter 25), involves the vertical deposition of small aliquots of filling agent (0.02 to 0.5 mL) at the supraperiosteal level using a 90-degree angle, with injections placed 2 to 3 mm apart.

Filling agent can also be "pushed" into the desired location manually. Bosniak et al. use topical anesthesia and a 27-gauge needle to inject two boluses of 0.25 mL HA less than 1 mm above the periosteum: the first in the lateral aspect of the tear trough just overlying the inferior orbital rim, and the second in the medial aspect taking care to avoid the infraorbital neurovascular bundle. After the needle is removed, the filler is pushed medially and superiorly along the surface of the inferior orbital rim to properly distribute material into the desired location.

Estimating the distance from the skin surface to the periosteum may be useful when selecting the most appropriate technique. El-Garem demonstrated that bolus

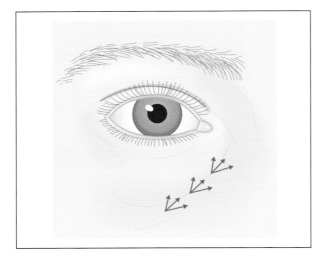

**Figure 18.3** The fanning technique.

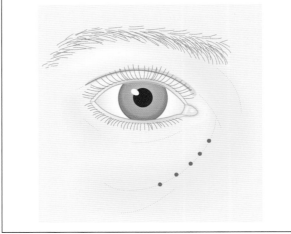

**Figure 18.4** Serial puncture in the infraorbital hollow.

injections led to better results in individuals with skin-to-periosteum depth greater than 0.5 cm, whereas serial injection was the more appropriate choice in patients with shallow depth (<0.5 cm).

## Posttreatment management and follow-up

After treatment, gentle pressure and the application of ice can minimize localized edema and erythema. The patient should be warned to expect swelling for up to 72 hours and bruising for up to 2 weeks; massage or manipulation of the area should be avoided until these effects subside. More specific aftercare procedures will vary according to the clinician but can include the avoidance of alcohol and exercise for up to 48 hours and the addition of *Arnica montana* tablets for 3 days.

### Pearl 2

*Arnica montana* tablets, slow injection, and application of ice may minimize ecchymosis and bruising in select patients, although this remains a common side effect in the infraorbital area.

Follow-up within 1 to 2 weeks of treatment allows evaluation of response and contour or volume irregularities. Touch-up injections or hyaluronidase may be required. HA in the IOH can last for a year or more; regular follow-up visits and touch-ups before the filling agent has dissipated will maintain the aesthetic effect.

### Pearl 3

Patients should be evaluated in animation throughout procedures to identify and correct bulging or dimpling that can occur with motion.

## Complications

Ecchymosis and edema are the most common injection-related side effects. Ecchymosis may last up to 10 days, while edema can last for up to 3 weeks or more depending on the causality. Visible irregularities in patients with thin or lax skin can be massaged away over several weeks. Superficial injection increases the risk of lumps that are often difficult to resolve without injections of hyaluronidase to dissolve the implant (Fig. 18.5).

Too superficial injections can yield the appearance of a bluish-gray tint secondary to the Tyndall effect, in which the injected filler, readily visible under thin skin, causes preferential scattering of blue light (Fig. 18.6). Overcorrection may lead to unnatural bulges and festooning or a "baggy" eyelid. It is critical to address other areas of deficit; undercorrection of the lateral orbit or mid-face will make the appearance of an augmented tear trough unappealing. Undercorrection or overcorrection can be assessed at follow-up and treated appropriately.

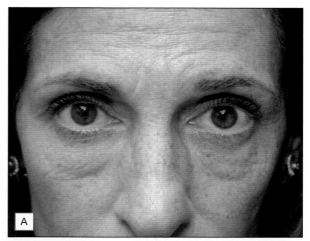

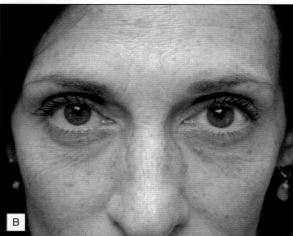

**Figure 18.5 A,** Edema in the lower lid following hyaluronic acid injection into the tear trough; **B,** edema resolved after a "watchful waiting" approach.

### Pearl 4

Remember the adage, "Less is more."

More serious but rare complications in the IOH include occlusion of the vascular supply (caused by compression, obstruction of the vessels with filler material, or direct injury to the vessels) leading to blindness, embolism, or stroke. Intravascular injection can be prevented by close attention to anatomy combined with careful injection techniques.

## Adjunctive therapy

Some patients are not suited to fillers alone and require adjuvant therapy for complete restoration of the IOH.

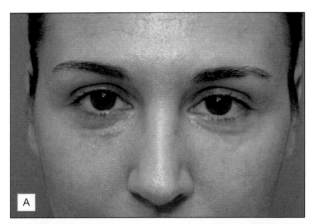

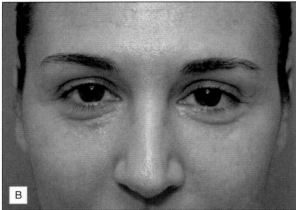

**Figure 18.6** Bluish-gray tint secondary to the Tyndall effect apparent **(A)** at rest and **(B)** smiling.

## Conclusion

The use of dermal fillers has become a common treatment to address hollowness of the periorbital region; however, it may be associated with significant complications. Best practice requires in-depth knowledge of regional anatomy, including the delicate and vascular nature of the surrounding tissues, careful patient selection, and precise injection techniques at target tissue planes likely to produce optimal results and avoid serious complications.

## Further reading

Bellman B. Complication following suspected intra-arterial injection of Restylane. *Aesthet Surg J.* 2006;26:304–305.

Bosniak S, Sadick NS, Cantisano-Zilkha M, Glavas IP, Roy D. The hyaluronic acid push technique for the nasojugal groove. *Dermatol Surg.* 2008;34:127–131.

Carruthers JD, Carruthers A. Facial sculpting and tissue augmentation. *Dermatol Surg.* 2005;31(11 pt 2):1604–1612.

Coleman SR. Avoidance of arterial occlusion from injection of soft tissue fillers. *Aesthet Surg J.* 2002; 22:555.

Donath AS, Glasgold RA, Meier J, Glasgold MJ. Quantitative evaluation of volume augmentation in the tear trough with a hyaluronic acid-based filler: a three-dimensional analysis. *Plast Reconstr Surg.* 2010;125:1515–1522.

Donofrio LM. Technique of periorbital lipoaugmentation. *Dermatol Surg.* 2003;29:92–98.

El-Garem YF. Estimation of bony orbit depth for optimal selection of the injection technique to correct the tear trough and palpebromalar groove. *Dermatol Surg.* 2015;41:94–101.

Goldberg RA, Fiaschetti D. Filling the periorbital hollows with hyaluronic acid gel: initial experience with 244 injections. *Ophthal Plast Reconstr Surg.* 2006;22:335–343.

Goldman MP. Superficial nodularity of hydroxylapatite filler to fill the infraorbital hollow. *Dermatol Surg.* 2010;36:822–824.

Hevia O. A retrospective review of calcium hydroxylapatite for correction of volume loss in the infraorbital region. *Dermatol Surg.* 2009;35:1487–1494.

Hill RH 3rd, Czyz CN, Kandapalli S, et al. Evolving minimally invasive techniques for tear trough enhancement. *Ophthalmic Plast Reconstr Surg.* 2015;31:306–309.

Hirmand H. Anatomy and nonsurgical correction of the tear trough deformity. *Plast Reconstr Surg.* 2010;125:699–708.

Hirsch RJ, Carruthers JDA, Carruthers A. Infraorbital hollow treatment by dermal fillers. *Dermatol Surg.* 2007;33:1116–1119.

Hirsch RJ, Cohen JL, Carruthers JD. Successful management of an unusual presentation of impending necrosis following a hyaluronic acid injection embolus and proposed algorithm for management of hyaluronidase. *Dermatol Surg.* 2007;33:357–360.

Hirsch RJ, Narurkar V, Carruthers JD. Management of injected hyaluronic acid induced Tyndall effects. *Lasers Surg Med.* 2006;38:202–204.

Lambros VS. Hyaluronic acid injections for correction of the tear trough deformity. *Plast Reconstr Surg.* 2007;120:745–805.

Lambros VS. Discussion: quantitative evaluation of volume augmentation in the tear trough with a hyaluronic acid-based filler: a three-dimensional analysis. *Plast Reconstr Surg.* 2010;125:1523–1524.

Lowe NJ Arterial embolization caused by injection of hyaluronic acid (Restylane). *Br J Dermatol.* 2003;148:379.

Morley AMS, Malhotra R. Use of hyaluronic acid filler for tear-trough rejuvenation as an alternative to lower eyelid surgery. *Ophthal Plast Reconstr Surg.* 2011;27:69–73.

Dark circles under the eye may be due to a number of variables; identifying the cause paves the way for appropriate treatment. Hyperpigmentation of the skin may respond to α-hydroxy acid chemical peels and agents that reduce pigment formation, such as topical kojic acid or hydroquinone combined with topical retinoids. Dark circles due to excessive pigmentation have also been successfully treated with various pigment lasers (such as the Q-switched Nd:YAG or alexandrite lasers). Skin laxity and tear trough deformity can be treated through ablative and non-ablative resurfacing, though the side effects associated with the former—prolonged erythema, pigmentary changes, infections, or even scarring—have led clinicians and patients to the less-invasive, nonablative, and light-based therapies. Dark shadows under the eye caused by a hypertrophic pretarsal orbicularis oculi can be improved by injections of botulinum toxin and/or surgery. Finally, excessive lower eyelid skin, laxity, or the appearance of significant fat herniation often requires surgical correction (blepharoplasty).

Pessa JE, Desvigne LD, Lambros VS, Nimerick J, Sugunan B, Zadoo VP. Changes in ocular globe-to-orbital rim position with age: implications for aesthetic blepharoplasty of the lower eyelids. *Aesthet Plast Surg.* 1999;23:337–342.

Roh MR, Chung KY. Infraorbital dark circles: definition, causes, and treatment options. *Dermatol Surg.* 2009;35:1163–1171.

Rohrich RJ, Arbique GM, Wong C, et al. The anatomy of suborbicularis fat: implications for periorbital rejuvenation. *Plast Reconstr Surg.* 2009;124:946–951.

Sadick NS, Bosniak SL, Cantisano-Zilkha M, Glavas IP, Roy D. Definition of the tear trough and the tear trough rating scale. *J Cosmet Dermatol.* 2007;6:218–222.

Saylan Z. Facial fillers and their complications. *Aesthet Surg J.* 2003;23:221–224.

Schanz W, Schippert W, Ultmer A, Rassner G, Fierlbeck G. Arterial embolization caused by injection of hyaluronic acid (Restylane). *Br J Dermatol.* 2002;146:928–929.

# 19

# Midface

## Ada R. Trindade de Almeida, André Vieira Braz

## Summary and Key Features

- Midface aging is a multifactorial process encompassing changes in bone, muscles, retaining ligaments, fat, and skin.
- Individual genetics and/or anatomic features can influence the precocity or delay of the appearance of the aging signs.
- Biodegradable fillers are optimal choices for nonsurgical rejuvenation of the midface because they are safe, effective, reversible, and provide natural-looking results.
- Proper knowledge of facial anatomy, including bone prominences, fat compartments, mimetic muscles, and risk areas are relevant to achieve better results and to avoid complications.
- The malar and zygomatic areas are the initial addressed locations, followed by the submalar region, if needed. The preauricular reflation helps to finalize the rejuvenation process, creating a frame for the midface.

## Introduction

The midface is considered the area between the lower eyelid and the oral commissure.[1] Since approximately 2006, from clinical practice to anatomic and tomographic imaging studies, the understanding of the midface aging process has evolved dramatically. It is now well recognized that a multifactorial process take place encompassing changes in bone (remodeling), muscles (increased resting tone or atrophy), retaining ligaments (elongation), fat (atrophy and/or displacement), and skin (discoloration, wrinkling, atrophy, etc.).[2–6]

Individual genetics and/or anatomic features can influence the precocity or delay of the appearance of the aging signs.

A young and attractive face is characterized by a well-contoured, anteriorly projected cheek,[7] with a smooth transition from and to the neighboring regions (e.g., no visible delimitation between the cheek and the lid, the Nasolabial Fold [NLF], and the jowls). The zygomatic arch is adequately covered. Deflation of this region impacts significantly in facial aging because instead of being convex,

reflecting light, the midface becomes flattened or even concave, forming shadows.

The advent of volumizing fillers shifted the paradigm of midface rejuvenation, becoming a safe and effective tool for nonsurgical facial reflation and reshaping.[1,2,8]

## Anatomical considerations

The subcutaneous fat tissue is compartmentalized by septal boundaries in superficial and deep portions, separated by the facial superficial muscular aponeurotic system (SMAS) and mimetic facial muscles.[2,4–6]

In the midface the superficial compartments are the nasolabial and the three malar portions: medial, intermediate and temporolateral, whereas the deep compartments are two portions located under the orbicularis oculi muscle (medial and lateral suborbicularis oculi fat [SOOF] or prezygomatic fat), and deep medial and lateral cheek fat portions[4–6] (Fig. 19.1A and B).

The knowledge of the fat compartments is important because volume replacement in the deep fat compartments results in structural support for midface rejuvenation.

Other important structures here are the retaining ligaments, such as the orbital retaining, the malar septum, or zygomaticocutaneous, and the MacGregor patch or zygomaticus. With volume loss they become elongated.[1]

The arteries of the face run along the borders of the superficial fat compartments but are located deep to them.[9,10] The facial artery is a main vessel that irrigates the midface directly or through derived branches, but several variations of its anatomic course have been described in recent papers.[10,11]

Usually it arises from the external carotid artery, crosses the lower border of the mandible anteriorly to the masseter muscle, and then continues its way up laterally to the nose, sending some ramifications (the lower and the upper lip branches, the lateral nasal branch). From the mouth corner to the NLF, the facial artery, now called as *angular artery*, runs in the subcutaneous plane, above facial muscles. From there it courses superiorly and may anastomose with the dorsal nasal, the infraorbital and transverse facial arteries, connecting external and internal carotid systems.[12]

Because of its location and anastomosis to other vessels, the angular artery is the vessel most likely to be compromised after filler injections to the midcheek, NLF, and periorbital area (Fig. 19.2).

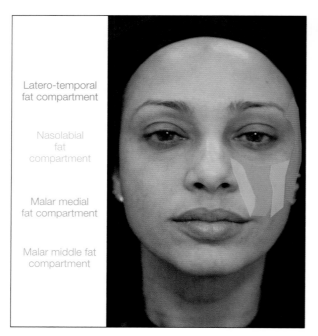

**Figure 19.1** Superficial and deep fat compartments of the face.

Latero-temporal fat compartment

Nasolabial fat compartment

Malar medial fat compartment

Malar middle fat compartment

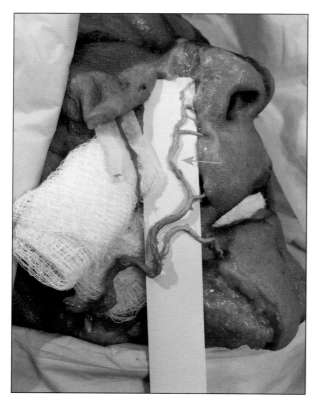

**Figure 19.2** The angular artery.

### Pearl 1

The angular artery is the vessel most likely to be compromised after filler injections to the midcheek, NLF, and periorbital area.[12]

The sensitive innervation of the midcheek is due to the maxillary branch of the trigeminal nerve, whereas the motor innervation is performed by the temporal and zygomatic branches of the facial nerve.

## Aesthetic goals

The ideal cheek contour follows the ogee curve. This S-shape curve was described many years ago and is formed by a concave arc going from the inferior lid, moving to a convex arc that includes the malar or cheek-bone prominence, and a gentle slide to the submalar hollow. Restoring this curve will help to achieve a natural-looking midface rejuvenation.[13]

Gender differences have to be borne in mind when planning to address the midface with fillers in order not to feminize the male subject. For the female patient the midface is stronger than the lower face, whereas for the male patient, the opposite is the ideal.

### Pearl 2

For the female patient the midface is stronger than the lower face, whereas for the male patient, the opposite is the ideal (Fig. 19.3A and B).

According to Remington and Swift, the female cheek is ovoid, with the apex angled and located high on the midface, below and lateral to lateral canthus.[13] The male cheek has a broader malar base, a more modest apex, located more inferomedial than the female cheek.[8] But for both genders, the transition from the lid–cheek junction to the midface, as well as from the cheek to the lower face, has to be smooth and even, without any abrupt changes in a young and attractive subject.

## Treatment areas

### Malar area

Reflating a retruded midface and recovering its natural contour, usually starts on the malar fat pads because it also helps to efface the lid–cheek junction and the upper nasolabial fold.

Before the procedure, all make-up is removed, the skin is cleaned with 4% chlohexidine gluconate, and some topical anesthesic cream may be applied to enhance patient comfort. After removal of the anesthetic cream, the area is cleaned again with 4% chlohexidine gluconate.

Outlining the best area for volume restoration is our first step. For this, we start tracing two lines: one linking the external corner of the eye to the labial commissure

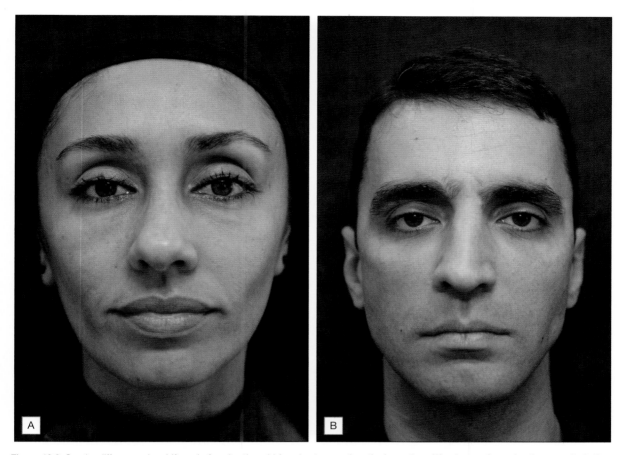

**Figure 19.3** Gender differences in midface. In females the mid face is stronger than the lower face **(A)**, whereas for males the opposite is the ideal **(B)**.

and another from the upper tragus to the superior part of the nasal ala. At the intersection of these two lines, our initial draw point, referred to as AB, is placed. This AB site points out the limit between the malar or zygomatic eminence and the maxilla bone (malar area) (Fig. 19.4, *blue circle*). From there, a concave line is traced in an upward direction, following the inferior limit of the tear trough, limited by the orbital rim (see Fig. 19.4, *superior black line*). A second concave line is traced starting from point AB downward, following the posteroinferior border of the malar bone (see Fig. 19.4, *lateral green line*). And finally, a convex line connecting the free corners of the two concave lines is traced, outlining the anterior limit of volume loss (see Fig. 19.4, *anterior brown line*). The convexity of this line is proportional to the area of volume loss.

To address the demarcated area we prefer to use 22- to 25-gauge 40-mm long cannulas to inject a three-dimensional (3D) hyaluronic acid (HA) filler with high G' and lift capacity already containing lidocaine. Alternatively, the filler can be mixed to external lidocaine using

a 30% proportion (0.3 mL of 2% lidocaine to a 1-mL HA filler syringe, connected by a sterile female-to-female connector and mixed by back and forward movements).

The filler is deposited in small boluses starting at the superior part of the demarcated area, followed by retroinjection tunnels and gentle molding massage. It can be deposited deep and also in the superficial fat compartments as needed (Fig. 19.5). The use of cannulas is recommended here to avoid the risk of inadvertent injection in the infraorbital foramen. Addressing the deep fat compartments helps to restore the structural support of the anterior cheek, whereas the superficial placement improves the natural projection.

The amount injected varies according to the degree of volume depletion, ranging from 0.5 to 2 mL per side (Fig. 19.6A [*before*] and B [*after*]).

## Zygomatic area

With senescence, the malar bone retrudes and loses volume, although in a smaller degree than the malar fat

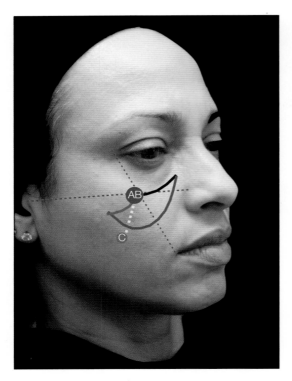

Figure 19.4 Markings for malar area augmentation with HA fillers.

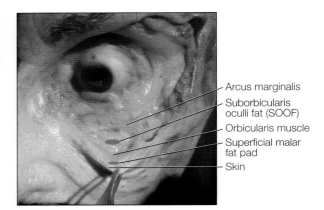

Arcus marginalis
Suborbicularis oculli fat (SOOF)
Orbicularis muscle
Superficial malar fat pad
Skin

Figure 19.5 Anatomic view of superficial and deep injection for malar area.

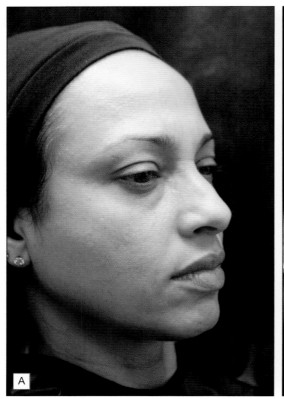

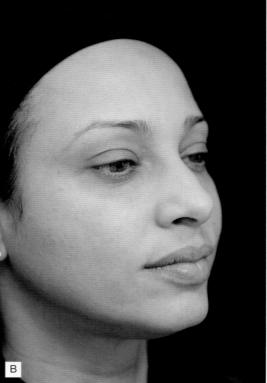

Figure 19.6. A, Before and B, after cheek augmentation.

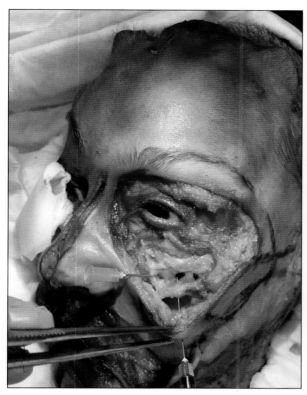

**Figure 19.7** Anatomic photo representing the filler deposits along the zygomatic arch.

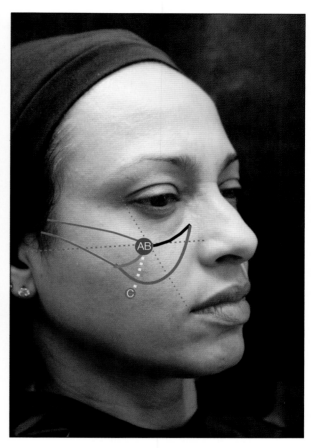

**Figure 19.8** Zygomatic area markings.

pad reduction. It may also be treated for a natural and refreshed look. To outline the optimum site for volume restoration, our technique is to first palpate the zygomatic bone. Beginning on point AB described earlier corresponding to the malar eminence, we draw two lines highlighting the superior and inferior margins of the zygomatic arch. The filler is placed between the two lines, deep to the bone using needles or cannulas, along the zygomatic arch ending at a point corresponding to the tail of the brow (Fig. 19.7, cadaver zygoma).[6–14] When injected in the supraperiosteal layer, the filler will be placed between the bone and the lateral SOOF.

Through a lifting action of the filler in these lateral zygomatic cheek areas, an improvement in the lower-eyelid appearance can be obtained[7,14] (Fig. 19.8).

## Submalar region

The aesthetic goal is that this region keeps a natural "shadow" to the midface to highlight the cheek apex and maintain the ogee curve. In some patients it will be improved after the treatment of other cheek areas but in subjects with very depleted cheek, especially athletes, there is a need for treatment. Another problem to be addressed here is the deep smile lines.

Reflation of the submalar region also helps to efface and lift the lower third of the NLF. Attention not to overfill this area or an appearance of overweight and round face instead of an oval ideal shape will be the result.

This area is prone to bruising. To allow a smooth transition from the upper cheek, the best option is to place an HA filler in the superficial subcutaneous plane in a fanning technique. In some very hollowed subjects, like runners, it is also necessary to inject in deeper layers to replace the volume loss. The subcutaneous plane depletion is better treated using 25- or 27-gauge cannulas, whereas for addressing the lines, our preference is for small-bore needles (27 to 31 gauge). For the lines, several techniques may be used, such as retrograde or anterograde linear threading, serial puncture, or fanning. The use of anterograde technique is preferable because, going ahead of the cannula or needle, the soft filler product expands the subcutaneous tissue, allows the anesthetic effect of the lidocaine mixed to the filler (more comfortable injection), and reduces the risk of inadvertent vascular damage.

After the procedure gentle massage to the overlying skin, as well as from the intraoral surface, is applied to obtain an even distribution of the filler (see Fig. 19.7A and B).

---

**Pearl 3**

Reflation of the submalar region also helps to efface and lift the lower third of the NLF.

---

## Preauricular or lateral cheek region

The plane to be addressed here is the lateral cheek superficial fat compartment and/or the skin. In some patients the loss of volume here will form a shadow located ahead of the preauricular area (Fig. 19.10).

Some relevant structures to remember are the parotid gland and duct and the transverse artery and vein, all of which are located below the SMAS, which is thicker in this region.

Lower or high G′ HA fillers can be used to replace the depleted volume here. The correct plane is subdermal, and our preference is for using cannulas to avoid damage of structures located below the SMAS and also surface irregularities. The cannula is introduced in the preauricular region and the filler is deposited in small aliquots in a fanning technique, forming a "star" (star lift) (Figs. 19.9 and 19.11). The idea is not only to fill but also to induce some lifting of the lateral part of the cheek, in continuation to the work performed in the anterior regions. Some defects may be difficult to correct due to parotid fascia attachments. Gentle massage would help to spread the product ensuring an even surface as a result.

The authors think that, after restoring the central areas of the cheek, correction of the preauricular region helps to finish the "frame" of the cheek, giving a natural-looking effect for the rejuvenation of the midface (Fig. 19.12).

## Conclusion

The midface aging is a multifactorial process that is manifested predominantly by volume loss. Biodegradable fillers are the best option for treatment because of their efficacy,

safety, versatility and reversibility, and long-lasting results. Proper training allows refinement of techniques to address this region, warranting natural-looking results, lower risk of complications, and higher patient and physician satisfaction.

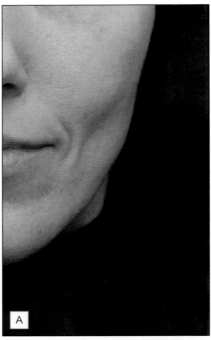

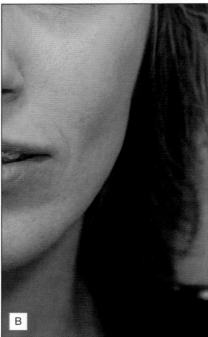

**Figure 19.10 A,** Before and **B,** after submalar filling.

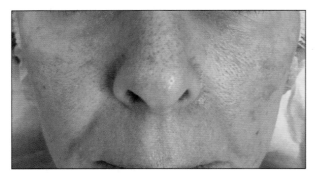

**Figure 19.9** Only left cheek was treated showing improvement of left lid–cheek junction and left nasolabial fold, compared with untreated right side.

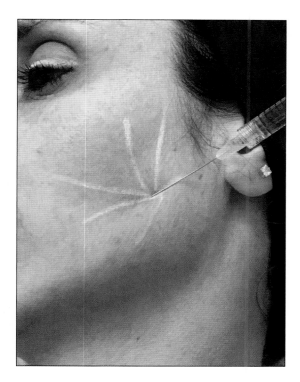

**Figure 19.11** The HA filler is deposited in a fanning technique, forming a "star," that helps to lift the lateral midface (star lift).

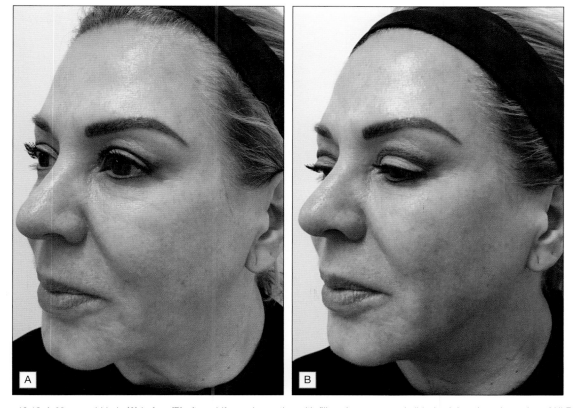

**Figure 19.12** A 60-year-old lady **(A)** before **(B)** after midface rejuvenation with fillers. Improvement in lid–cheek junction, shortening of NLF, and lifting of lateral cheek.

# References

1. Lam S, Glasgold R, Glasgold M. Analysis of facial aesthetics as applied to injectables. *Plast Reconstr Surg*. 2015;136:11s–21s.
2. Sadick N, Dorizas A, Krueguer N, Nassar A. The facial adipose system: its role in facial aging and approaches to volume restoration. *Dermatol Surg*. 2015;41:s333–s339.
3. Wong C, Medelson B. Newer understanding of specific anatomic targets in the aging face as applied to injectables: aging changes in the craniofacial skeleton and facial ligaments. *Plast Reconstr Surg*. 2015;136:44s–48s.
4. Rohrich RJ, Pessa JE. The fat compartments of the face: anatomy and clinical implications for cosmetic surgery. *Plast Reconstr Surg*. 2007;119(7):2219–2227.
5. Rohrich RJ, Pessa JE, Ristow B. The youthful cheek and the deep medial fat compartment. *Plast Reconstr Surg*. 2008;121:2107–2112.
6. Ramanadhan S, Rohrich R. Newer understanding of specific anatomic targets in the aging face as applied to injectables: superficial and deep fat compartments—an evolving target for site-specific facial augmentation. *Plast Reconstr Surg*. 2015;136:49S–55S.
7. Braz AV, Sakuma T. Midface rejuvenation: an innovative technique to restore cheek volume. *Dermatol Surg*. 2012;38(1):118–120.
8. Goodman G, Swift A, Remington K. Current concepts in the use of Voluma, Volift and Volbella. *Plast Reconstr Surg*. 2015;136:139S–148S.
9. Schaverien MV, Pessa JE, Rohrich RJ. Vascularized membranes determine the anatomical boundaries of the subcutaneous fat compartments. *Plast Reconstr Surg*. 2009;123:695–700.
10. Pilsl U, Anderhuber F, Neugebauer S. The facial artery—the main blood vessel for the anterior face? *Dermatol Surg*. 2016; 42:203–208.
11. Furukawa M, Mathes DW, Anzai Y. Evaluation of the facial artery on computed tomographic angiography using 64-slice multidetector computed tomography: implications for facial reconstruction in plastic surgery. *Plast Reconstr Surg*. 2013;131(3):526–535.
12. Beleznay K, Carruthers J, Humphrey S, Jones D. Avoiding and treating blindness from fillers: a review of the world literature. *Dermatol Surg*. 2015;41:1097–1117.
13. Swift A, Remington K. Beautiphication™: a global approach to facial beauty. *Clin Plast Surg*. 2011;38:347–377.
14. Cotofana S, Schenck T, Trevidic P Sykes J et al. Midface: clinical anatomy and regional approaches with injectable fillers. *Plast Reconstr Surg*. 2015;136:219s-–234s.

# 20

# Nose

Kyle Koo-Il Seo

## Summary and Key Features

- Filler rhinoplasty is a safe and effective technique to augment and reshape the nose without social downtime.
- Nasal dorsum augmentation is indicated for patients with a mild hump, short nose, saddle nose, flat nose, and irregularity of nasal dorsum at lateral view.
- Tip rotation or correction of the acute nasolabial angle is indicated for patients with a nasal hump, columella recession, droopy nasal tip (plunged tip), and inadequate tip projection. To raise the tip of the nose, the injection should be made between the footplates of the medial crura and the anterior nasal spine or in the columella, as opposed to the nasal lobule itself.
- A weak and overly narrow nasal lobule and a bifid tip can be corrected by placing fillers into the interdomal area of the nasal tip.
- Subcutaneous injection of fillers into the columella helps to project the columella recession frequently seen in Asians and Africans.
- Hyaluronic acid (HA) fillers high in viscoelasticity are recommended for filler rhinoplasty because any inadvertent irregularity can be readily reversible by hyaluronidase.
- The use of a cannula has definite benefits over using a needle in filler rhinoplasty because it can prevent risks of unwanted bruising, as well as embolization.
- When the cannula is used for filler rhinoplasty, the entry point for the blunt cannula should be made at the infratip lobule of the nasal tip by a 21-gauge sharp needle.
- The blood supply to the nasal dorsum is principally supplied by the lateral nasal artery (LNA) and dorsal nasal artery (DNA), a branch of the ophthalmic artery. Because these arteries form broad-based anastomosis among themselves at the nasal dorsum, fillers injected inadvertently into the DNA and even LNA may migrate in reverse direction to the ophthalmic artery, causing blindness.

## Introduction

The nose represents the central feature of the face, with an aesthetically profound effect on the overall balance of and descriptions of the other facial features. Accordingly, enhancing a flat, poorly defined nose can give definition to the face and refine its overall appearance. For this reason, augmentation rhinoplasty has long been practiced as a well-established procedure among Asians, who have relatively smaller noses than whites. Significantly, the ability to conveniently reshape the nose without undergoing surgery is a key benefit of filler rhinoplasty, which has made it one of the most popular filler procedures among Asian patients.

Although some drawbacks of filler rhinoplasty versus conventional surgery are the need for repeat treatments and the unsuitability for reduction rhinoplasty (e.g., sharpening a bulbous nose or narrowing a wide nasal base), the countervailing advantages are numerous and compelling: it ensures minimum social downtime compared with surgery; in terms of its safety profile, filler rhinoplasty does not entail any of the potential risks arising from surgery, such as unnatural contractural pull and distortion; and filler rhinoplasty is capable of making the shape appear more natural by allowing the creation of arches extending from the medial brows to the dorsum of nose.

This chapter aims to provide an overview of the concept, techniques, useful tips, and precautions involved in performing filler rhinoplasty.

## The attractively proportioned nose and face

An ideal nose is generally characterized as one with a high dorsum and projected tip despite specific variations according to ethnic preferences. However, it is also true that there is no set standard for an ideal nose that works for every face because aesthetic standards tend to vary among different ethnicities, between the genders, as well as evolving over time. Just as importantly, facial beauty is a function of the balance among various facial features, including the nose. Thus efforts have been directed at identifying the ideal facial and nasal proportions and effecting changes that afford better proportionality and harmony to the overall face. This notion of facial

**Figure 20.1** Topographical facial landmarks and ideal facial proportion.

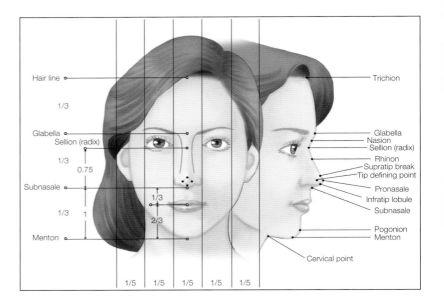

proportion also assists the field of filler rhinoplasty in the planning of the treatment strategy for a given patient.

The nose is divided into several subportions, including the dorsum, sidewall, nasal tip, ala nasi, and columella. In addition, there are certain topographic landmarks of the nose used for describing the cosmetic and reconstructive procedures. Recognized topographical facial landmarks are shown in **Fig. 20.1**. Although the term "nasion" is sometimes confusingly used to refer to the deepest point of the nasal root, it represents the median anterior tip of the nasofrontal suture. Rather, the sellion represents the deepest point of the nasal bone or the nasofrontal angle (NFrtA). Because the sellion is also the bony landmark, corresponding to surface anatomy, the term "radix" is used for the deepest point of the nasal root. Rhinion refers to the osteocartilaginous junction, whereas pronasale is the most prominent point of the nasal tip and the subnasale represents the junction between the columella and the philtrum.

On the frontal view a balanced white face should divide into equal vertical thirds and equal horizontal fifths, as shown in **Fig. 20.1**. The ideal length of the nose in proportion to the face is three-quarters the length of the lower one-third of the face, from the subnasale to the mentum. Meanwhile, the ideal nasal width at the alar base is believed to correspond to the intercanthal distance, which equals one-fifth of the facial width. The width of the body of the nose should be 80% of the width of the nose at the alar bases. The narrowest point of the nasal dorsum is at the radix, where the width at the radix approximates the height of the palpebral fissure. A gentle curve emanating from the medial brow courses along the lateral border of the nasal dorsum to end at the ipsilateral tip-defining point. Any irregularities of this line will be easily noticeable as deviations from the

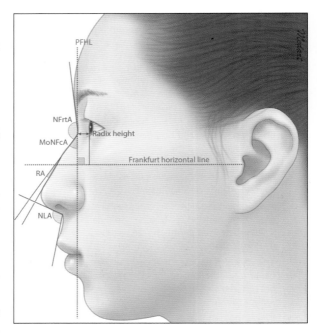

**Figure 20.2** Anthropometric factors related to the nose. *MoNFcA*, Modified nasofacial angle; *NFrtA*, nasofrontal angle; *NLA*, nasolabial angle; *RA*, rhinion angle. *Reproduced with permission from Seo K. Filler for Asians. Seoul Medical Publishing Ltd.: Jeju; 2016.*

contralateral line, thereby contributing to asymmetry and unsightly appearance.

On the lateral view there are certain anthropometric factors related to the nose that deserve special mention in evaluating filler rhinoplasty patients (**Fig. 20.2**). The glabella-to-radix line intersecting with the radix-to-tip line forms the NFrtA. Ideally this angle should be within 115 to 130 degrees. Meanwhile, the nasofacial angle represents the angle between the nasal dorsum line and the glabella-to-pogonion line. However, considering that the glabella-to-pogonion line is subject to change in case the patient underwent any forehead and/or chin augmentation, the line perpendicular to the Frankfurt horizontal line (PFHL) is more advisable than the glabella-to-pogonion line as the reference. The resulting angle between the nasal dorsum line and the PFHL is the modified nasofacial angle (MoNFcA). The aesthetic ideal for MoNFcA is 35 to 40 degrees. Meanwhile, the nasolabial angle (NLA), which is useful for assessing the effectiveness of nasal tip rotation, represents the angle formed by the line tangent to the columella intersected by the subnasale-to-labial limb line. The ideal aesthetic range for NLA should be 90 to 110 degrees.

For assessing nasal radix augmentation and nasal dorsum augmentation, radix height increment (RHI) can be used. RHI represents the rate of increase (%) in the distance between the radix and the line parallel to the PFHL drawn at the anterior margin of the lower eyelid measured before and after treatment. To assess the efficacy of nasal hump correction, rhinion angle (RA), the angle between the nasal dorsum line intersected by the rhinion-to-nasal tip line, is measured.

## Ethnic differences

The typical features of a white nose, leptorrhine (tall and thin), have been described previously. The African platyrrhine (broad and flat) nose is characterized by a low radix, short concave dorsum, widened alae base, a bulbous and an underprojected tip, flared alae with round nostril, and extremely thick skin. The Asian mesorrhine (intermediate) nose is characterized as a blend of the above two; it is typically characterized by a low broad dorsum, short nasal bones, a round underprojected and underrotated tip, columellar recession, somewhat rounded nostrils, and moderately thick skin. The nasal tip is unilobular instead of having definite nasal tip definition. Understanding these ethnic differences is useful for tailoring filler rhinoplasty to the needs and characteristics of the different ethnic groups.

However, one must also take note of the increased intermingling among different racial groups, and the difference among races even within the same ethnic group. Moreover, as the standard of beauty becomes increasingly universal, applying a strict ethnic classification would be less meaningful.

## Vascular patterns of the nose (Fig. 20.3)

The blood supply to the external nose is largely divided into the ophthalmic artery, a branch of the internal carotid system, and the facial artery, a branch of the external carotid system. The dorsum of the nose is principally supplied by the lateral nasal artery (LNA), a branch of the angular artery branching out from the facial artery, with

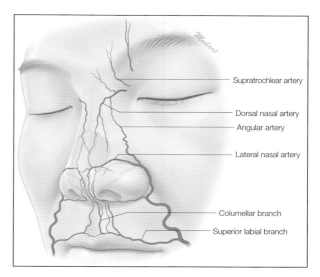

**Figure 20.3** Vascular patterns of the nose.

a contribution over the upper part of the dorsum of the nose by the dorsal nasal artery (DNA), a branch of the ophthalmic artery. Meanwhile, the columellar is supplied by the columellar branch of the superior labial artery, which branches off from the facial artery. The blood supply to the nasal tip originates primarily from the LNA or the DNA and to some extent from the columellar branch of the superior labial artery. These arteries form broad-based anastomosis among themselves at the nasal dorsum.

## Appropriate filler for nose

Considering the thin skin at the dorsum of the nose and that the subtle change of nose may affect the overall balance of other facial features, practitioners are advised to apply only hyaluronic acid (HA) fillers for nose filler because any unsatisfactory results are readily reversible by using hyaluronidase. Among various HA fillers, it is advisable to use HA fillers high in viscoelasticity and on the contrary less in water-absorbing capacity from surrounding tissue to retain the enhanced nasal shape and also to maintain the initial nasal shape. Good examples include large particle HA fillers, such as Restylane SubQ® or Yvoire® contour. For making fine corrections, use of HA fillers with fine particles, such as Restylane® and Belotero Balance®, is recommended.

## Anesthesia

When using the needle, topical anesthetic cream applied 20 to 30 minutes in advance is sufficient for reducing the pain. If a cannula is used, prior injection of local anesthetic is advised to help to minimize the potential discomfort caused by the large size of the cannula. For dorsum augmentation, the anesthetic is to be injected subcutaneously at three different points, including the radix, rhinion, and infratip lobule of the nasal tip, wheras local anesthetic must be injected additionally into the columella and subnasale for the tip rotation. To minimize incidental volume change effected by the injected anesthetic itself, the amount of local anesthetic should be limited to no more than 0.1 mL per point. Local anesthetics containing lidocaine with 1:100,000 epinephrine are to be injected at the infratip lobule, the entry point for the cannula to minimize the bruising.

## Injection technique (Fig. 20.4)

Although some practitioners use only the needle for filler rhinoplasty, others prefer the cannula; it is a matter of personal preference. However, as a general rule, when augmentation is performed on the entire nasal dorsum or whole nose, including the columella, using a cannula has some definite benefits over using a needle because it can prevent risks of unwanted bruising, as well as embolization. Regarding the size of cannula, 23 gauge is required for Restylane SubQ® because of its large particle size. When the cannula is used, an entry point for the cannula should be made at the infratip lobule of the nose tip by a 21-gauge sharp needle.

The cannula is to be inserted into the entry point and pushed all the way up to point just above the sellion for dorsum augmentation or posteriorly to the nasal spine in the case of tip elevation. The depth of the cannula insertion should be at the deep subcutaneous layer. Using the retrograde threading technique, inject the filler in volumes sufficient to raise the dorsum or nasal tip to the desired height. The needle is also recommended for making any contemporaneous fine corrections following filler placement with the cannula.

However, use of the needle is also acceptable in simpler cases involving, for example, mild hump corrections, small amount injections, or superficial injection to the nasal tip, or when the patient has a low tolerance for pain from local anesthetic injection. It bears noting, however, that, when the procedure calls for the use of the needle, an aspiration test for blood should be performed prior to each injection of fillers so as to avoid any unwanted intravascular injection.

Massaging is essential throughout the treatment to ensure a smooth contour regardless of cannula technique or needle technique.

## Injection techniques by nasal region

### Nasal dorsum augmentation (Fig. 20.5)

Dorsum augmentation is indicated for patients with a nasal hump, flat and short nose, saddle nose, irregularity of the nasal dorsum at lateral view and other issues relating to the nasal dorsum. Here, the filler is injected along the nasal dorsum from the radix to the nasal tip to increase both the nasal length and height. This effect is equivalent to the surgical implant of nasal dorsum. Additional filler injection from the radix to the glabella area may also be necessary during dorsum augmentation to create a curvilinear arch extending from the medial brow to the dorsum of the nose, particularly in patients with a deep glabellar frown line. This gives a more appealing and natural appearance to the nasal dorsum.

Standing in front of the patient, the cannula is pushed all the way up to the point just above the sellion, along the midline of the nasal dorsum radix, gently pinch the dorsum of the nose to prevent the filler from spreading laterally upon injection. The filler should be injected continuously in a retrograde manner so as to build a "column" to the desired height. Subsequent filler injections are made on either side of the "column" to the desired width to even out the contour. Although the radix in an Asian face typically sits on the intercanthal line, the injection of fillers into the sellion relocates the radix to sit 3 to 5 mm above its original position in line with the eyelashes. As to the lower portion of the nose, fillers may be injected either as far down to the nasal lobule where augmentation of the nasal tip is required, or otherwise only cephalic to the supratip break.

When using the needle, filler injection also begins at the radix. Piercing the skin just 2 to 3 mm cephalic to the rhinion in the midline of the nasal dorsum, advance the needle along the dorsum at a depth where it reaches the periosteum above the sellion. Inject the filler in a retrograde manner to the desired height. Subsequently, inject the lateral sides of the injected filler to smoothen out the contours on the sidewalls. Repeat the above-mentioned threading injections two or three times in the region between the rhinion and the nasal tip to achieve alignment with the previously injected filler in the nasal dorsum.

For a curvilinear arch from the medial brow to the radix, standing behind the patient, pierce the skin at the glabellar and advance the needle to the newly formed radix at the deep subcutaneous level. Inject the filler to ensure the appropriate NFA in accordance with the heightened midline of the upper nasal dorsum. Next, inject the filler in the same manner to create an arch from the medial brow to the dorsum. This process is particularly essential in patients with a deep glabellar frown line. The average amount of filler is 0.8 ± 0.4 mL for nasal dorsum augmentation and 0.3 ± 0.2 mL for curvilinear arch.

### Pearl 1

Caution should be taken against placing excessive amounts of fillers for dorsum augmentation, which may lead to an overly thick and broad dorsum. Such outcomes can be prevented by using the double-layer technique, whereby fillers are first injected deep into the subcutaneous layer to build up and heighten the nasal dorsum, followed by superficial injection in smaller amounts made additionally in the subdermal layer.

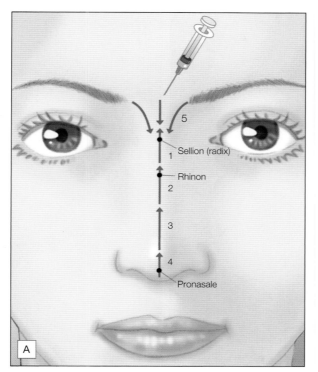

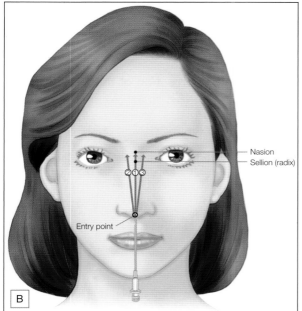

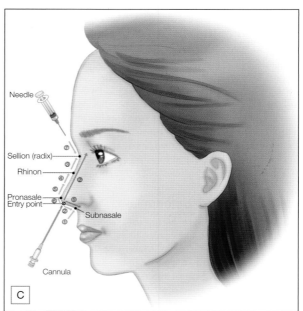

**Figure 20.4** Injection technique for filler rhinoplasty: **(A)** needle technique; **(B)** cannula technique; **(C)** lateral view of needle and cannula technique.

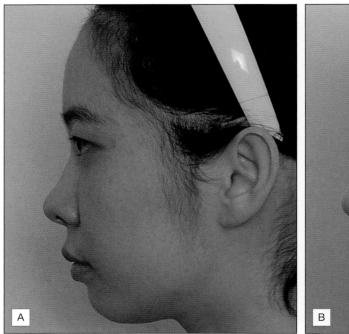
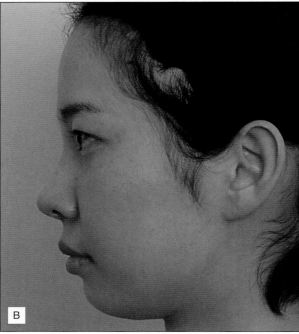

**Figure 20.5** Dorsum of the nose was augmented from the nasal tip to the arch connecting the medial brow (before **[A]** and after **[B]**).

## Correction of the nasal tip

A weak and overly narrow nasal lobule can be corrected by placing fillers into the interdomal area. Augmenting the lobule by filling the interdomal area also helps in cases in which the overlying skin or the subcutaneous fat above the alar cartilage is too thin, causing the alar cartilage to become overly visible. A bifid tip can also be successfully treated with filler injection into the nasal tip. Conversely, filler injection into the interdomal area is not advised for patients with a large nasal lobule because they would end up instead with a prominently bulbous nose.

## Correction of the columella

Columella recession is frequently seen in Asians and Africans. From the side, too little columella show is undesirable; instead a slight protrusion of the columella helps to create a much more sophisticated appearance. Subcutaneous injection of fillers in volumes ranging from 0.2 to 0.5 mL into the columella readily helps to project the retracted columella.

Holding the syringe vertically, pierce the nasal tip just above the infratip lobule and advance posteriorly along the midline of the columella. Use of the cannula would be preferable when concurrent injection into the NLA is required. Using the threading technique, inject the filler until the columella show is visible on the profile view.

However, precaution should be taken when using a cannula for this procedure because the filler may overspill through the needle entry point if excess volumes are injected.

## Tip rotation or correction of the acute nasolabial angle (Fig. 20.6)

The NLA is known to range 90 to 95 degrees for men and 95 to 110 degrees for women, whereas the corresponding angle in Asians in many cases falls below 90 degrees. Tip rotation or correction of acute NLA is indicated for patients with a nasal hump, columella recession, droopy nasal tip (plunged tip), and inadequate tip projection. During the tip rotation the filler is injected mainly into the columella and around the anterior nasal spine at the nasolabial junction. This opens the acute NLA to beyond 90 degrees and causes the cephalic rotation of the nasal tip, allowing for a more refined lateral view of the face. This procedure is equivalent to a columellar strut insertion in surgical rhinoplasty.

Insert the cannula into the entry point, and push posteriorly to the nasal spine. Inject the filler between the footplates of the medial crura and the anterior nasal spine in volumes sufficient to improve the previously acute NLA to more than 90 degrees. When using a needle for this procedure, directly insert the needle into the nasolabial junction and advance it to the nasal spine. Concomitantly with this the columella should be corrected. A total of 0.7 ± 0.3 mL of HA filler is required for this indication.

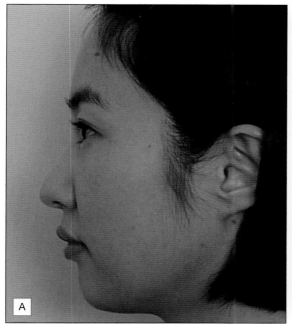
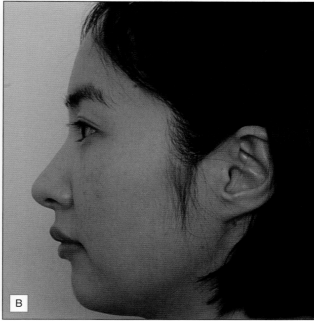

**Figure 20.6** Inadequate tip projection was corrected by enhancing the nasolabial angle and the columella (before **[A]** and after **[B]**).

### Pearl 2

It must be noted that fillers injected in excess volumes may add unwanted bulk to the upper portion of the philtrum. It also bears noting that this procedure is contraindicated in patients with an upturned, overrotated nose with excessive nostril show or who generally do not desire nostril show.

### Pearl 3

Effectiveness of the tip rotation can be simulated by pinching the nasolabial junction right under the columella and observing the corresponding degree of elevation in the nasal tip. Generally speaking, a hard and thick nasal tip consisting of abundant fibrous tissue will not lift well, whereas a small and softer tip tends to lift up more readily. With patients exhibiting any anxiety or doubts about the outcomes of filler rhinoplasty, a useful approach would be to inject non-cross-linked HA into the nose to demonstrate to them what the actual results may look like before they commit to the treatment.

## Hump (Fig. 20.7)

A mild nasal hump is easily corrected by retrograde injection of fillers, starting from the nasion down to the depression just above the hump, using a needle; however, in patients with a severe hump, concurrent tip rotation by using a cannula is required for the appropriate nasofrontal and nasofacial angles. When undertaking such concomitant tip rotation, it bears mention that fillers must also be placed in the saddle created between the elevated nasal tip and the rhinion to straighten the nasal profile.

## Wide nasal base (Fig. 20.8)

Filler injection for tip rotation can also reduce the width of the nasal base to some extent by elongating the columella. Furthermore, the dorsum augmentation can give the optical illusion of a slimmer nose. The appropriate ratio of nasal length to width is considered to be 1 : 1.4 to 1.5.

### Pearl 4

Basically no filler is able to make the bulbous tip of the nose become sharpened. However, nose filler can give subtle sharpness to the nasal tip, leveraging the optical illusion of a narrower nose, which can be effected by increasing the length of the nose with the dorsum augmentation as in the case of a wide nose. Moreover, the tip rotation would actually bring about the reduction of the nasal base width by elongating the columella as is the case with columellar strut. Lastly, injection of filler into the pronasale is also recommended for effecting subtle definition to the nasal tip in the bulbous tip by injection of very small amounts of fillers. Injection of filler intradermally and subdermally into the pronasale. Injection of fillers directly into the nasal lobule should be avoided in patients with a bulbous tip because this would only serve to add bulk and bulbosity to the nose.

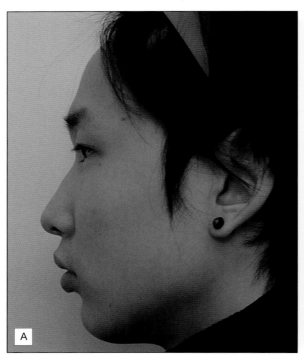 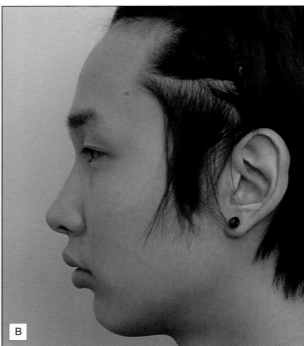

**Figure 20.7** A mild nasal hump and irregularity of nasal dorsum at lateral view was corrected by injection of fillers into the depression just above the hump along with elevation of the nasal tip by injection into the nasolabial junction and columella (before **[A]** and after **[B]**).

## Deviated nose

### Concavely or convexly bent nose

The bent nose at the frontal view can be straightened by filling out the concave side in the midportion of the nasal dorsum, while filling the opposite side at each of the radix and the lower part of the nasal dorsum. Precaution should be taken to avoid creating an overly thick nasal dorsum.

### Slanted nose (deviation to one side)

Fillers should be injected into the point opposite to the deviated side between the rhinion and the nasal lobule, to compensate for the asymmetry. Precaution should be taken to avoid creating an overly thick nasal dorsum.

---

### Pearl 5

Compared with other regions on the face, longevity of nose filler, especially dorsum augmentation at radix, lasts more than 2 to 3 years by only one session of injection. This seems to be because radix is limited space without sufficient surrounding host tissue, which means less chance of attacking by host hyaluronidase. However, longevity of nose filler at other nasal regions, such as the columella and subnasal area, lasts much less than dorsum augmentation.

Therefore touch-up for these regions is recommended at approximately 6-month intervals for sustained effect.

---

## Adverse effects

Although there are several mild, transient adverse effects, such as bruising, headache, swelling, erythema, and infection after nose filler, the most serious adverse effect is vascular complication. The causes of vascular complication are largely twofold (i.e., vascular compression caused by fillers injected into limited space and intravascular embolization by the injected filler material). Vascular complication may happen more frequently in patients with a history of previous nose surgery because previous nose surgery may not only compromise their vascular circulation but also fix the vessels by the scar tissue, which makes the vessels more vulnerable to puncture by needle. Therefore keen attention should be paid to patients with previous nose surgery, a procedure popular among Asians. Vascular complications at their worst can bring about skin necrosis and even blindness, whereas mild cases may fortunately end up with only multiple mottled erythematous patches over nose, glabellar area, and even forehead for 1 to 4 weeks (Fig. 20.9). However, in the early stage of severe cases, infection can be mistakenly suspected because patients usually show erythematous swelling with multiple pustules on the nose instead of crust (see Fig. 20.9).

Blood supply to the nasal dorsum is mainly provided by the DNA, a branch of the ophthalmic artery, and the LNA. These arteries form broad-based anastomosis among

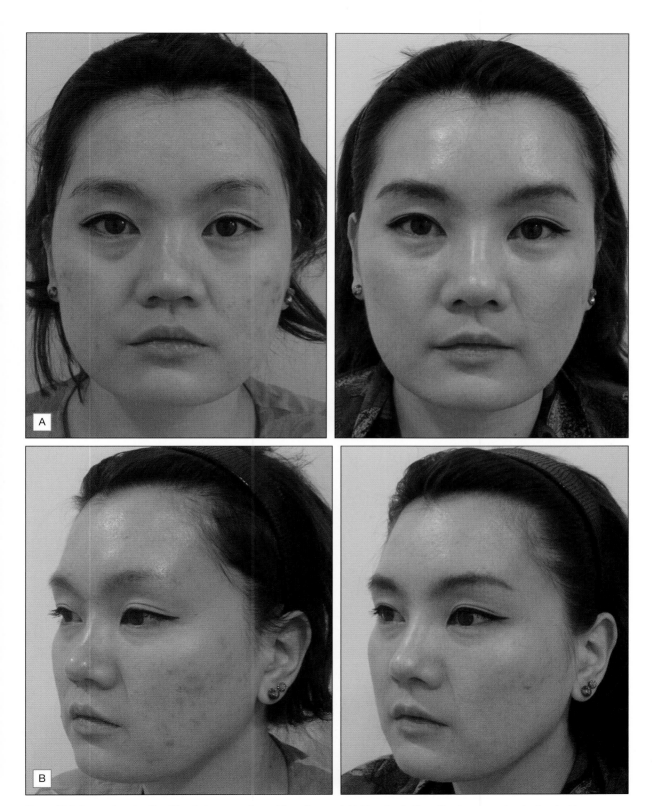

**Figure 20.8** Comprehensive filler rhinoplasty was performed from the nasolabial junction to the sellion to augment a short and wide nose: **(A)** front view, **(B)** 45-degree view, **(C)** bottom view. The elongated nostril is also observed along with the elevation of the nasal tip in the bottom view.

*Continued*

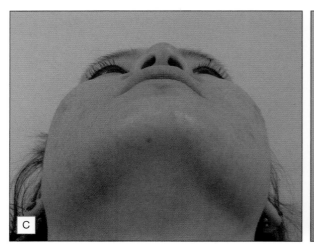
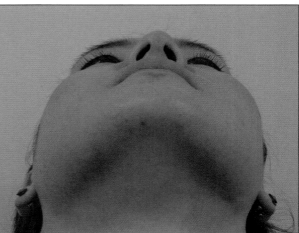

**Figure 20.8, cont'd**

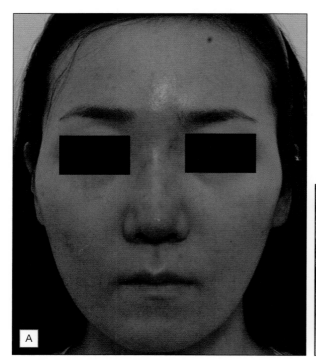
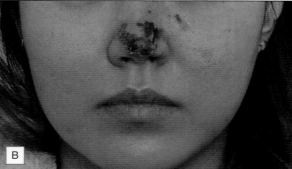

**Figure 20.9 A,** Mild cases may show only multiple mottled erythematous patches over nose, glabellar area, and even forehead for 1 to 4 weeks. **B,** Severe cases show even skin necrosis in the nasal tip. *Reproduced with permission from Seo K. Filler for Asians. Seoul Medical Publishing Ltd.: Jeju; 2016.*

themselves at the nasal dorsum. Therefore, fillers injected inadvertently into the DNA and even LNA may migrate in a reverse direction to the ophthalmic artery, causing occlusion to the branches of the ophthalmic artery, such as the retinal artery and the posterior ciliary artery, which in turn may lead to blindness.

As a key prevention strategy against intravascular injection, the routine use of the cannula is recommended instead of a needle. Where needles are used, inevitably, blood aspiration tests should be performed before injection. However, because of the thin vessels of the nose, the blood aspiration test may present false-negative results upon intravascular puncture, depending on the filler type, needle gauge, and vessel size. Therefore it is important to select the right needle of adequately large gauge for the blood aspiration test. In addition, slower injection speed, smooth progression of the cannula, the use of large cannulas of at least 23-gauge, and retrograde injection technique can help to reduce the risk of vascular complications.

Practitioners should also pay close attention to any ischemic signs, such as pain following filler injection, blanching during or immediately after the injection, as well as any subsequent violaceous or grayish discoloration, in which case timely and adequate intervention is required. The first-line treatment for vascular complications in the case of HA fillers is the subcutaneous injection of hyaluronidase into the ischemic lesion and adjacent areas as soon as possible (within 1 day). For this reason, HA filler should be considered the preferred filler type for treating areas particularly vulnerable to intravascular injection, such as the nose, glabella, nasolabial fold, and forehead. Intake of sublingual nitroglycerin and oral aspirin (100 mg), facilitating peripheral blood circulation, is also prerequisite. Steroids and antibiotics also help to reduce the risk of inflammation and any possible secondary infection. Subject to availability, hyperbaric oxygen treatment is also recommended as a well-known treatment modality for various peripheral ischemic diseases.

Other adverse effects include temporary redness, which may on occasion persist over several months. Such a complication is presumed to arise from vascular dilatation triggered as a secondary reaction to compensate for the impaired circulation from vascular compression caused by injection of fillers into a confined space. Symptoms persisting for several months can be reversed by injecting hyaluronidase only if HA fillers were used.

---

### Pearl 6

For patients who already have implants placed in the nose from a previous surgical rhinoplasty, filler rhinoplasty would basically be a contraindication, given that the skin is left thinner, the space for filler injection is more limited, and blood circulation is already compromised by the previous surgery. However, when the inserted implant has left unsightly linear depression between radix and nasion, small amounts of filler may be placed in the radix to straighten irregularity.

---

### Further reading

Behrbohm H, Tardy ME. *Essentials of Septorhinoplasty. Philosophy—Approaches—Techniques*. New York, NY: Thieme; 2004.

Carruthers J, Carruthers A, eds. *Soft Tissue Augmentation*. Philadelphia, PA: Elsevier; 2005.

Dhong ES, Han SK, Lee CH, Yoon ES, Kim WK. Anthropometric study of alar cartilage in Asians. *Ann Plast Surg.* 2002;48:386–391.

Gunter JP, Rohrich RJ, Adams WP. *Dallas Rhinoplasty; Nasal Surgery by the Masters*. Missouri, MO: Quality Medical Publishing; 2007.

Larrabee WF, Makielski KH, Henderson JL. *Surgical Anatomy of the Face*. Philadelphia, PA: Lippincott Williams & Wilkins; 2004.

Tanaka Y, Matsuo K, Yuzuriha S. Westernization of the Asian nose by augmentation of the retropositioned anterior nasal spine with an injectable filler. *Eplasty.* 2011;11:e7.

Tardy ME, Brown RJ. *Surgical Anatomy of the Nose*. New York, NY: Raven Press; 1990.

Tebbetts JB. *Primary Rhinoplasty: Redefining the Logic and Techniques*. Philadelphia, PA: Mosby Elsevier; 2008.

# 21

# Perioral and mandibular filling: framing the lips

## Jean Carruthers, Ada R. Trindade de Almeida

### Summary and Key Features

- The underlying neurovascular anatomy in the perioral region is extremely important.
- The retrusion of perioral bone and fat and descent of the cutaneous envelope with jowl formation give the desired treatment algorithm to attempt to reverse these changes.
- Biodegradable reversible fillers are preferred in the perioral region.
- Adjuvant therapy with neuromodulators helps to lift areas of descent (e.g., mouth corners) as well as increase the longevity of the fillers.
- Adjuvant treatments with energy-based devices that also recontour the lower face and upper neck are ideal partners in achieving the best aesthetic results.

## Introduction

The face is our unique individual and deeply personal calling card. Its remarkable transformation over time is determined by the repetitive interplay of both extrinsic and intrinsic factors. Surface changes in the turgor and draping of the skin, as well as actinic changes in vascularity and pigmentation, have been well understood for years as signs of aging.

More recent imaging studies have demonstrated predictable related changes in the facial skeleton, with the frontal bone moving inferiorly, the maxilla moving posteriorly and superiorly, the orbital and the piriform apertures widening, and the mandible reducing in both height and length.[1]

The perioral area is no different. From the frontal perspective, it is considered the lower third of the face. This highly mobile region suffers the impact of deep volume loss, from bone reabsorption especially those of dental origin (maxilla and mandible), fat atrophy and/or displacement, and elongation of the retaining ligaments from both local and neighboring areas.[2–4]

Nasolabial folds become more etched and folded, secondary to fat pad atrophy from cheek compartments, as well as to enlargement of the piriform aperture from recession of the medial edge of the maxilla. The oral commissures turn downward, and become deeper marionette lines. The bony mandible loses definition, and the chin fat compartments become atrophic too, permitting the mentalis to develop a pebbled appearance. With the emergence of the jowls, the prejowl sulcus becomes evident. All the described changes shorten the size of the lower face in the middle-aged and older subject.

The addition of the newer volumizing fillers to repair the loss of support from the lost facial fat pads and the age-related retrusion of the bony facial skeleton is particularly effective in restoring the desired natural soft look. The almost continuous movement of the lower facial mimetic musculature tends to reduce the length of time a nonpermanent filler can last if unaided by judicious use of neuromodulators.

## Anatomic considerations

In the past the perioral area was considered to extend from the subnasal region and nasolabial folds to the lower border of the soft tissue contour of the chin (the menton). Because many people are bothered by their immediate submental region as their periocular region,[5] the public consider the submental region as an important part of the lower face. Now that noninvasive treatment modalities are available for the submental area, we suggest that cryolipolysis and chemolipolysis also be discussed with our patients when considering lower facial rejuvenation and restoration treatments.

## Neocollagenesis

Research in human skin has shown that the injection of soft tissue augmenting agents, such as hyaluronic acid (HA), can help to stimulate neocollagenesis.[6,7] The underlying mechanism may be that stretching of human skin with the filler activates the aged "resting" fibroblasts with neocollagenesis seen after 1 month and lasting for 3 months.

The injection of botulinum toxin is also associated with dermal neocollagenesis.[8] Procollagen type 1 carboxyterminal peptide (PIP) levels increased in dermal fibroblasts with upregulation of type 1 collagen and reduction of matrix metalloproteinase (MMP) production. These effects may explain the surface "glow" seen in neuromodulator- and filler-treated human skin.

It is now realized that the combination of three-dimensional (3D) volumizing fillers with neuromodulators and noninvasive skin tightening permits the most optimal aesthetic result.[9] This improvement is also recognized by the subjects.[10]

## Treatment modalities

We prefer to use nonpermanent cross-linked fillers, such as HA (Juvéderm Voluma group of fillers [HA-V], Belotero HA-PDM, Restylane NASHA group), in the entire perioral region because they are long-lasting, easily molded, well tolerated, and with the use of hyaluronidase, reversible. For the jawline we have used also calcium hydroxylapatite (CaHA) (Radiesse).

We have used both onabotulinumtoxinA (Botox Cosmetic, Allergan Pharmaceuticals, Irvine, CA) and incobotulinumtoxinA (Xeomin, Merz Aesthetics) to treat masseters, depressor anguli oris, mentalis, orbicularis oris, and platysma.

### Pearl 1

In the perioral area, fillers that are soft and malleable give the most aesthetic and functional result.

## Treatment

Reflation and restoration of the lower face begins with a complete history from the patient and an understanding of the areas that are of aesthetic concern. Simultaneous evaluation with the subject looking at his or her face on the mirror while animating and relaxing their facial muscles must be followed by standardized photography. It is important to show the photos to the subject prior to treatment so they can be more aware of preexisting asymmetries, etc. It is also helpful for them when they are showing their friends and family.

## Pain management

Strategies for pain management have progressed from direct nerve blocks, which alter the muscular function of the perioral region, to patient education, which reduces anxiety, topical anesthetic creams, and ice, and cold roller anesthesia, none of which alter the underlying facial expressivity.

Should maxillary and mandibular blocks be considered, it is wise to see the subjects again in a few days to check for posttreatment symmetry and proportion.

## Injection technique

Both needle and cannula can be excellent injection techniques both from the points of view of efficacy and safety. There is controversy only about relative safety, but it should be noted that vascular occlusion has been reported with both methods.[11]

Our opinion is that the safest injection technique using either modality is that performed by an experienced physician who has an excellent knowledge of 3D facial anatomy, including the neurovascular anatomy in the subcutaneous preperiosteal space. Some excellent human anatomy courses are available through such organizations as the American Society for Dermatologic Surgery (www.ASDS.net) and the American Academy of Dermatology (www.aad.org).

It is also very important that the issue of potential vascular complications also be disclosed to each patient verbally and in the physician consent form so that subjects can give their full informed consent.

Many physician injectors are used to injecting using the retrograde technique, in which the needle or cannula is advanced and then the plunger on the syringe is depressed as the injecting instrument is withdrawn. Both authors prefer to use anterograde injection technique so that the plunger is depressed as soon as the injecting instrument is subdermal so that the soft fluid filler product (whether injected by needle or cannula) ballottés the subcutaneous tissues gently away, thus reducing the chance of accidental vascular perforation.

## Treatment regions

### Nasolabial folds

The lower extent of the nasolabial fold is in the perioral region. When the subject smiles, the vertical lines at the lateral border of the mouth can become etched and obvious. Superficial injection of a malleable soft HA filler can nicely soften this appearance.

An interesting technique to address the upper nasolabial fold is to volumize the malar area and this often effaces the upper nasolabial fold so that no injections are required (Fig. 21.1).

In some selected cases in which recession of perinasal maxillary bone has occurred, a 3D filler can be carefully deposited in a small pocket in the supraperiosteal plane, near the piriform aperture. This helps to soften the nasolabial groove and also corrects the retruded alar base.[12,13]

### Pearl 2

Pay attention to avoid injecting in the subcutaneous layer lateral to the ala, where the angular artery is most commonly located and the risk of vascular occlusion is higher.[11]

### Marionnette lines and "mouth frown"

With the aging process, atrophy of subcutaneous fat and bone along with actinic and intrinsic changes in the perioral skin allows the mouth corners to turn downward, giving a sad, bitter expression, the "mouth frown." Simultaneous 3D filling with higher-viscosity HA fillers in the deeper

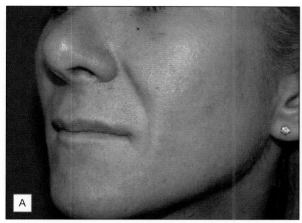

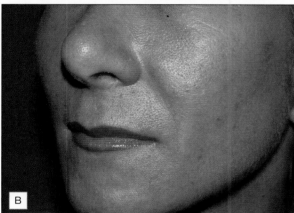

**Figure 21.1 A, B** Before and after: Reflating the malar area with 3D filling can efface the upper nasolabial fold without elongating the upper lip.

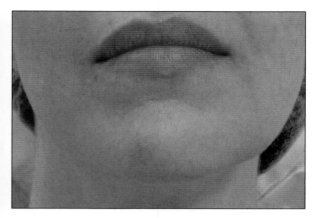

**Figure 21.2** Photograph taken to show the aesthetic difference that lifting both the mouth corner and lateral mentum together make. Left side treated; right side about to be treated.

tissue to apply a "tent pole" to the lateral commissure and the lateral lower lip area with superficial filling of fine lines is helpful.

Starting from the mandibular border to the mouth corner, the filler is placed deep inferiorly (near the mandible), in the subcutaneous layer in the half of the way up and in the dermis near the oral commissure. In this location, to achieve eversion, one option is to inject in a superficial fanning technique with three lines forming an inverted tripod with the base located at the mouth corner (Fig. 21.2).

Simultaneous use of neuromodulator to the depressor anguli oris and mentalis and platysma below the mandibular margin[14] allows the lateral oral commissure to elevate, restoring a more harmonious expression.

## Chin retrusion

The chin shape and contour is determined by the position of the mandible and the amount of overlying soft tissues.

It has superficial and deep fat compartments that deflate over time along with bone reabsorption. This way, with aging, the chin "deflates" like other facial areas, impacting the size of the lower face. The objective of the treatment is to reflate and/or project the chin in addition to the correction of the prejowl sulcus, to achieve a uniform and smooth surface from the lower lip to the mandibular border in the frontal view and a naturally projected and sharper jawline transition from the lateral view (Fig. 21.3).

Our technique of preference is to inject 3D filler in the center of the mentum, between the two vascular arcades of the mental arteries. This usually requires 0.5 to 1 mL of HA filler centrally and perpendicularly into the mentum at its point. After this, gentle molding is performed so the contiguous marionette filler can be blended with filler injected laterally in the prejowl sulcus and marionette lines. In addition, 0.2 to 0.4 mL of filler material can be injected subdermally into the regions superior and lateral to the mentum. Deep locations are better addressed by needles, whereas more superficial placement can be performed using cannulas. We suggest using relatively large-bore 27-gauge cannulas and 27/28-gauge needles. The combined use of HA-V and onabotulinum can last remarkably well in the perioral area (Fig. 21.4).

Calcium hydroxyapatite is a viscous product well suited to the thicker skin of the mentum. We dilute the product 100% with 0.3% lidocaine with 1/200,000 epinephrine with preserved saline using 20 back-and-forth movements across the female-to-female Luer-Lock so that the product is more malleable. We inject with anterograde technique, and we are careful not to inject too much so we do not masculinize the female jawline. To ensure appropriate gender differentiation in this area, a tip is to limit the width of the female chin to the width of the treated woman's nose. For the man, where a stronger and more protruded chin is expected, the comparison is made to the mouth width.

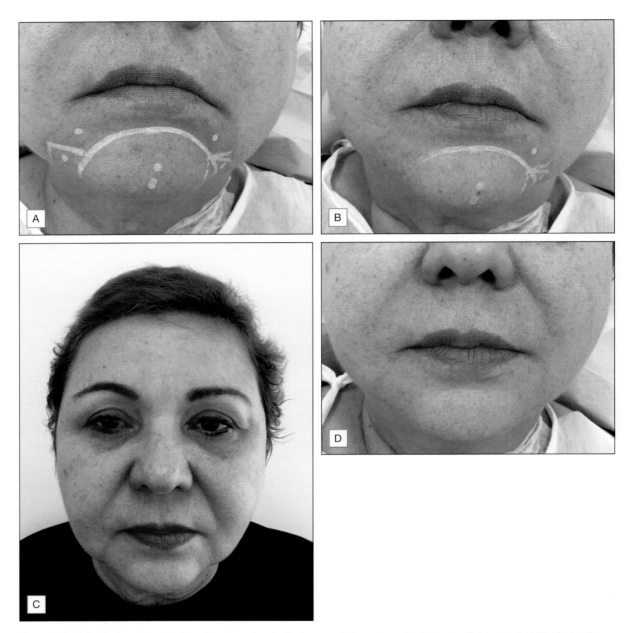

**Figure 21.3** Perioral rejuvenation with filler: Injections at prejowl sulcus, mentalis, and mandibular border. Total amount of filler (Voluma): 2 mL. **A.** Mental crease and melomental folds marked pre treatment. **B.** After right side treated. **C.** Surface after treatment. **D.** closeup of post perioral filling using Juvederm Voluma.

## Jawline and mandibular margin

The contour of the mandibular margin changes with time, starting at age 25 in women and 45 in men.[4] The reduced definition of the jawline associated with the retrusion of the chin, descent of the jowls and the addition of submental fat gives an impression of weakness and lack of decisiveness (Fig. 21.5).

## Anatomy

Important neurovascular landmarks include the antigonal notch, where the facial artery and vessels pass over the jawline just anterior to masseter. Ask the subject to clench the jaw, and feel at the anterior border of masseter. The notch may be easier to feel in older subjects, but the facial artery pulsation is easily palpated in all ages.

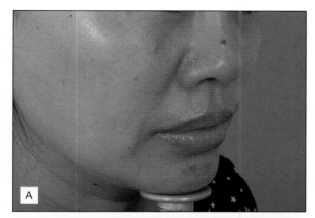

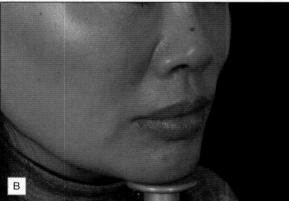

**Figure 21.4** Injection of HA-V into the menton centrally to enhance the projection of the chin, blended with filling of the lateral submental region to create a uniform smooth contour. **A.** Before treatment. **B.** After treatment.

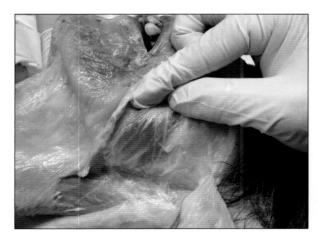

**Figure 21.5** Getting the subject to project the platysma by saying "eeee" permits the injecting physician to identify the lateral platysmal band that is depressing the cervicomental junction.

### Injection technique

Support along the jawline is helpful using a higher G′ filler, such as an HA or CaHA. We suggest pinching the skin up away from the periosteum during anterograde injection, both for comfort and for safety because the underlying vasculature is vulnerable.

Because it is easier to inject the lateral mandibular margins from their respective side, we suggest frequent moments of observation from the anterior aspect to achieve symmetry.

## Upper neck

A lifted midface and lower face and smooth jawline pair beautifully with a more acute cervicomental angle. The Nefertiti lift was described in 2007.[14] This was a landmark paper showing the muscular effect of platysma was not just on the neck as had commonly been presumed. The platysma also acts as a co-depressor of the corners of the mouth with the depressor anguli oris, so that when it is selectively weakened, the platysmal depressing effect is weakened, allowing a more elegant and refined less obtuse cervicomental angle to appear. There are several techniques used. From the described technique: four intradermal points at the mandibular border, 1 to 2 cm apart, and four intramuscular points along the upper part of the posterior platysmal band, several experts have been using their own technical variation. One of us (JC) prefers to use a single injection of onabotulinum of 20 to 30 units in the lateral platysmal band, which becomes prominent when the subject says "eeeeeee" (see **Fig. 21.5**). This relaxes the downward pull of the platysma and allows the cervicomental junction to be elevated and more acute.

The submental fat deposit, which is frequently seen in our patients, responds well to both cryolipolysis (Zeltiq)[15] and to injection chemolipolysis.[16] In the former a specially designed suction tip applicator is applied to the prominent submental fat pocket, and the subject is treated for an hour, with substantial reduction in fat and also tightening of the submental skin.

In our experience many submental fat deposits are less full and do very well with injection lipolysis. Sodium deoxycholate (Belkyra in Canada; Kybella in the United States) is injected into the preplatysmal fat using a temporary tattoo grid to ensure even deposition of the product.

The combination treatment of using fillers in the lower face and lipolysis in the submental area with neuromodulators in the perioral and platysmal musculature gives the most acceptable aesthetic reversal of the aging changes seen in the perioral region.

## Conclusions

The perioral area deflates faster than other facial regions because of its important functional characteristics: it is highly mobile and the local bones (maxilla and mandible) have dental origin and a higher tendency to reabsorb with function and aging. The fat compartments are also less prominent than other regions, such as the midface.

The combination of 3 dimensional fillers with BoNTA and energy based devices is more successful than using any single treatment alone.[9,10]

Combination with other skin-tightening treatment modalities* is helpful also in recontouring the cutaneous lower facial envelope.[17]

## References

1. Agrawal VS, Kapoor S, Bhesania D, Shah C. Comparative photographic evaluation of various geometric and mathematical proportions of maxillary anterior teeth: a clinical study. *Indian J Dent Res.* 2016;27(1):32–36.
2. Wong C, Medelson B. Newer understanding of specific anatomic targets in the aging face as applied to injectables: aging changes in the craniofacial skeleton and facial ligaments. *Plast Reconstr Surg.* 2015;136:44S–48S.
3. Ramanadhan S, Rohrich R. Newer understanding of specific anatomic targets in the aging face as applied to injectables: superficial and deep fat compartments—an evolving target for site-specific facial augmentation. *Plast Reconstr Surg.* 2015;136:49S–55S.
4. Shaw RB Jr, Katzel EB, Koltz PF, et al. Aging of the facial skeleton: aesthetic implications and rejuvenation strategies. *Plast Reconstr Surg.* 2011;127(1):374–383.
5. *ASDS Consumer Survey on Cosmetic Dermatologic Procedures.* Rolling Meadows, IL: American Society for Dermatologic Surgery. <https://www.asds.net/_Media.aspx?id=8963>;2015. Accessed 05.08.15.
6. Wang F, Garza L, Kang S, et al. In vivo stimulation of de novo collagen production caused by cross linked HA dermal filler injections in photodamaged human skin. *Arch Dermatol.* 2007;143:155–163.
7. Quan. T, Wang F, Shao Y, et al. Enhancing structural support of dermal microenviroment activates fibroblasts, endothelial cells, and keratinocytes in aged human skin in vivo. *J Invest Dermatol.* 2013;133:658–667.
8. Oh S, Lee Y, Seo Y, et al. The potential effect of botulinum toxin type a on human dermal fibroblasts: an in vitro study. *Dermatol Surg.* 2012;38:1689–1694.
9. Carruthers A, Carruthers J, Monheit GD, Davis PG, Tardie G. Multicenter, randomized, parallel-group study of the safety and effectiveness of onabotulinumtoxinA and hyaluronic acid dermal fillers (24-mg/ml smooth, cohesive gel) alone and in combination for lower facial rejuvenation. *Dermatol Surg.* 2010;36(Suppl 4):2121–2134.
10. Carruthers J, Carruthers A, Monheit GD, Davis PG. Multicenter, randomized, parallel-group study of onabotulinumtoxinA and hyaluronic acid dermal fillers (24-mg/ml smooth, cohesive gel) alone and in combination for lower facial rejuvenation: satisfaction and patient-reported outcomes. *Dermatol Surg.* 2010;36(Suppl 4):2135–2145.
11. Beleznay K, Carruthers JD, Humphrey S, Jones D. Avoiding and treating blindness from fillers: a review of the world literature. *Dermatol Surg.* 2015;41:1097–1117.
12. Goodman GJ, Swift A, Remington BK. Current concepts in the use of Voluma, Volift, and Volbella. *Plast Reconstr Surg.* 2015;136(5 Suppl):139S–148S.
13. Pavicic T, Few JW, Huber-Vorländer J. A novel, multistep, combination facial rejuvenation procedure for treatment of the whole face with incobotulinumtoxinA, and two dermal fillers—calcium hydroxylapatite and a monophasic, polydensified hyaluronic acid filler. *J Drugs Dermatol.* 2013;12:978–984.
14. Levy P. The 'Nefertiti lift': a new technique for specific re-contouring of the jawline. *J Cosmet Laser Ther.* 2007;9:249–252.
15. Kilmer SL, Burns AJ, Zelickson BD. Safety and efficacy of cryolipolysis for noninvasive reduction of submental fat. *Lasers Surg Med.* 2016;48(1):3–13. doi:10.1002/lsm.22440.
16. Jones D, Carruthers J, Joseph J, et al. REFINE-1, a multicenter, randomized, double-blind, placebo-controlled, phase 3 trial with ATX-101, an injectable drug for submental fat reduction. *Dermatol Surg.* 2016;42(1):38–49.
17. Carruthers J, Fabi S, Weiss R. Monopolar radiofrequency for skin tightening: our experience and a review of the literature. *Dermatol Surg.* 2014;40(Suppl 12):S168–S173.

---

*Microfocused Ultrasound (MFU) (Ulthera), Radiofrequency (MRF) devices (Thermage, Exilis system; BTL Aesthetics, Prague, Czech Republic) and Pelleve (Ellman International, Inc., Oceanside, NY, ThermiTight; ThermiAesthetics, Southlake, TX, Trusculpt by Cutera, Ulthera.

The addition of sodium deoxycholate injections (Kybella, Belkyra, Allergan Pharmaceuticals, Dublin, Ireland) in the submental region serves to clarify the lower facial boundaries, thus framing the lower facial enhancement and the lips.[16]

# 22

# Lip augmentation

Isabela Tollini Jones, Sabrina Guillen Fabi, Jean Carruthers

## Summary and Key Features

- The lips are a defining feature of the face; enhancement of lip volume and structure through the use of fillers is a commonly requested cosmetic procedure.
- Ethnic variations and aesthetic preferences should be considered in the evaluation and treatment planning for lip augmentation.
- Hyaluronic acids are commonly used filler products for lip rejuvenation; their safety profile coupled with their potential reversibility using hyaluronidase makes them a frequent choice for treatment of the lips. Semipermanent and permanent fillers, such as calcium hydroxylapatite, poly-l-lactic acid, silicone, and polymethylmethacrylate, have higher incidences of nodule and granuloma formation and should therefore be avoided in the lips.
- Injection of filler product into the rolled border of the lip will produce definition of the lip. Injection of filler product along the wet–dry junction of the lip will augment the volume of the lips.
- Bruising and swelling are common, temporary side effects of lip augmentation. Small-volume injections can minimize these effects. Touch-up treatments 1 to 2 weeks later may be necessary.
- Multimodality treatments including soft tissue fillers, botulinum toxins, and resurfacing techniques can be incorporated into treatment of the lips and perioral area.

## Introduction

The lips are a defining feature of youth and beauty. Although they may represent a small portion of the face based on size, they can have a substantial effect on a person's overall appearance. Unfortunately, as we age, lips undergo some of the most dramatic changes of the entire face. These changes are a natural part of the aging process, but they can be softened or reversed to give a more youthful and rejuvenated appearance.

## The aging process on the lips

Although this chapter will focus specifically on the rejuvenation of the lips, it is important to consider the lips in the larger context of the perioral region, demarcated by the nasal base, cheeks, and chin. There are a multitude of causes and effects of the aging process in the lower face. In addition to intrinsic aging, ultraviolet radiation can cause photoaging of the skin, resulting in mottled dyspigmentation and irregular texture. Collagen fibers diminish, elastic tissue is degraded, and there is a loss of subcutaneous fat and bone. These changes result in an overall drooping of the perioral region, which may call attention to the lips. Therefore, to truly rejuvenate the lips, it may be necessary to address the entire perioral region, including the nasolabial folds, melomental creases, and chin. These topics are covered elsewhere in this book but should be considered in any cosmetic consultation.

### Pearl 1

When rejuvenating the lips, it may be necessary to address other components of the perioral region. Multimodality approaches, including the use of soft tissue fillers, botulinum toxin, and resurfacing, may be necessary to achieve the best outcomes.

The lips specifically are dramatically redefined by an overall loss of lip volume and structure throughout the aging process: the upper lip becomes thin and elongated, and the lower lip becomes thin and rolls inward. There is blunting of the appearance of the pink vermilion of the lip and a sagging of the corners of the mouth, which is further accentuated by the activity of the depressor anguli oris muscle. The result is a loss of show of the upper teeth, with an increase in the show of the lower teeth. The Cupid's bow—the area defined by the two high arched points of the upper lip—becomes effaced and flattened; the two philtral columns of the upper lip also loose definition. Over time, the beautiful, defined, arched structure of the upper lip is lost, and in its place a thin, poorly defined upper lip develops. In conjunction with the overall loss of lip volume, there is also the chronic effect of activity of the orbicularis oris muscle, leading to the formation of radiating deep perioral rhytides. Patients often complain that these rhytides cause "bleeding lipstick" lines and are a frequent issue of discussion in cosmetic consultations.

**Figure 22.1** Validated lip fullness grading scale. *Reprinted with permission from Carruthers A, Carruthers J, Hardas B, et al. A validated lip fullness grading scale. Dermatol Surg. 2008;34(Suppl 2):S161–S166.*

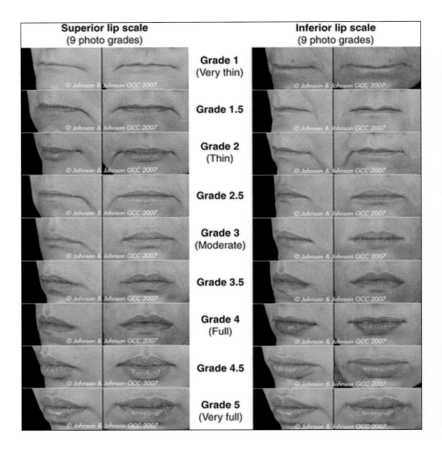

Multiple assessment scales have been developed to quantify these changes. Validated scales include the five-point Medicis Lip Fullness Scale (MLFS) by Carruthers et al. (Fig. 22.1), the five-point Allergan Lip Fullness Scale by Werschler et al., the Perioral Lines at Rest (POL), Perioral Lines at Maximum Contraction (POLM) and Oral Commissures Severity (OCS) scales by Cohen et al., the facial fold assessment scale by Narins et al., the Catherine-Knowles-Clarke (CKC) scale by Downie et al. (Table 22.1), and the photonumeric grading scale for assessing lip volume and thickness by Rossi et al. These scales may be of benefit in the initial assessment of patients and their clinical improvement following lip augmentation.

When done well, lip augmentation and rejuvenation can dramatically address many of these changes associated with aging lips to both replace the volume loss and redefine the lip structure. Numerous studies have shown that for a majority of patients, injection of HA fillers to the lips produces significant improvement in lip fullness and investigator- and patient-assessed global appearance (via the Global Aesthetic Improvement Scale).

However, in some cases, simply injecting soft tissue fillers into the lips alone may not achieve the best results. Judicious use of low-dose botulinum toxins around the lips may improve perioral rhytides, whereas botulinum toxin injections into the depressor anguli oris muscles may reduce the downturning of the oral commissures and enhance the longevity of the fillers. However, although reported in the literature, these are off-label uses of botulinum toxin not approved by regulatory authorities, such as the US Food and Drug Administration (FDA), Health Canada, or European regulatory authorities. In severe cases, resurfacing of the perioral skin with lasers or chemical peels may be necessary. Although this chapter will focus on the use of soft tissue fillers, in many cases a multimodality approach may be beneficial for patients to achieve optimal rejuvenation.

## An approach to patient evaluation

The first issue to address with lip augmentation is to determine the treatment goals of the patient. Does the patient seek enhancement or restoration of the lips? Younger patients typically seek enhancement, whereas older patients typically seek restoration.

If the patient is seeking enhancement of the lips, are they satisfied with their existing lip shape but desiring fuller lips, or is the patient seeking an entirely different shape of his or her lips? It is then important to perform a

**Table 22.1** The CKC lip evaluation scale. Reprinted with permission from Downie J, Mao Z, Lo WR, et al. A double-blind, clinical evaluatino of facial augmentation treatments: a comparison of PR 1, PR 2, Zyplast® and Perlane®. *J Plast Reconstr Aesthet Surg.* 2009;62:1636-1643.

| Size | | | |
|---|---|---|---|
| Score | Letter | Description | |
| −2 | V | Very thin | ≤1:15 |
| −1 | T | Thin | 1:15 to 1:10 |
| 0 | M | Medium-sized | 1:10 to 1:7 |
| 1 | F | Full | 1:7 to 1:4 |
| 2 | E | Extremely full | >1:4 |

| Vermilion body | |
|---|---|
| Score | Description |
| −1 | Tight almost unlined |
| 0 | Rounded with natural lines |
| 1 | Less rounded with fine lines |
| 2 | Flattening with moderate wrinkles |
| 3 | Severe wrinkles |

| Vermilion border | |
|---|---|
| Score | Description |
| −1 | Protruding and/or creating perioral shadow |
| 0 | Distinct and intact, with/without shadow from mid-lower lip |
| 1 | Distinct but broken by fine lines, with/without shadow from mid-lower lip |
| 2 | Indistinct and broken by moderate lines with/without shadow from mid-lower lip |
| 3 | Indistinct and severely lined, with/without shadow from mid-lower lip |

careful assessment of the appropriateness of that desired look in proportion to the rest of the patient's face. Lip volume enhancement not only increases the vertical height of the vermilion but also increases lip volume circumferentially, potentially resulting in the undesirable "duck lip" appearance. To prevent an unnatural look, the forward projection of the lip should barely graze a line drawn from the mid-columella to the chin (Steiner line), not projecting beyond 1 to 2 mm beyond the top of the lower lip. We advocate small-volume treatments, especially for

first-time treatments, with potential touch-up procedures 1 to 2 weeks later to achieve the best outcome and limit the potential for overcorrection.

For patients seeking lip restoration, it is important to determine their specific concerns. Are the lips asymmetric at baseline? Has the patient lost the overall structure of the lips? Are they having trouble with "lipstick bleed"? A single concern may necessitate multiple treatments, while at times one treatment may achieve various objectives. Treatments do not need to occur in a single session; indeed it is often better to schedule multiple visits with gradual treatments in order to better assess the effects of previous sessions on the overall restoration goal.

Aside from individual preferences, morphologic differences between racial groups and ethnic variations should also be considered to optimize results and achieve patient satisfaction. Many ethnic patients seek lip augmentation based on their cultural and racial background rather than obtaining a more Westernized appearance. For example, individuals of African descent tend to have fuller lips, but as they age volume loss occurs, particularly of the upper lip. Therefore, the goal of lip augmentation would focus more on upper lip enhancement rather than on upper and lower lip restoration.

Aside from discussion goals during the pretreatment consultation, existing asymmetries should be pointed out, and frontal, oblique and lateral photos taken before any intervention is performed. Counsel the patient on expected side effects and downtime.

## Filler products

When performing lip rejuvenation, temporary fillers are the treatment of choice. Historically, collagen was the gold standard product for lip augmentation. At this time, collagen is longer commercially available in the United States and HA products have become the most frequently used products for lip rejuvenation. These HA fillers are cross-linked to extend their longevity to 6 to 12 months. Restylane (Medicis Aesthetics Inc., Scottsdale, Arizona), Resytlane-L, Restylane Silk, Juvéderm Ultra XC (Allergan Inc., Irvine, California) and Juvéderm Volbella XC were approved by the FDA for lip enhancement in patients older than 21 years of age 2011, 2012, 2014, 2015, and 2016, respectively. Restylane Silk, Juvéderm Ultra XC, and Juvéderm Volbella XC, in addition to Belotero Balance (Merz North America, Greensboro, North Carolina), are also FDA-approved for perioral rhytids. Many of these products are premixed with lidocaine to reduce discomfort during injections.

In 2007 a multidisciplinary group of experts in aesthetic treatments (the Facial Aesthetics Consensus Group) developed recommendations for lip augmentation and rejuvenation (Carruthers et al.). Of the available HA products, the faculty typically used Restylane, Juvéderm Ultra, or Juvéderm Ultra Plus for lip and perioral rejuvenation. The majority of the faculty (67%) used 1.0 mL of

HA while the remainder (33%) used 2.0 mL to reshape the vermilion border and rejuvenate the lips. In a study of Restylane, Glogau et al. showed that using more than 3 mL of filler was associated with a significant increase in moderate-to-severe adverse events.

Although a full discussion of filler properties is beyond the scope of this chapter, a few notable differences should be considered. Restylane and Restylane Silk are biphasic particulate gels that create a greater surface area for water binding, which may result in more postprocedure edema. Restylane Silk is even more hydrophilic than Restylane and Restylane-L because it has a greater number of particles, which are also smaller. Juvéderm Ultra and Juvéderm Ultra Plus are nonparticle monophasic gels that contain long-chain HA cross-linked via Hylacross technology. In contrast, Juvéderm Voluma, Volbella, and Volift are viscous nonparticle gels made using Vycross technology, which incorporate both long and short chains of HA, producing more cross-linking and longer duration in tissue. In addition, their lower HA concentration results in less water absorption.

Semipermanent fillers, such as calcium hydroxylapatite and poly-L-lactic acid, can be used to rejuvenate the perioral area, including the nasolabial folds and jowls, but have an increased risk of adverse effects and nodule formation. Permanent fillers, such as polymethylmethacrylate and liquid injectable silicone, have been used for lip rejuvenation. However, these permanent fillers have an increased risk of granulomas, foreign body reaction, extrusion, recurrent chronic inflammation, and possible permanent scarring when injected into the lips. As a result, semipermanent and permanent fillers are not recommended for lip augmentation.

## Injection techniques for lip rejuvenation

Most patients feel mild-to-moderate discomfort during lip injections. Although HA products premixed with lidocaine can reduce the discomfort, some patients may still prefer to have either topical anesthesia or a small nerve block. The nerve block should be placed near the infraorbital foramen (midpupillary line, lateral to nasal ala) and the mental foramen (angle of jawline, inferior to the corners of the mouth) and can be injected via an intraoral approach or through the skin. Alternatively, a small amount of lidocaine can be placed as a bleb at the junction where the gum and mucosa join. It is important to remember that, if lidocaine is used, the minimal amount of lidocaine should be injected to avoid distorting the lip architecture, which would make the aesthetic correction more difficult to assess. In our experience, these blocks are often not necessary.

There are many different techniques for injecting soft tissue fillers, including tunneling, serial puncture, threading, cross-hatching, and fanning. In our experience the exact location and volume of product injected is most important to the outcome.

**Pearl 2**

In general, injections in the rolled border of the lip produce definition, whereas injections in the body will augment the volume of the lips. Pushing in an anterograde fashion or "tunneling" the filler in a single injection from lateral to medial and allowing it to "flow" into the potential space just under the dermis can result in a smooth effect and avoid lumpiness associated with serial injections.

Overall, many patients require slightly more volume in the lower lip than in the upper lip, but the exact volume and proportions must be individualized for each patient. The ideal vertical height ratio of the upper lip to the lower lip is 1 : 1.6 in whites. African American patients may require greater volume injections into the upper lip than in the lower lip to achieve their ideal outcome.

Typically, when rejuvenating the upper lip, the vermilion border is treated first to define the Cupid's bow and vermilion border prior to volumizing the body of the lip (Fig. 22.2A and B). The needle is inserted at the lateral edge of the upper lip, and tunneled lateral to medial along the vermilion border to the G-K points in the Cupid's bow. A small amount of filler is placed into the Cupid's bow to define this area. The remainder of the product is then injected in a retrograde fashion as the needle is withdrawn. Alternatively, the filler can be "pushed" anterograde along the border in the superficial to mid dermis. Applying gentle traction to the surrounding skin can make needle insertion more comfortable. Injection should be stopped before the needle exits the skin to prevent filler from being placed too superficially. Although most physicians use hypodermic needles, Fulton et al. showed that blunt-tip microcannulas can be used to inject the vermillion border of the lips. The authors in the study recommend a 38-mm, 27-gauge microcannula for this area.

If the patient's philtral columns are poorly defined, the filler can also be used to redefine these points. A highly cross-linked cohesive filler will be best for the philtral columns. The needle should be inserted at the G-K points and then advanced superiorly along the philtral column in a mid-dermal plane. Again, the product is placed with a retrograde injection technique. A small amount of filler is sufficient to redefine each column; a slightly greater amount of the should be placed towards the inferior aspect to maintain the natural contour and appearance of the philtral column. If the patient desires volume enhancement of the upper lip, filler can be placed along the body of the lip using a serial puncture or linear threading technique, focusing on maintaining the fullness of the tubercles by adding more product in these areas. After any injection, it is important to palpate the treated area and massage any lumps to create a smooth contour.

The lower lip is similarly treated. We recommend inserting the needle at the lateral edge of the lower lip, and then either pushing the filler in an anterograde fashion

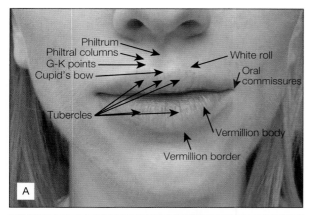

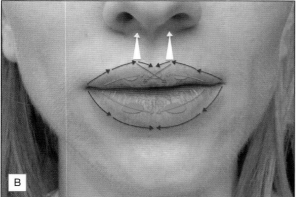

**Figure 22.2 A,** Anatomic landmarks of the lips. **B,** Location of injections for the lips. *Blue lines* represent the vermillion border. *White lines* signify the philtral columns; more filler should be placed in the inferior aspect. *Pink lines* indicate injection technique for the medial upper lip. *Green lines* denote the area of injection of the body of the lips; more filler should be placed in the tubercles (*green circles*).

If the patient's lips are symmetric prior to augmentation, it is important to ensure that an equal amount of product is placed into each side of the lip to maintain this symmetry. Frequently, patients have asymmetrical lips requiring a slightly different amount to be injected to each side of the lips. It should be noted that sometimes a small amount of filler (0.1 to 0.3 mL) can make an enormous difference in the appearance of the lips.

In addition to rejuvenating the lips themselves, it is often necessary to buttress the corners of the mouth to prevent or reverse downturned corners of the lips. This can be easily accomplished by injecting filler product underneath the lateral corners of the mouth, providing a scaffolding to support the remainder of the lips. This effect can be further enhanced by injecting botulinum toxin into the depressor anguli oris muscles to help to turn the corners of the mouth up, thereby rejuvenating the lips and mouth.

Finally, the patient may desire treatment of perioral rhytides. These lines can be improved with soft tissue augmentation. The needle should be inserted at one end of the rhytides, and then tunneled along the depression. Very small amounts of filler are placed in a relatively superficial plane. Alternatively, microdroplets can be injected along the line using a microdroplet technique. Botulinum toxin can also be administered to relax the orbicularis oris muscle and help to prevent or reduce these rhytides. In severe cases a chemical peel or laser resurfacing may be necessary to provide better improvement.

**Pearl 3**

Place filler inferior to the commissures of the mouth to provide a buttress to elevate and turn up the corners of the mouth, which relax and turn downward with age.

**CASE STUDY 1**

A patient presented for lip rejuvenation (**Fig. 22.3A**). On examination, upper lip is thin and flat, with a loss of the Cupid's bow. The philtral columns are not well defined. There are multiple perioral radiating rhytides. The lower lip is also small and lacks definition.

The patient underwent lip rejuvenation with 1 mL of HA product (see **Fig. 22.3B**). Following the augmentation, note the reshaped and defined Cupid's bow; there is also greater definition of the inferior aspects of the philtral columns. The overall volume of the upper and lower lips is increased slightly as well. Finally, there is a reduction in the appearance of the radiating perioral rhytides.

**Potential side effects**

Bruising and swelling are the most common side effects following lip augmentation. These are typically mild and

in the subdermal space or tunneling the needle along the vermilion border to the midpoint of the lower lip and injecting in a linear retrograde fashion. If augmentation is also desired, product can be injected along the body of the lower lip.

Lee et al. examined the course of the superior labial artery in 36 cadavers. They found that in most cases, the artery ran superior to the lateral vermilion border under the orbicularis oris muscle at a minimum depth of 3 mm. Prior to approaching the peak of Cubid's bow, the artery courses inferior to the vermillion border. Twenty-one percent of the superior labial arteries examined contained a nasal septal branch that ramified in the sagittal midline and coursed above the orbicularis muscle. The authors concluded that to safely treat the upper lip, injections should not be deeper than 3 mm. Because the inferior labial artery courses in the cutaneous lower lip between the orbicularis oris and the lip depressors, injections above the muscle are considered safe.

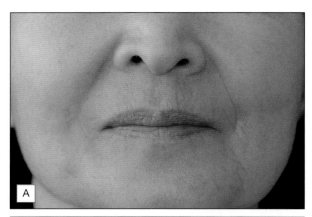

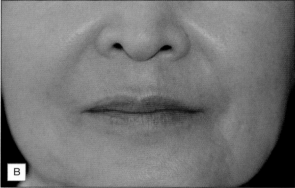

**Figure 22.3 A,** Patient presented complaining of thin lips, a loss of structure and shape on the upper lip, and radiating perioral rhytides. **B,** Following lip rejuvenation with 1 mL of hyaluronic acid product, note the defined Cupid's bow and vermilion border of the lip. There is also enhanced volume and a reduction in the appearance of the radiating perioral rhytides.

**CASE STUDY 2**

A 40-year-old female patient presents for lip augmentation. The upper lip is augmented with 0.3 mL of HA to define the rolled border. The lower lip is augmented with 0.5 mL of HA, with injections along the rolled border and into the wet–dry junction of the lip. At the conclusion of the procedure, the lips are slightly swollen but appear symmetric. Two days later, the patient calls the office upset that her lips are "huge and overcorrected." She requests treatment with a reversing agent to undo the augmentation. What should the treating physician do next?

The patient should be reassured and instructed to return to the office. Swelling following the augmentation is very common and may require several days to resolve. Hyaluronidase will remove the product but will not improve bruising or swelling associated with the injections themselves. Patients often benefit from massage of the area to smooth down any nodules or lumpiness. Patients should then be instructed to ice the areas and wait for any swelling associated with the procedure to resolve before judging the final result. Translucent lumps still present after swelling has subsided can represent superficial collections of filler. An 18 or 22-gauge needle can be used to pierce the center of the collection and manually express filler. The patient in this case study returned to the office, had a good response to massage, and 1 week later was thrilled with the appearance of her augmentation.

approach may be necessary to complete the rejuvenation of the perioral area.

self-resolve within the first week. Small-volume injections reduce these side effects and the likelihood of overcorrection and asymmetry; potential touch-up procedures 1 to 2 weeks after the initial treatments can be performed as needed. Although rare, there are reports of filler migration to the surrounding perioral skin, herpes simplex virus reactivation, and late-onset nodule and granuloma formation, even with HA filler. There is no evidence of the risk of postinflammatory pigment alterations, hypertrophic scarring, or keloid formation in ethnic patients following treatment.

## Conclusion

The lips are a dramatic and defining feature of the face. Unfortunately, the aging process denies patients of the beautiful structure and volume of the lips. Lip rejuvenation and augmentation is a safe, simple, and effective procedure to reverse these changes. HA fillers are the treatment of choice to both redefine and restore volume to the lips. In more advanced cases a multimodality

## Further reading

Alam M, Gladstone H, Kramer EM, et al with the Guidelines Task Force. ASDS Guidelines of care: injectable fillers. *Dermatol Surg.* 2008;34:S115–S148.

Beer K, Glogau RG, Dover JS, et al. A randomized, evaluator-blinded, controlled study of effectiveness and safety of small particle hyaluronic acid plus lidocaine for lip augmentation and perioral rhytides. *Dermatol Surg.* 2015;41(suppl 1):S127–S136.

Carruthers J, Glogau R, Blitzer A, and the Facial Aesthetics Consensus Group Faculty. Advances in facial rejuvenation: botulinum toxin type A, hyaluronic acid dermal fillers, and combination therapies—consensus recommendations. *Plast Reconstr Surg.* 2008;121(suppl 5):S5–S30.

Cohen JL, Thomas J, Paradkar D, et al. An interrater and intrarater reliability study of 3 photographic scales for the classification of perioral aesthetic features. *Dermatol Surg.* 2014;40(6): 663–670.

Custis T, Beynet D, Carranza D, et al. Comparison of treatment of melomental fold rhytides with cross-linked hyaluronic acid combined with onabotulinumtoxinA and cross-linked hyaluronic acid alone. *Dermatol Surg.* 2010;36(suppl 3):S1852–S1858.

Dayan S, Bruce S, Kilmer S, et al. Safety and effectiveness of the hyaluronic acid filler, HYC-24L, for lip and perioral augmentation. *Dermatol Surg.* 2015;41(suppl 1):S293–S301.

Dougherty AL, Rashid RM, Bangert CA. Angioedema-type swelling and herpes simplex virus reactivation following hyaluronic acid injection for lip augmentation. *J Am Acad Dermatol.* 2011;65(1):e21–22.

Downie J, Mao Z, Lo TWR, et al. A double-blind, clinical evaluation of facial augmentation treatments: a comparison of

PRI 1, PRI 2, Zyplast® and Perlane®. *J Plast Reconstr Aesthet Surg*. 2009;62:1636–1643.

Eccleston D, Murphy DK. Juvéderm® Volbella™ in the perioral area: a 12-month prospective, multicenter, open-label study. *Clin Cosmet Investig Dermatol*. 2012;5:167–172

Fulton J, Caperton C, Weinkle S, Dewandre L. Filler injections with the blunt-tip microcannula. *J Drugs Dermatol*. 2012;11(9):1098–1103.

Glogau RG, Bank D, Brandt F, et al. A randomized, evaluator-blinded, controlled study of the effectiveness and safety of small gel particle hyaluronic acid for lip augmentation. *Dermatol Surg*. 2012;38(7 Pt 2):1180–1192.

Ibher N, Kloepper J, Penna V, Bartholomae JP, Stark GB. Changes in the aging upper lip—a photomorphic and MRI-based study (on a quest to find the right rejuvenation approach). *J Plast Reconstr Aesthet Surg*. 2008;61:1170–1176.

Jacono AA. A new classification of lip zones to customize injectable lip augmentation. *Arch Facial Plast Surg*. 2008;10(1):25–29.

Lee SH, Gil YC, Choi YJ, Tansatit T, Kim HJ, Hu KS. Topographic anatomy of the superior labial artery for dermal filler injection. *Plast Reconstr Surg*. 2015;135(2):445–450.

Narins RS, Carruthers J, Flynn TC, et al. Validated Assessment Scales for the Lower Face. *Dermatol Surg*. 2012;38(2 Spec No.):333–342.

Rossi AB, Nkengne A, Stamatas G, Bertin C. Development and validation of a photonumeric grading scale for assessing lip volume and thickness. *J Eur Acad Dermatol Venereol*. 2011;25(5):523–531.

San Miguel Moragas J, Reddy RR, Hernández Alfaro F, et al. Systematic review of "filling" procedures for lip augmentation regarding types of material, outcomes and complications. *J Craniomaxillofac Surg*. 2015;43(6):883–906.

Shahrabi Farahani S, Sexton J, Stone JD et al. Lip nodules caused by hyaluronic acid filler injection: report of three cases. *Head Neck Pathol*. 2012;6(1):16–20.

Talakoub L, Wesly NO. Differences in perceptions of beauty and cosmetic procedures performed in ethnic patients. *Semin Cutan Med Surg*. 2009;28:115–129.

Tansatit T, Apinuntrum P, Phetudom T. A typical pattern of the labial arteries with implication for lip augmentation with injectable fillers. *Aesthet Plast Surg*. 2014;38(6):1083–1089.

Werschler WP, Fagien S, Thomas J, Paradkar-Mitragotri D, Rotunda A, Beddingfield FC. Development and validation of a photographic scale for assessment of lip fullness. *Aesthet Surg J*. 2015;35(3):294–307.

Wong WW, Davis DG, Camp MC, et al. Contribution of lip proportions to facial aesthetics in different ethnicities: a three-dimensional analysis. *J Plast Reconstr Aesthet Surg*. 2010;63:2032–2039.

# 23

# Soft tissue augmentation of the hands

## Heidi A. Waldorf, Jason J. Emer

**Summary and Key Features**

- Extrinsic and intrinsic factors cause skin laxity, dyspigmentation, and fat loss in the hands.

- Soft tissue augmentation with a variety of fillers and autologous fat has been well studied and shown to be safe and efficacious to camouflage exposed tendons and vessels and improve lipoatrophy of the hands.

- The most common fillers for the hands are calcium hydroxylapatite, hyaluronic acid, and autologous fat.

- Poly-L-lactic acid has fallen out of favor for hand augmentation because of the risk of visible nodules under lax skin.

- Use of disposable blunt-tipped cannulas has improved the ease and reduced the side effect profile for hand filling.

- In addition to standard postfiller instructions, such as ice and elevation, patients should be told to massage the hand after treatment.

- Potential complications of hand augmentation include visible product, Tyndall effect, persistent edema and pain, and inflammatory reactions or nodules.

- Combination therapies, such as lasers, radiofrequency, microneedling, and platelet-rich plasma, may improve outcomes and give sustained results in addition to fillers for volumization.

## Introduction

Throughout a person's life, hands are exposed to multiple extrinsic factors. Ultraviolet radiation, temperature variations, and friction forces exacerbate the signs of aging. The result is excessive skin laxity, erythematous and pigmented background dyschromias, and the development of distinct neoplasms, such as lentigines and actinic keratoses. Textural and pigmentary concerns can be treated by numerous therapies, including chemical peels, intense pulsed light, pigment-specific lasers, and fractional resurfacing. However, these therapies do not address the increasing visibility of underlying bones, tendons, and veins as the dermis thins and fat is lost. Volume restoration with fat

and long-lasting dermal fillers has become a standard of care for this purpose. The ideal filler for extremities must be moldable enough to provide smooth volume around underlying structures but also be durable enough to persist despite repeated movement and pressure. Treatment modalities must also address pain anticipated in these highly innervated areas. This chapter will discuss risks, benefits, and techniques for augmentation of the hands.

## Soft tissue augmentation of the hands

### Calcium hydroxylapatite

Calcium hydroxylapatite (CaHA, Radiesse, Merz Aesthetics) has become the most commonly recommended filler for rejuvenation of the aging hand. Specific approval for hand rejuvenation was obtained in Canada in 2010 and in the United States in 2015.

As an opaque, white substance, CaHA has the advantage of acting as both a filler and camouflage for underlying anatomic architecture. However, its use for hand rejuvenation was initially limited by the product's high viscosity and pain upon injection. In 2007 Busso and Applebaum reported a novel approach that overcame both issues. Using a Luer-to-Luer lock connector (Fig. 23.1), the authors mixed 0.1 mL 2% lidocaine without epinephrine with 1.3 mL of CaHA (the standard syringe volume at that time). After tenting the skin of the central dorsal hand to separate it from underlying large vessels and tendons, they injected a single bolus of 0.5 to 1.4 mL of the lidocaine-CaHA mixture into the space created between the subcutaneous layer and the superficial fascia. The bolus was then massaged and molded into a cosmetically smooth appearance. The addition of lidocaine reduced both the viscosity and pain.

**Pearl 1**

Mix 1:1 or 1.5:1.0 dilution of CaHA with 1% or 2% lidocaine without epinephrine using a Luer-to-Luer connector.

Since this initial report, physicians have modified the technique by increasing the volume of lidocaine used for dilution (e.g., the 2009 study by Edelson). In 2010 Marmur et al. published the first organized institutional review board-approved study of CaHA filler for hand

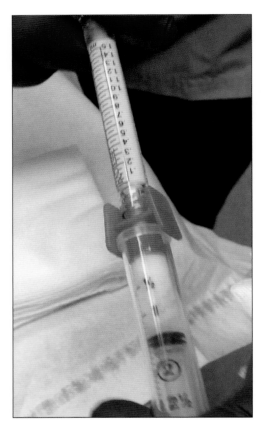

**Figure 23.1** Technique to mix CaHA with anesthetic: 1.5 mL of 1% lidocaine without epinephrine in a Luer Lock syringe, attached to a syringe containing 1.5 mL of CaHA via a disposable Luer-to-Luer lock connector and mixed.

rejuvenation. They mixed 2.0 mL of 2% lidocaine without epinephrine per 1.3 mL syringe of CaHA. A total of 0.3 to 1.0 mL of the product was injected interdigitally using a 25-gauge 1.5-inch (3.75 cm) needle at three to five insertion points, as opposed to a single bolus injection. They reported high patient satisfaction rates with only a few short-term side effects, such as persistent edema requiring oral corticosteroids for resolution.

Several larger studies by Busso et al., Bank, and Marmur et al. have supported the safety and efficacy of CaHA as an anti-aging hand filler. Busso et al. published a multicenter, randomized controlled trial of 101 patients followed over 6 months and established a new hand volume severity scale to assess results. Following administration of a lidocaine bolus preoperatively, CaHA was administered as a bolus into the dorsal hand using a 27-gauge, 0.75-inch (20-mm) needle. Aside from reporting statistically significant improvement in the treatment group, the study also found that adverse events, including bruising, itching, pain, redness, and swelling (**Fig. 23.2**), were frequent yet short in duration and did not affect overall patient function significantly.

From 2013 to 2014 another prospective, randomized controlled study was performed in 114 patients who were randomized and received immediate or delayed treatment, which validated the primary findings supporting US Food and Drug Administration (FDA) approval. The Global Aesthetic Improvement Scale (GAIS) was used to evaluate effectiveness from "worse" to "very much improved." The Merz Hand Grading Scale (MHGS) Cohen, et al. Dermatol Surg. 2015 Dec;41 Suppl 1: S384-8, a five-point photonumeric scale, was used to objectively rate the severity of aging in the hand from 0 (no loss of fatty tissue) to 4 (very severe loss of fatty tissue; marked visibility of veins and tendons) (**Fig. 23.3**).

**Figure 23.2** Postoperative swelling. Two weeks after injection of CaHA-lidocaine mixture the patient had clinical improvement but complained of persistent pain at rest and with movement. Her symptoms resolved after 1 month with oral corticosteroids and massage: (A) before treatment and (B) 10 days after treatment.

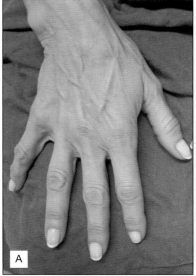

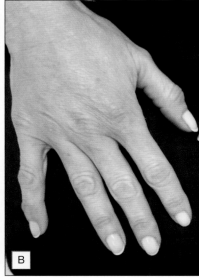

# Hand Grading Scale

*Please rate the Hand by using the following scale*

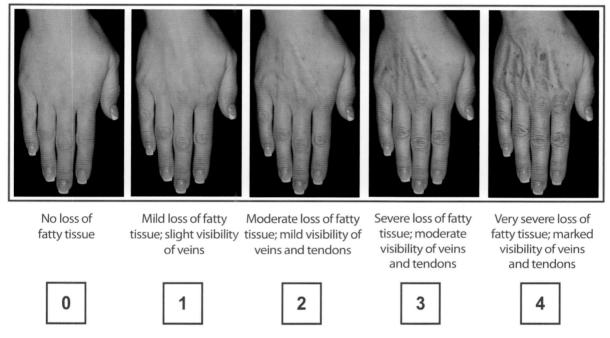

| No loss of fatty tissue | Mild loss of fatty tissue; slight visibility of veins | Moderate loss of fatty tissue; mild visibility of veins and tendons | Severe loss of fatty tissue; moderate visibility of veins and tendons | Very severe loss of fatty tissue; marked visibility of veins and tendons |
|:---:|:---:|:---:|:---:|:---:|
| 0 | 1 | 2 | 3 | 4 |

*Please indicate your choice by checking the appropriate box*

©2009 Merz Pharmaceuticals

**Figure 23.3** Merz Hand Grading Scale (MHGS). *Copyright 2016 Merz North America, Inc. All rights reserved.*

Results of the FDA trial revealed a similar adverse effect profile as prior studies (Table 23.1). All adverse events reported in this study resolved completely.

**Pearl 2**

Warn patients that they may have 1 to 4 weeks of mild-to-moderate swelling and soreness.

**Pearl 3**

Start with no more than 0.8 mL per hand CaHA (predilution).

**Pearl 4**

Consider the use of a blunt cannula instead of a needle.

**Pearl 5**

Using massage, compression, and ice after treatment is necessary, but avoid aggressive massage to limit immediate postprocedural swelling.

The availability of disposable blunt-tipped, small-gauge cannulas has revolutionized the procedure by reducing the number of puncture sites required, patient discomfort, and postoperative bruising. A study evaluating blunt-tipped cannula injection technique to the FDA-approved needle injection showed a comparable safety profile and interestingly showed no differences in participant satisfaction. The authors recommend delivering boluses or linear threads with one entry point at the dorsal wrist (Fig. 23.4), although an alternate approach from proximal web spaces can be used. The product is massaged until smooth. Patients are instructed to massage several times daily and use topical ice packs for the first 48 hours. A small latex-free examination glove can be applied immediately with a thin ice pack or plastic bag with frozen gauze between the glove and the treated hand (Fig. 23.5). Despite these interventions, some patients complain of severe pain, which limits range of motion. Therefore small boluses should be limited to 0.2 to 05 mL/bolus with no more than 0.5 mL injected per bolus and no more than 3 mL of injectable product per hand at any given treatment session. The authors have found that dividing the treatment into planned sessions using approximately

**Table 23.1** (A) Physician-reported adverse events over a 12-month period (*N* = 113 subjects)

| Adverse event type | # of subjects with event (% total) | Maximum severity (N, % with event) | | |
|---|---|---|---|---|
| | | Mild | Moderate | Severe |
| Bruising | 21 (18.6) | 13 (61.9) | 6 (28.6) | 2 (9.5) |
| Swelling | 23 (20.4) | 7 (30.4) | 14 (60.9) | 2 (8.7) |
| Redness | 9 (8.0) | 5 (55.6) | 4 (44.4) | 0 (0.0) |
| Itching | 4 (3.5) | 3 (75.0) | 1 (25.0) | 0 (0.0) |
| Pain | 7 (6.2) | 4 (57.1) | 2 (28.6) | 1 (14.3) |
| Hematoma | 0 (0.0) | 0 (0.0) | 0 (0.0) | 0 (0.0) |
| Nodule, bumps/lumps | 7 (6.2) | 7 (100.0) | 0 (0.0) | 0 (0.0) |
| Difficulty performing activities | 2 (1.8) | 2 (100.0) | 0 (0.0) | 0 (0.0) |
| Loss of sensation | 0 (0.0) | 0 (0.0) | 0 (0.0) | 0 (0.0) |
| Other | 13 (11.5) | 7 (53.8) | 5 (38.5) | 1 (7.7) |
| Total | 50 (44.2) | 24 (48.0) | 21 (42.0) | 5 (10.0) |

*Other adverse events reported that were related to the device include vagal response, dry skin, hypersensitivity, and needle pricks.
*Copyright 2016 Merz North America, Inc. All rights reserved.*

(B) Physician-reported total number of adverse events onset after initial treatment (*N* = 117 events)

| Adverse event type | All first onset (N, % total) | Reported adverse events (N, % with event) | | | | |
|---|---|---|---|---|---|---|
| | | Week 1 | Week 2 | Week 3 | Week 4 and beyond | Weeks 1 and 2 combined |
| Bruising | 26 (22.2) | 23 (88.5) | 0 (0.0%) | 0 (0.0) | 3 (11.5) | 23 (88.5) |
| Swelling | 39 (33.3) | 28 (71.8) | 10 (25.6) | 1 (2.6) | 0 (0.0) | 38 (97.4) |
| Redness | 15 (12.8) | 14 (93.3) | 1 (6.7) | 0 (0.0) | 0 (0.0) | 15 (100.0) |
| Pain | 11 (9.4) | 5 (45.5) | 2 (18.2) | 1 (9.1) | 3 (27.3) | 7 (63.6) |
| Itching | 7 (6.0) | 5 (71.4) | 0 (0.0) | 0 (0.0) | 2 (28.6) | 5 (71.4) |
| Hematoma | 0 (0.0) | 0 (0.0) | 0 (0.0) | 0 (0.0) | 0 (0.0) | 0 (0.0) |
| Nodule, bumps/lumps | 3 (2.6) | 2 (66.7) | 0 (0.0) | 0 (0.0) | 1 (33.3) | 2 (66.7) |
| Difficulty performing activities | 4 (3.4) | 2 (50.0) | 2 (50.0) | 0 (0.0) | 0 (0.0) | 4 (100.0) |
| Loss of sensation | 0 (0.0) | 0 (0.0) | 0 (0.0) | 0 (0.0) | 0 (0.0) | 0 (0.0) |
| Other | 12 (10.3) | 4 (33.3) | 0 (0.0) | 0 (0.0) | 8 (66.7) | 4 (33.3) |
| Total | 117 (100.0) | 83 (70.9) | 15 (12.8) | 2 (1.7) | 17 (14.5) | 98 (83.8) |

[†]Radiesse injectable implant instructions for use for the dorsum of the hand.

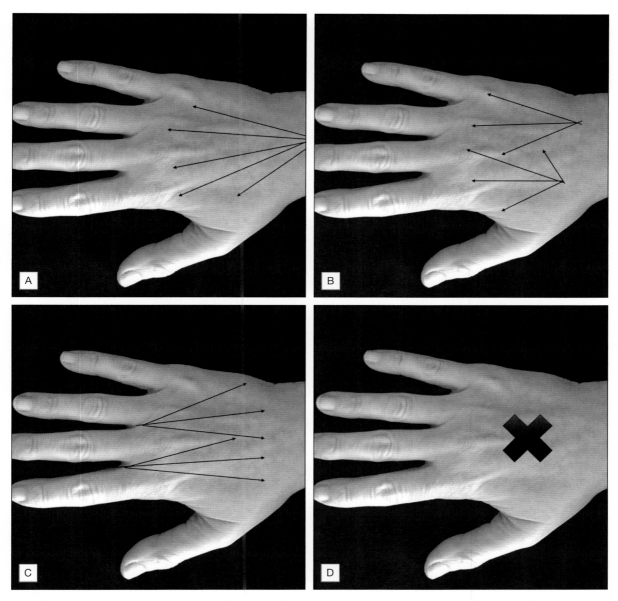

**Figure 23.4** Injection technique using a cannula: (A) using a single proximal entry point at the wrist (*arrows*), (B) using two distal entry points between metacarpals (*arrows*), (C) intradermal bolus of 1% lidocaine with epinephrine on the dorsal wrist made with a 21-gauge needle. While tenting skin away from underlying structures, a 22-gauge 2.0-inch blunt-tipped cannula (SoftFil) was introduced and CaHa placed via combination of bolus and retrograde linear injection, then massaged, and (D) pretreatment photo of hand.

half the diluted product of one syringe per hand at 2- to 4-week intervals has reduced the incidence of significant pain and/or swelling and made the treatment viable for patients who work with their hands. Oral gabapentin, corticosteroids, and diuretics can help to speed resolution but is typically not needed.

## Poly-L-lactic acid

Poly-L-lactic acid (PLLA) was initially considered to be a good filler for hand rejuvenation, but its use has gone out of favor for this purpose. PLLA (Sculptra) was approved

by the FDA in 2004 for the treatment of HIV-associated lipoatrophy and was largely used off-label cosmetically in the United States until cosmetic facial approval in 2009. Vleggaar in 2006 reported soft tissue augmentation of the hands with PLLA, lasting up to 2 years. Redaelli published a study of 27 patients treated in Italy in 2004–2005 with 150 mg of PLLA diluted with 0.5 mL of 3% mepivacaine in water to a final volume between 5 and 8 mL. The patients were treated with 1.5 to 2 mL of PLLA mixture over several sessions, with multiple intermetacarpal injections using 25- to 27-gauge needles for the first three sessions

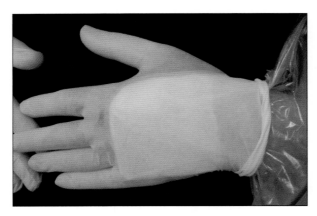

**Figure 23.5** Postoperative hand care: a flat ice pack composed of wet gauze frozen in a plastic bag is slid under a fingerless snug examination glove. Prior to gloving, an antibacterial ointment (mupirocin) is applied to the insertion sites and a glycerin serum applied to the dorsal hand.

at monthly intervals and evaluations for treatment every 3 months thereafter. Despite postoperative massage, both of these European articles noted nodule formation as late as 1 year after the last injection as a potential complication of therapy.

Sadick et al. in 2008 described the experience of three clinical practices that treated the hands of 26 patients with PLLA diluted with 5 to 6 mL sterile water and 2 to 5 mL of 1% lidocaine. Therapy was performed with a 25-gauge 1.5-inch needle at 1-month intervals for a total of two or three treatments and resulted in a high rate of patient satisfaction. Although 46% of patients reported adverse events, such as bruising or swelling (30.8%), pain (15.4%), itching (3.8%), and arterial spasm (3.8%), they were minor and resolved within a few days of treatment. No nodule formation postoperatively was noted, although an "uneven result" was reported with a low incidence of 3.8%. As with facial use of PLLA, higher dilutions of 8 to 10 mL of sterile water plus lidocaine (as opposed to the 5 mL sterile water dilution written in the package insert) have been recommended by Rendon et al. to try to reduce the risk of nodule formation. However, unlike in the face, injection depth is limited for the dorsal hands so that any nodules that develop will be noticeable, and this has limited its usefulness for this area.

## Fat transplantation

Autologous fat grafting was used as early as the 1980s by Coleman for soft tissue augmentation of the dorsal hands. Though considerable difference still exists regarding harvesting and transplant, many experts report positive results with this modality. The "Coleman technique" involves anesthetic infiltration into the donor fat site (i.e., lower abdomen) through a blunt infiltrator. Through the same incision site a blunt-tip harvesting cannula is connected via a Luer Lock syringe to aspirate the fat. The hand is subsequently prepared through preoperative regional

blocks, and then through a limited number of incisions, fat is injected via a 1-mL Luer Lock syringe and cannula in 0.02- and 1-mL aliquots.

Some sources claim longevity of a year or beyond, although others, such as Haq et al., claim that multiple treatment sessions may be needed and that duration is not easy to predict; a publication by Giunta et al. estimated 69% residual injection volume at 6 months postoperatively following hand rejuvenation with autologous fat transplant. Fat transfer for hand augmentation is a great long-term solution for those who seek a more permanent treatment option or even better suited for patients seeking fat reduction at donor areas and those for whom fat transfer will also be used for facial augmentation. In one author's clinical practice (JE) fat transfer is used first for large-volume change and any touch-up procedures are performed with dermal fillers, such as CaHA.

### Pearl 6

Hyaluronic acid fillers can be used for volume repletion and wrinkle reduction of the hands.

## Hyaluronic acid

Although hyaluronic acid (HA) fillers are the most commonly used category of dermal filling agents worldwide, there are fewer supporting studies and reports of their use for hand augmentation than for the therapies described previously. The only FDA-approved HAs are Belotero, Juvéderm Ultra, Juvéderm Ultra Plus, Juvéderm Voluma, Restylane, Restylane Silk, and Restylane Lyft. Man et al. in 2008 published a study comparing 10 patients randomized to receive either 1.4 cm³ HA or 2.0 cm³ human collagen for rejuvenation of the dorsal hands; HA was superior in terms of decreasing signs of intrinsic aging. More recently, Sattler et al. published a study comparing the efficacy of CaHA filler with HA filler in hand augmentation (Juvéderm Ultra 4). Thirty-seven female patients demonstrated significant improvement from baseline on the hand grading scale for both fillers, but the HA filler-treated side required more touch-up treatments ($n = 3$) and the CaHA-treated sides had more transient adverse events related to the injection ($n = 6$).

Despite safety and efficacy, hand augmentation with HA products is limited by the Tyndall effect, the blue hue that results when a clear gel filler is placed superficially or beneath thin skin. Lax, aged, and photoaged dorsal hand skin tends to be particularly thin and transparent and therefore more prone to this effect. A blue discoloration in this area can simulate or aggravate the appearance of solar purpura.

### Pearl 7

Combine multiple modalities, such as lasers, peels, and fillers, to get improved and sustained results in the aging hand.

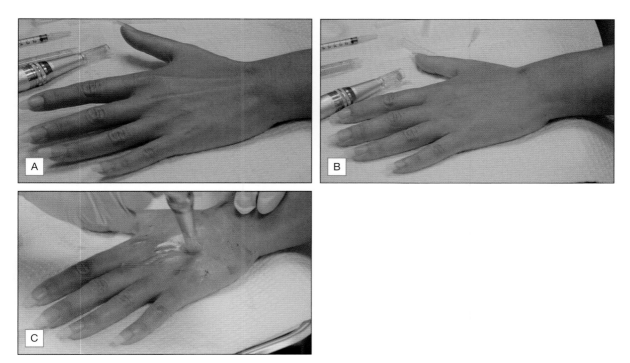

**Figure 23.6** Combination therapy (A) before treatment, (B) immediately after filler (C) with microneedling (1.0 mm depth) with PRP.

## Combination therapies

Just like the aging face, the aging hand requires rejuvenation that addresses multiple factors, such as dyschromia, lentigines, textural changes, volume loss, laxity, and visibility of superficial veins and tendons. Fillers can address improvements in volume and visibility of veins and tendons, with minimal changes to laxity and wrinkling, and with no effect on textural changes and dyschromias. Synergistic combinations can give better outcomes and prolong the effect of any given single modality. Narurkar published a combination of nonablative fractional resurfacing, radiofrequency, and CaHA for sustained improved results in hand rejuvenation. All three procedures can be performed on the same day or in stages. From this study and others, it is clear that laser resurfacing does not reduce efficacy of dermal fillers or fat. Indeed, combination protocols such as this one will theoretically increase neocollagenesis synergistically with the immediate and delayed effects of dermal fillers, such as CaHA. In one author's (JE) clinical practice, fillers or autologous fat injections to the hands are routinely combined with laser or radiofrequency treatments and microneedling on the same day, followed immediately by the topical application of platelet-rich plasma (PRP) and/or PLLA. The PRP and/or PLLA are "dripped" on to the treated skin and occluded for 24 hours to speed healing time and further promote neocollagenesis (Fig. 23.6A to D). Further studies are needed to determine

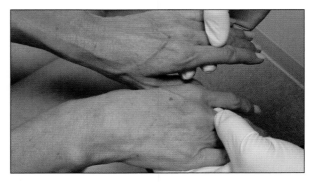

**Figure 23.7** One hand combination therapy at 1 month with 1.5 mL CaHA followed by Fraxel Dual (1550 20 mJ, TL 8, passes 6; 1927 10 mJ, TL 4, passes 2), microneedling (1.0 mm depth) with PRP. See the distinct difference in volume, vein, and tendon show, as well as fine wrinkling as compared with the opposite hand.

the best combinations for sustained improvements with regard to the treatment of all aspects of aging, not solely volume change (Fig 23.7).

## Further reading

Balkin SW, Kaplan L. Silicone injection management of diabetic foot ulcers: a possible model for prevention of pressure ulcers. *Decubitus* 1991;4(4):38–40.

Bank DE. A novel approach to treatment of the aging hand with Radiesse. *J Drugs Dermatol.* 2009;8(12):1122–1126.

Beck M. Toe the line: doctors fight cosmetic foot surgery. *Health J.* 2010; <http://online.wsj.com/article/>.

Bertucci V, Solish N, Wong M, Howell M. Evaluation of the Merz Hand Grading Scale after calcium hydroxylapatite hand treatment. *Dermatol Surg.* 2015;41(suppl 1):S389–S396.

Busso M, Applebaum D. Hand augmentation with Radiesse (calcium hydroxylapatite). *Dermatol Ther.* 2007;20(6): 385–387.

Busso M, Moers-Carpi M, Storck R, Ogilvie P, Ogilvie A. Multicenter, randomized trial assessing the effectiveness and safety of calcium hydroxylapatite for hand rejuvenation. *Dermatol Surg.* 2010;36(s1):790–797.

Butterwick KJ. Rejuvenation of the aging hand. *Dermatol Clin.* 2005;23:515–527.

Butterwick KJ, Bevin AA, Iyer S. Fat transplantation using fresh versus frozen fat: a side-by-side two-hand comparison pilot study. *Dermatol Surg.* 2006;32(5):640–644.

Coleman SR. Hand rejuvenation with structural fat grafting. *Plast Reconstr Surg.* 2002;110(7):1731–1744; discussion 1745–1747.

Edelson KL. Hand recontouring with calcium hydroxylapatite (Radiesse). *J Cosmet Dermatol.* 2009;8(1):44–51.

Giunta RE, Eder M, Machens HG, Muller DF, Kovacs L. Structural fat grafting for rejuvenation of the dorsum of the hand. *Handchir Mikrochir Plast Chir.* 2010;42(2):143–147.

Gubanova EI, Starovatova PA. A prospective, comparative, evaluator-blind clinical study investigating efficacy and safety of two injection techniques with Radiesse® for the correction of skin changes in aging hands. *J Cutan Aesthet Surg.* 2015;8(3):147–152.

Gutowski KA. Current applications and safety of autologous fat grafts: a report of the ASPS fat graft task force. *Plast Reconstr Surg.* 2009; 124(1):272–280.

Haq S, Storck R, Martine B, et al. Multinational, multipatient study of calcium hydroxylapatite for treatment of the aging hand: European cosmetic physician group on hand augmentation. *Dermatol Surg.* 2010;36(s1):782–789.

Hartmann V, Bachmann F, Plaschke M, et al. Hand augmentation with stabilized hyaluronic acid (Macrolane VRF20 and Restylane Vital, Restylane Vital Light). *J Dtsch Dermatol Ges.* 2010;8(1):41–44.

Man J, Rao J, Goldman M. A double-blind, comparative study of nonanimal-stabilized hyaluronic acid versus human collagen for tissue augmentation of the dorsal hands. *Dermatol Surg.* 2008;34(8):1026–1031.

Marmur ES, Al Quran H, De Sa Earp AP, Yoo JP. A five-patient satisfaction pilot study of calcium hydroxylapatite injection for treatment of aging hands. *Dermatol Surg.* 2009;35(12):1978–1984.

Narurkar V. Combination therapy of the aging hand using non-ablative fractional resurfacing radiofrequency and calcium hydroxylapatite in clinical practice. *J Drugs Dermatol.* 2014;9(4):s20–s22.

Pu LL, Coleman SR, Cui X, et al. Autologous fat grafts harvested and refined by the Coleman technique: a comparative study. *Plast Reconstr Surg.* 2008;122(3):932–937.

Redaelli A. Cosmetic use of polylactic acid for hand rejuvenation: report on 27 patients. *J Cosmet Dermatol.* 2006;5(3):233–238.

Rendon MI, Cardona LM, Pinzon-Plazas M. Treatment of the aged hand with injectable poly-L-lactic acid. *J Cosmet Laser Ther.* 2010;12(6):284–287.

Sadick NS. A 52-week study of safety and efficacy of calcium hydroxylapatite for rejuvenation of the aging hand. *J Drugs Dermatol.* 2011;10(1):47–51.

Sadick NS, Anderson D, Werschler WP. Addressing volume loss in hand rejuvenation: a report of clinical experience. *J Cosmet Laser Ther.* 2008;10(4):237–241.

Sattler G, Walker T, Buxmeyer B, Blwer B. Efficacy of calcium hydroxylapatite filler versus hyaluronic acid filler in hand augmentation. *Akt Dermatol.* 2014;40:445–451.

Vleggaar D. Soft-tissue augmentation and the role of poly-L-lactic acid. *Plast Reconstr Surg.* 2006;118(3 Suppl):46S–54S.

Werschler PBM, Busso M. Prepackaged injectable soft-tissue rejuvenation of the hand and other nonfacial area. *Body Rejuvenation* 2010;7:221–225.

# 24

# Neck and chest

Monique Vanaman Wilson, Sabrina Guillen Fabi, Steven H. Dayan

## Summary and Key Features

- Patient demand and options available for aesthetic rejuvenation of the neck and chest are expanding rapidly.
- Dermal fillers and biostimulatory products can be used safely and effectively in these areas.
- Combining soft tissue augmentation with such techniques as lasers/energy devices, fat sculpting, and neuromodulators is often the ideal method of achieving optimal outcomes.

The neck and chest are not immune to the cumulative effects of intrinsic aging and chronic environmental exposures. Like the face, they gradually demonstrate the changes associated with aging: dyschromia, volume loss, wrinkles, and laxity. As patients increasingly achieve a more youthful facial appearance with the wide variety of rejuvenation procedures on the market, they also seek options for enhancing the appearance of their neck and chest. Fillers and biostimulatory products can be used safely and effectively in this area to achieve a patient's desired aesthetic outcome, especially when combined with other rejuvenation modalities, such as lasers/energy devices, fat sculpting, and neuromodulators.

## Neck

The neck is an area that is particularly prone to laxity and wrinkling. This is largely attributable to volume loss in the face, as well as collagen degradation and loss of elasticity, which result in thinning of the skin.[1] Although this chapter will focus specifically on rejuvenation of the neck and chest, it is important to consider the neck in the larger context of the upper body and as an extension of the lower face. Therefore to truly rejuvenate the neck, it may be necessary to address the mid- and lower face. Volume replacement along the mandible and chin, as well as in the midface, will provide structural support to the overlying soft tissue and secondarily improve the appearance of redundant, lax neck skin. These topics are covered elsewhere in this book but should be considered in any cosmetic consultation involving the neck.

Dermal fillers can also be used to address discrete rhytides of the neck, whereas biostimulatory products may be more useful in improving skin texture and laxity.

### Hyaluronic acid

One of the most noticeable skin changes of the aging neck is the appearance of horizontal neck lines. A 2008 study found that 27% of surveyed faculty address these lines with platysmal neuromodulator injections, but deeply etched horizontal neck lines can be further corrected with highly cross-linked, cohesive polydensified hyaluronic acid (HA) gel (Belotero Balance; Merz Aesthetics, Raleigh, NC), often diluted 1:1 with 1% lidocaine (Fig. 24.1). However, consensus recommendations caution regarding the use of dermal fillers to correct horizontal neck lines in persons of color, due to the increased risk of hyperpigmentation.[2]

### Poly-L-lactic acid

Injectable poly-L-lactic acid (PLLA) (Sculptra, Sanofi-Aventis, Bridgewater, NJ) is a biocompatible, biodegradable, immunologically inert, semipermanent synthetic soft tissue biostimulator. PLLA produces a gradual aesthetic correction via induction of neocollagenesis by fibroblasts. Since its initial approval by the US Food and Drug Administration (FDA) in 2004 for treatment of human immunodeficiency virus (HIV)-associated lipoatrophy, PLLA has gained additional approval for correction of shallow-to-deep nasolabial folds, contour deficiencies, and other facial rhytides. PLLA is typically injected into the reticular dermis and subcutaneous tissue planes, providing long-lasting correction for 2 years or longer.[3]

PLLA can be used in the anterior neck to treat flaccidity and rhytides because it improves skin quality by increasing collagen production and improving dermal thickness.[4,5] Mazzuco described the treatment of 36 patients using PLLA to the neck with an average of 1.8 sessions per patient, and 3.9 mL injected per session. The product was reconstituted with 10 mL of sterile water 2 to 3 days prior to injection. Immediately prior to treatment, 0.1 mL of lidocaine 2% was added to 0.9 mL of reconstituted PLLA. At the end of treatment, 91.6% of patients stated they were pleased with their results and would have the procedure done again. The majority of patients also demonstrated sustained improvement at 18 months post

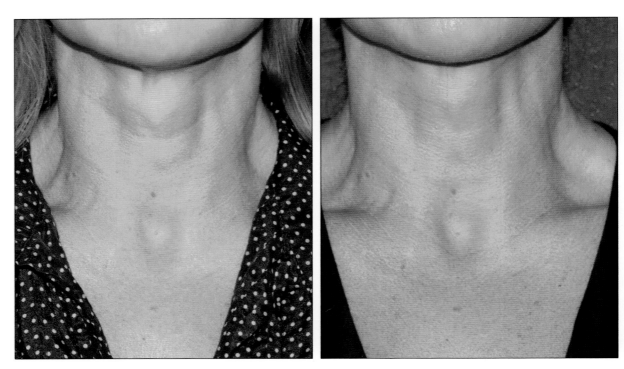

**Figure 24.1** A 40-year-old female (*left*) before and (*right*) 2 weeks after undergoing injection of half a syringe of cohesive polydensified matrix gel (Belotero Balance) at a 1 : 1 dilution with 1% lidocaine without epinephrine into horizontal neck lines.

injection when judged by three independent evaluators. One patient, who reported that she did not follow post-treatment massage instructions, developed subcutaneous nodules in the anterior neck. These were successfully treated with injection of sterile water, vigorous massage, and intralesional triamcinolone.[4]

Of note, the authors do not use PLLA to treat the neck because the incidence of nodules is greater in areas where PLLA is able to aggregate in the muscle. This includes highly mobile or dynamic areas, such as the perioral and periocular regions, as well as the hands. The neck is also a high-risk area due to the proximity between the platysma and the skin.[6]

## Platelet-rich plasma

Platelet-rich plasma (PRP) was initially used in maxillofacial and orthopedic specialties, but it has more recently demonstrated some promise in cosmetic applications. Like PLLA, PRP is thought to produce a gradual aesthetic improvement via stimulatory mechanisms rather than immediate filling. PRP is easily and inexpensively generated through centrifugation of whole autologous blood, which separates the components of blood and concentrates platelets in the plasma. PRP can be injected subdermally or applied to the face after procedures, such as fractional ablative lasers or microneedling. Though

there are small studies that suggest benefit when PRP is used for rejuvenation of the neck,[7] data demonstrating sustained significant benefit are lacking.

## Chest

Like the face and neck, the chest is subjected to both intrinsic aging and the aging effects of environmental exposures. The chest is also prone to the development of rhytides because of chronic positional influences on the breast tissue. The severity of chest rhytides can be objectively graded using the Fabi-Bolton Chest Wrinkle Scale (F-B scale), a five-point scale that grades chest wrinkle severity from grade 1 to 5.[8] Chest rhytides can be addressed using both traditional dermal fillers and injectable biostimulatory products with excellent cosmetic outcomes.

## Poly-L-lactic acid

Several authors have described the use of a 16 mL dilution of PLLA for the correction of chest rhytides with excellent correction and minimal adverse events. This technique uses a 25-gauge, 1.5-inch needle (or cannula to minimize reticular vein puncture) to perform injections starting with rhytides centrally between the breasts then proceeding laterally and superiorly in the plane of

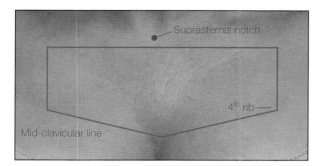

**Figure 24.2** The boundaries of the treatment area when using PLLA in the chest are the suprasternal notch superiorly, the mid-clavicular line laterally, and the fourth rib inferiolaterally.

the subcutaneous fat, using a retrograde linear threading technique. The boundaries of the treatment area are the suprasternal notch superiorly, the mid-clavicular line laterally, and the fourth rib inferiolaterally (Fig. 24.2). The total product administered varies based on the severity of rhytides and volume loss but classically is 16 mL (1 vial) per treatment session. It is important to avoid overcorrection because the treatment effect is gradual and will be more apparent as neocollagenesis progresses. The chest is then vigorously massaged to ensure equal dispersion of the PLLA microparticles. Injections are administered at least 4 weeks apart, for a total of 3 to 4 treatments as needed.[9,10]

A retrospective review of 28 patients who underwent this technique for treatment of chest rhytides demonstrated a one- to two-point improvement on the F-B scale at 6 months post treatment without adverse events.[10]

Perhaps the best described complication of PLLA injection is the formation of subcutaneous nodules. Several techniques to reduce the incidence of nodule formation have been suggested. Use of dilutions greater than 5 mL, overnight reconstitution, and vigorous post-treatment massage are of particular importance in this technique.[4,6,11,12]

## Hyaluronic acid

If injecting an HA filler in the chest, a 22.5 mg/mL monophasic HA filler (Belotero Balance, Merz, Frankfurt, Germany) provides excellent cosmetic outcomes. This product is a cohesive polydensified matrix HA with a low viscosity and a resultant tendency to integrate evenly into tissue, making it an ideal product for use in areas with thin skin, such as the chest.[13] Prior to injection, the product is mixed with 0.5 to 1.0 mL of 1% lidocaine without epinephrine. Using either a 30- or 32-gauge needle, a serial puncture or retrograde linear threading technique is used to inject the filler into the superficial dermis. When compared with more viscous HA products, the 22.5 mg/mL monophasic HA filler intercalates into the dermis more completely, giving the patient an even, smoother cosmetic appearance without Tyndall effect.[14]

Restylane Vital Light (Galderma, Uppsala, Sweden) is available in parts of Europe and Asia for enhancement of the neck, chest, and dorsal hands. This product contains 12 mg/mL of HA, rather than the 20 mg/mL found in the other Restylane injectables (Q-med, Uppsala, Sweden), and is injected in the mid- to deep dermis. Restylane Vital Light is available in an autoinjector that is preloaded with 2 mL of the filler and dispenses aliquots of 10 μL per injection, resulting in a total of 200 doses per autoinjector. The manufacturer claims this microdroplet deposition, in a procedure commonly referred to as "skin boosting," provides a more uniform deposition of HA at the correct depth, thus decreasing the incidence of nodules (http://www.q-medpractitioner.com/International/Restylane/Product-Range/Skin-rejuvenation-skinboosters/Restylane-Injector/, accessed March 2016).

In the United States a 20 mg/mL, 250,000 gel particles/mL HA (Restylane Silk, Galderma) can be used in place of Restylane Vital Light, and the authors commonly mix the product with 0.5 mL of 1% lidocaine without epinephrine prior to injection. A serial puncture or retrograde linear threading technique using a 30- or 32-gauge needle is used to inject the product into the deep dermis.

When compared with PLLA, correction of chest rhytides with HA requires more syringes and is shorter-lived, with results typically lasting for 6 to 8 months.[15] Thus, for most patients it is more cost-effective to use fewer syringes of PLLA to achieve excellent correction for up to 2 years or longer without a touch-up (Fig. 24.3). In the authors' experience, PLLA also results in fewer nodules and surface irregularities than HA, likely due to the depth of injection.

## Calcium hydroxylapatite

The authors are currently investigating the safety, efficacy, and patient satisfaction associated with the use of one syringe of calcium hydroxylapatite (CaHP) with lidocaine (Radiesse, Merz Aesthetics) diluted 1:2 with bacteriostatic saline for treatment of chest rhytides. In the study, one treatment arm will be treated with CaHP alone and the other with the combination of microfocused ultrasound plus visualization (MFU-V) immediately followed by CaHP to determine if a synergistic effect can be achieved when both a collagen-stimulating injectable and energy-based device are combined, as has been seen clinically and histologically in previous studies.[15,16]

In this procedure, a 27-gauge, 3/4-inch needle or a 25- to 27-gauge cannula is used to deliver CaHP along the subcutaneous plane using a retrograde linear threading technique.

## Summary

Soft tissue augmentation of the neck and chest is useful in addressing the volume loss, skin thinning, and rhytides characteristic of aging in these aesthetically important areas. HA fillers and PLLA can be used safely and

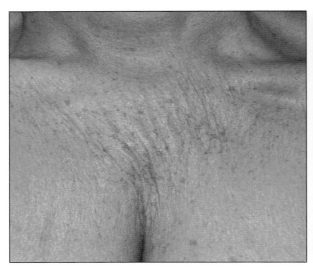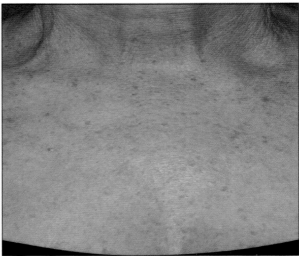

**Figure 24.3** A 49-year-old female (*left*) before and (*right*) 3 years after undergoing treatment with three vials of PLLA for rhytides and two intense pulsed light (IPL) sessions for dyschromia.

effectively to achieve the cosmetic rejuvenation that patients seek. CaHP may also prove to be a safe and effective treatment modality for chest rhytides. Because aging is a multifaceted process, it is important for the treating physician to keep in mind that a multimodal approach is often ideal; combining various techniques, such as lasers, energy devices, fat sculpting, and neuromodulators, with soft tissue augmentation is the best method of achieving the optimal aesthetic outcome.

## References

1. Fisher GJ, Varani J, Voorhees JJ. Looking older: fibroblast collapse and therapeutic implications. *Arch Dermatol.* 2008;144:666–672.
2. Carruthers JD, Glogau RG, Blitzer A. Facial aesthetics consensus group faculty. Advances in facial rejuvenation: botulinum toxin type a, hyaluronic acid dermal fillers, and combination therapies—consensus recommendations. *Plast Reconstr Surg.* 2008;121(5 Suppl):5S–30S.
3. Butterwick K, Lowe NJ. Injectable poly-L-lactic acid for cosmetic enhancement: learning from the European experience. *J Am Acad Dermatol.* 2009;61:281–293.
4. Mazzuco R, Hexsel D. Poly-L-lactic acid for neck and chest rejuvenation. *Dermatol Surg.* 2009;35:1228–1237.
5. Valantin MA, Aubron-Olivier C, Ghosn J, et al. Polylactic acid implants (New-Fill) to correct facial lipoatrophy in HIV-infected patients: results of the open-label study VEGA. *AIDS* 2003;17:2471–2477.
6. Palm MD, Woodhall KE, Butterwick KJ, Goldman MP. Cosmetic use of poly-l-lactic acid: a retrospective study of 130 patients. *Dermatol Surg.* 2010;36:161–170.
7. Redaelli A, Romano D, Marcianó A. Face and neck revitalization with platelet-rich plasma (PRP): clinical outcome in a series of 23 consecutively treated patients. *J Drugs Dermatol.* 2010;9:466–472.
8. Fabi SG, Bolton J, Goldman M, Guiha I. The Fabi-Bolton chest wrinkle scale: a validation study. *J Cosmet Dermatol.* 2012;11:229–234.
9. Peterson JD, Goldman MP. Rejuvenation of the aging chest: a review and our experience. *Dermatol Surg.* 2011;37:555–571.
10. Bolton J, Fabi SG, Peterson J, Goldman M. Poly-L-lactic acid for chest rejuvenation: a retrospective study of 28 cases using a 5-point chest wrinkle scale. *Cosmet Dermatol.* 2011;24:278–284.
11. Fitzgerald R, Vleggaar D. Using poly-L-lactic acid (PLLA) to mimic volume in multiple tissue layers. *J Drugs Dermatol.* 2009;8:S5–S14.
12. Narins RS. Minimizing adverse events associated with poly-L-lactic acid injection. *Dermatol Surg.* 2008;34:S100–S104.
13. Flynn TC, Sarazin D, Bezzola A, Terrani C, Micheels P. Comparative histology of intradermal implantation of mono and biphasic hyaluronic acid fillers. *Dermatol Surg.* 2011;37(5):637–643.
14. Sundaram H, Cassuto D. Biophysical characteristics of hyaluronic acid soft-tissue fillers and their relevance to aesthetic applications. *Plast Reconstr Surg.* 2013;132(4 Suppl 2):5S–21S.
15. Casabona G, Michalany N. Micro-focused ultrasound with visualization and fillers for increased neocollagenesis: clinical and histological evaluation. *Dermatol Surg.* 2014;40(Suppl 12):S194–S198.
16. Ascher B, Talarico S, Cassuto D, et al. International consensus recommendations on the aesthetic usage of botulinum toxin type A (Speywood Unit)—Part II: wrinkles on the middle and lower face, neck and chest. *J Eur Acad Dermatol Venereol.* 2010;24(11):1285–1295.

# 25

# Buttocks

## Ada R. Trindade de Almeida, Raúl Alberto Banegas

### Summary and Key Features

- The waist–hip ratio is a measure of beauty and sexual attractiveness in females. Fat grafting, increasing the gluteal volume, and narrowing the waist, enable patients to approach this proportion.
- Fat grafting with growth factors derived from platelet-rich plasma and adipocyte stem cells induces angiogenesis and consequently improves fat tissue survival.
- Biodegradable fillers, such as stabilized hyaluronic acid and poly-L-lactic acid, can also be used in the gluteal region.

There is a growing demand for gluteal aesthetics because this region plays an important role in an ideal of physical attractiveness.

Globally pleasing gluteal features include homogeneous skin tone and texture, smooth round projection and contour, lateral thighs following the shape of the buttocks without excess fat, infragluteal folds ending before mid-thigh line and waist–hip ratio between 0.6 and 0.7.[1]

With aging, women tend to develop a more centralized fat distribution, accumulating subcutaneous adipose tissue at the waist, losing the smooth inward sweep of the lumbosacral area and waist. As the buttocks lose their projection, the infragluteal fold becomes longer. The main gluteal complaints from patients are flaccidity, loss of projection, depressions (traumatic or "cellulite-derived"), asymmetries, and striae distensae.

In recent years, the search for procedures to provide a more appealing body contour, improving buttock volume, firmness, and/or shape, has been increasing. Currently the major procedures available are buttock lifting, silicone implants, autologous fat transfer, and injection of biodegradable fillers.

The gluteal aesthetic landmarks are summarized in Box 25.1.

## Gluteal augmentation with fat grafting

Although many products have being used, fat tissue continues to be the most reliable material in terms of abundance, safety, easy of harvesting, lower cost, and long-lasting results.

When planning a gluteal augmentation with fat grafting, selection of the donor area is very important because of its contribution to the final shape of the buttocks. The waist–hip ratio between 0.6 and 0.7 in females is a measure of beauty and sexual attractiveness in many cultures. Increasing the gluteal volume and narrowing of the waist are surgical corrections that enable patients to approach this proportion.[2] Fat may be obtained as a single process associated with regional or circumferential liposculpture. This way, while liposuction defines the limits and shape of the buttocks, lipotransference improves its projection.

### Pearl 1

Fat extraction is performed using 3- to 4-mm blunt-tipped cannulas.

Fat injection must end when it begins to exit through the incision holes to avoid excessive local pressure that may induce graft low irrigation and oxygenation.

Table 25.1 describes the tumescent solution used for gluteal augmentation.

## Fat preparation for injection

Fat extraction is performed using 3- to 4-mm blunt-tipped cannulas to avoid the destruction of the adipocyte and collected in a sealed vial ("no touch technique"). For minor procedures 10-, 20-, or 60-mL syringes may be used.

After the fat is harvested, there are several methods to process it. The technique proved most effective is centrifugation to concentrate the fat fraction.[3] Removal of deleterious components improves outcomes by decreasing the inflammatory response to the graft. In our clinic (RB), we use centrifugation at 900 rpm for 1 minute.

## Fat grafting with growth factors

Although adipose transfer has been widely used in different clinical cases, high variability in long-term results has been reported, mainly due to unpredictable degrees of reabsorption and volume loss.

Because of that, the need arises to increase the survival rate of the transplanted fat by the addition of growth factors obtained from platelet-rich plasma (PRP) and adipocyte stem cells (ASCs). There are demonstrated synergistic effects of both factors on adipose transplanted tissue survival.[4] One of the findings is the beneficial effect on angiogenesis. Neovascularization in the early stage of fat transplantation is essential to keep the viability of implanted cells and newly formed tissues, as well as to provide a potential solution for reabsorption problems during soft-tissue reconstruction.

---

**Box 25.1**
**Gluteal aesthetic landmarks**

- **Lateral depressions**.
- **Infragluteal fold:** long = ptotic buttock; short = young buttock.
- **Supragluteal fossettes:** depressions at each side of the sacral region.
- **Triangle or V-shaped fold**.
- **Waist–hip ratio:** ideally between 0.6 and 0.7.

---

**Table 25.1** Klein tumescent solution used for gluteal augmentation

| | |
|---|---|
| 0.9% Saline solution | 1000 mL |
| 2% Lidocaine | 25 mL |
| 1/1000 Epinephrine | 1 mL |
| 8.4% Sodium bicarbonate | 12.5 mL |

Adipocyte survival is also improved when deposited in the intramuscular tissue, where the irrigation is higher. But it also increases the morbidity of the procedure, enhancing the risk of vascular damage. Some fatal cases of fat embolic problems were described after gluteal lipoinjections, especially when performed in the deep muscular layers. Therefore it is a procedure that should be performed very carefully to avoid injury to the deep gluteal vessels.[5]

## Injection technique

It is important to perform the infiltration of fat tissue in multiple layers, aiming to maximize the number of normally irrigated cells. The fat is injected using 10- to 60-mL syringes adapted to 2- to 4-mm blunt cannulas with lateral hole tips. According to the treatment area, the fat is injected in a retrograde fashion in the two layers of the subcutaneous tissue, as well as in the muscular plane, to ensure higher irrigation. It is important to avoid injecting in the "dangerous triangle" area, formed by the trochanter (tip of the triangle) and the external borders of the sacral bone (base of it). This triangle points out the emergence of the superior and inferior gluteal arteries, where there is a higher risk of intravascular injection and fat embolism (Fig. 2z5.1).

The best recipient locations, in terms of shape and volume, are the upper poles of the buttocks. They are identified by taking a meridian line drawn between both trochanters, with the upper limit following the edge of the posterior iliac crest.

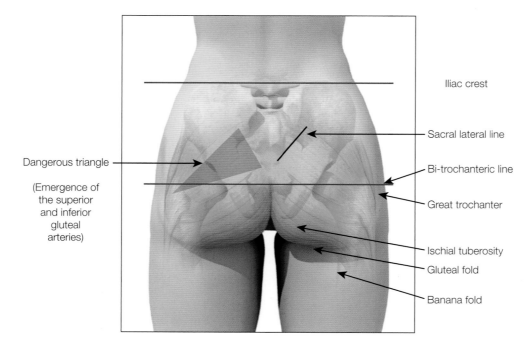

**Figure 25.1** Buttocks landmarks and the dangerous triangle area, point of emergence of superior, and inferior gluteal arteries.

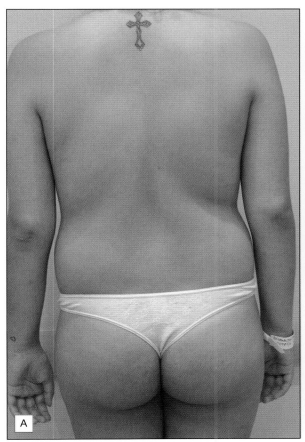 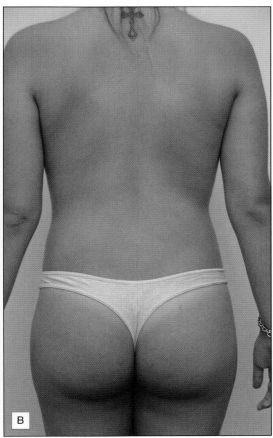

**Figure 25.2** Liposuction of flanks and 360 mL of fat grafting in each side, mixed with growth factors in different layers of the buttocks: intramuscular and superficial and deep fat tissue, in a 21-year-old woman. **A,** Preoperative condition. **B,** Eight months after the procedure.

The amount of fat tissue used to increase the volume and projection of the buttocks has changed over time. We began by using 30 to 40 mL per side, but we are currently using 300 to 500 mL per treatment session.

To prevent embolic problems, bed rest is not recommended and patients are instructed to walk during the first 2 or 3 days, returning to normal activities within a week and to sports after 30 days.

The main advantages of fat grafting are the long-lasting results and possibility to treat large areas, whereas the need of donor material and the surgical procedure itself are the drawbacks. **Figs. 25.2** and **25.3** illustrate two treated cases.

## Gluteal enhancement with biodegradable fillers

Some subjects are not suitable for fat grafting because of insufficient donor areas, small defects to correct, or not wanting a surgical procedure.

For these cases our choice is for nonpermanent fillers, such as hyaluronic acid (HA) gels or poly-L-lactic acid (PLLA), that are safe, effective, and long-lasting, allowing for retreatment when necessary.

## Hyaluronic acid gels

Stabilized HA gels, similarly to implants and fat grafts, add volume simply by occupying space within the tissue. The best option is a large-particle product developed specifically for body shaping: Macrolane Volume Restoration Factor (VRF), manufactured using the non-animal stabilized hyaluronic acid (NASHA) technology (Q-Med AB, Uppsala, Sweden). It comes in two versions: Macrolane VRF 30, for deep subcutaneous deposition, and Macrolane VRF 20, for more superficial subcutaneous injections. Both products are available in 10-mL syringes and are currently approved in some countries of the European Union, Brazil, Mexico, Israel, Taiwan, Singapore, Malaysia, and Hong Kong.

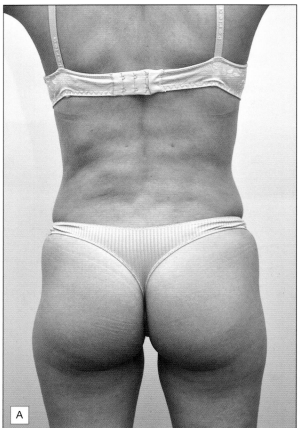 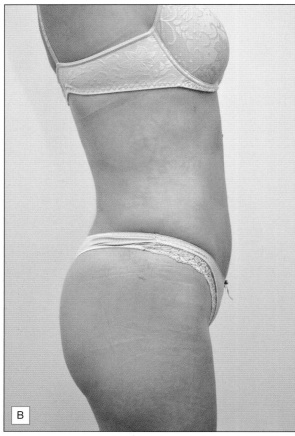

**Figure 25.3** Liposuction of flanks, waist, inner part of the legs and abdomen, and fat grafting (300 mL/side) mixed with growth factors in a 48-year-old woman. The fat graft was injected in several layers, improving the buttocks' shape and also volume. Preoperative and 14 months after. **A,** Back. **B,** Right side.

Its use offers several advantages: a minimally invasive procedure performed in an outpatient basis, no requirement of a donor site, little downtime, reversibility, and the safety record of the NASHA products. However, like for other regions, the injection technique requires proper training. When large amounts of the product are needed, the cost would be a concern.

So far, several publications have demonstrated its safety and efficacy for various body indications, such as scars, concavities, and asymmetries, as well as shaping or augmentation of calves, buttocks, and chest.[6,7] For breast augmentation, stabilized HA gel is no longer marketed or indicated due to an ongoing debate on radiologic imaging issues for breast cancer screening.

For gluteal indications, an international, multicenter study evaluated 61 subjects for buttocks augmentation, followed for 24 months. Macrolane VRF30 was injected into the deep subcutaneous fat layer, using a multitunneling technique. The mean injected volume was 340 mL (200 to 400 mL). No unexpected or serious treatment-related adverse events occurred. They concluded that "although the substance degrades over time, a good proportion of subjects still rated their buttocks as improved (40%) and expressed satisfaction (33%) 24 months after treatment."

Another study used Macrolane for correcting body irregularities from several causes (after liposuction, trauma, or surgery) in 56 patients. The mean injected volume was 20 mL; there were no serious adverse events. Investigators found persistence of improvement after 12 months in 57% of patients.

## Injection technique

The gluteal depressions are marked with the patient in a standing position. After that, the treatment area is cleaned with 4% chlorhexidine gluconate, and incision sites are infiltrated by small amounts of anesthetic solution, as described in Table 25.2. Additional infiltration can be added to painful adherent locations.

Before injection, an 18-gauge (G), 70-mm long blunt disposable cannula is filled with the product, until a droplet is visible at the tip. Entry incisions are performed

**Table 25.2** Anesthetic solution used for Macrolane injections

| | |
|---|---|
| 0.9% Unpreserved saline | 180 mL |
| 2% Lidocaine | 20 mL |
| Epinephrine | 0.4 mL |

using an 18G needle. An average of two incision sites is planned per side.

Prior to injecting the filler, we perform some undermining, releasing dermal fibrous attachments that sometimes are strong, with the cannula. After that, in each previous demarcated defect, the filler is deposited deep in the subcutaneous layer in multiple passes. Small amounts are released in each pass, avoiding the formation of large-volume pockets. The nondominant hand follows the procedure, palpating the treated area.

At the end of the procedure, each incision site has its borders carefully everted and these are closed directly with adhesive tape (Micropore). Patients are advised to wear a mild compressive garment, to avoid excessive physical activity, and to be careful with their sitting position for 1 to 2 weeks.

Some swelling, tenderness, and bruising may be expected after the procedure. A mild bluish discoloration can appear, lasting approximately 30 days. Because the undermining before injection is performed using a blunt cannula, instead of using a sharp instrument, bleeding is minimal, recovery is fast, and no postinflammatory hyperpigmentation is observed, even in dark-skinned subjects. The product may also be aspirated through an 18G needle or drained, or, if complete removal is desired, hyaluronidase may be used.

The majority of the patients are treated in only one session. After 1 month, if the final aesthetic correction proves suboptimal, touch-up injections may be planned. Fig. 25.4 illustrates two treated cases.

As patients continue to opt for nonsurgical procedures that offer predictable results, HA for body enhancement offers the cosmetic surgeon a new tool.

---

**Pearl 2**

Inject small amounts of Macrolane deep into the subcutaneous plane in multiple passes.

---

**Pearl 3**

Using a cannula to release fibrous attachments instead of a sharp instrument reduces the risk of bruises and postinflammatory hyperpigmentation.

A summary of the recommendations for stabilized HA injection to the gluteal area is presented in Box 25.2.

---

**Box 25.2**
**Recommendations for macrolane gluteal injections**

- **Markings:** mark areas to be treated with the patient standing up.
- **Antisepsis:** chlorhexine gluconate.
- **Anesthesia:** minimal amount of anesthetic solution (see Table 25.2).
- **Macrolane preparation:** Add 1 mL of diluent to each 10-mL syringe.
  Diluent: 0.3 mL 2% lidocaine + 0.7 mL 0.9% saline.
- **Material:** 18-gauge needle for entry and 18-gauge cannulas for injections.
- **Technique:** Begin with gentle release of fibrous attachments, followed by injection of small HA amounts, deep into the SQ, in multiple passes.

---

## Poly-L-lactic acid

PLLA, known as Sculptra (Galderma Pharma SA, Galderma Lausanne. Switzerland), has been widely used for many years, as a gradual volume restoration for facial treatment with the added effect of collagen stimulation.[8] This latter effect is supposed to be due to the inflammatory reaction responsible for degradation of the PLLA particles inducing neocollagenesis and gradual correction of lipoatrophies and/or age-related changes. It is frequently injected in the deep dermis and subcutaneous layers and was demonstrated to improve dermal volume loss and bony deficits in multiple tissue layers.[9] Despite this, the product is biocompatible and has minimal risk of immune reactions. However, it usually needs multiple treatment sessions for the biostimulatory effect to reach its optimal result.

A review of the literature highlighted the relationship between dilution volumes and the presence of posttreatment nodules, finding reduced risk of this adverse effect, when higher dilutions are used.[8] This way, dilutions higher than 7 mL are recommended.

After the face, PLLA was used in hands, neck, chest, thighs, and buttocks, with success. Another review[10] resumed some of the published studies of PLLA cosmetic body indications: Coimbra and Amorim, treating sagging arms, and Vleggaar and Shulman for chest indications (pectus excavatum, and thoracic deformity secondary to breast reconstruction, respectively).[10] For the décolletage, some authors described the use of PLLA alone, reconstituted to 10 to 16 mL, or associated to other procedures.[9]

For gluteal enhancement, although being used in clinical practice, we found only a case report letter, from Mazzuco and Sadick.[11] They treated two female subjects: the first received three treatments, with four vials each, spaced 1 month apart. The second, treated with three vials in each of two monthly sessions. The aim was to improve buttocks projection, skin laxity, and cellulite depressions. They used a 12-mL dilution (10 mL of sterile water plus

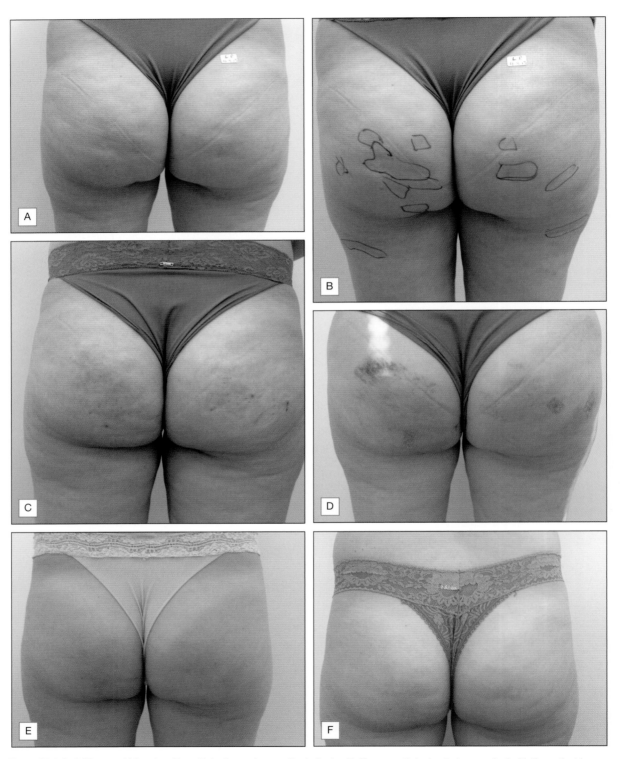

**Figure 25.4 A,** A 30-year-old female with multiple depressions on the buttocks. **B,** The areas to be treated are marked with the patient in an upright position. **C,** Immediate postoperatory result, after 40 mL of Macrolane VRF30. **D,** Twenty-four hours post operation, with some visible bruises. **E, F** Before and after 3 and 12 months.

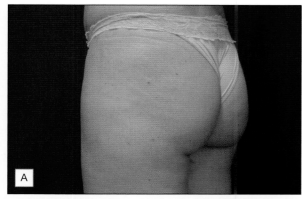

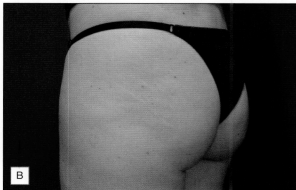

Figure 25.5 A, B Before and after 1 month of first session of poly-L-lactic acid (PLLA) injections. Mild improvement in flaccidity and buttock projection. *Courtesy of Dr. Marisa Gonzaga, MD, Brazil.*

2 mL of lidocaíne). The gluteal area was divided into three thirds and markings were performed mainly in the upper two thirds. Using a 3-mL Luer Lock syringe and 27G needles, PLLA was injected in a retrograde manner, 1.5 to 2.5 cm below the skin surface, at a 60-degree angle, in 0.1 mL aliquots, spaced 1 cm apart. Patients were asked to massage the treated area for 5 minutes, 3 times a day, for 7 days and to avoid rigorous exercising for 2 weeks (Fig. 25.5).

Despite the small number of publications for corporal indications, PLLA is gaining acceptance for body treatment in clinical practice. A review of the literature shows that the majority of authors prefer dilution volumes between 8 and 20 mL.

## Technical considerations for gluteal poly-L-lactic acid injections

PLLA (Sculptra) comes as a lyophilized powder. The consensus recommendations are dilutions higher than 7 mL, at least 24 hours prior to use. The vast majority of physicians prefer to reconstitute the Sculptra with bacteriostatic water because it reduces patient discomfort

> **Box 25.3**
> **Recommendations for poly-L-lactic acid gluteal injections**
>
> - **Reconstitution:** at least 2 h prior to use, preferably 24 h.
> - **Dilution:** 8 mL 0.9% saline the day before and 2% lidocaine prior to use.
> - **Amount:** 10 mL/vial; 1 to 2 vials per buttock side.
> - **Vigorous agitation:** manually or vortex.
> - **Markings:** mark areas to be treated with the patient standing up.
> - **Antisepsis:** chlorhexidine gluconate.
> - **Material:** 27-gauge needles and 1-mL syringes.
> - **Injections:** Retrograde. 0.1 mL aliquots in the SQ plane.
>   Deep depressions receive crossed injections.
> - **Massage:** Firm just after the procedure and at home following the "5-5-5" rule: for 5 min, 5 times per day, for 5 days.
> - **Retreatments:** 3 to 6 sessions may be necessary, spaced monthly.

during application. For the same reason one of us (ARTA) prefers to use saline solution. The product needs agitation prior to use, performed manually or by a vortex, as described in the literature.[8]

In our office, we use a 10-mL dilution for corporal indications. The vial is prepared the day before the procedure, with the addition of 8 mL of saline solution. Just prior to injection, 2 mL of 2% lidocaine is added, followed by vigorous agitation; 1 mL Luer Lock syringes, and 27G, 1.5-inch needles are used for injections. After cleaning with 4% chlorhexidine gluconate, retrograde deposits of 0.1 mL are placed in linear lines over the marked sites in the superficial subcutaneous layer. Deep depressions receive crossed injections to allow higher deposits but not in the same place. The total amount injected varies according to the severity of the problem, most patients receiving one to two vials per treatment session.

Immediately after the procedure, firm massage is administered. The patient is counseled to do the same at home, following the 5-5-5 rule: for 5 minutes, 5 times per day, for 5 days.[12] Results are expected to appear after three to six treatment sessions, according to the amount of product injected and patient response.

A summary of the recommendations for PLLA injections is presented in Box 25.3.

As patients continue to opt for nonsurgical procedures, the use of PLLA seems to be a promising and safe option to add to our cosmetic armamentarium. The product could be used solely or associated with other procedures for patients seeking less invasive means of achieve gluteal improvement.

## References

1. Toledo L. Gluteal augmentation with fat grafting: the Brazilian technique: 30 years' experience. *Clin Plast Surg.* 2015;42(2):253–261.

2. Rosique R, Rosique M, De Moraes C. Gluteoplasty with autologous fat tissue. Experience with 106 consecutive cases. *Plast Reconstr Surg.* 2015;135(5):1381.

3. Salinas HM, Broelsch GF, Fernandes JR, et al. Comparative analysis of processing methods in fat grafting. *Plast Reconstr Surg.* 2014;134(4):675.

4. Li F, Guo W, Li K, et al. Improved fat graft survival by different volume fractions of platelet-rich plasma and adipose-derived stem cells. *Aesthetic Surg J.* 2015;35(3):319–333.

5. Cárdenas-Camarena L, Bayter J, Aguirre-Serrano H, Cuenca-Pardo J. Deaths caused by gluteal lipoinjection: what are we doing wrong? *Plast Reconstr Surg.* 2015;136(1):58–66.

6. Hedén P, Sellman G, Von Wachenfeldt M, Olenius M, Fagrell D. Body shaping and volume restoration: the role of hyaluronic acid. *Aesthetic Plast Surg.* 2009;33:274–282.

7. De Meyere B, Mir-Mir S, Peña J, Camenisch C, Heden P. Stabilized hyaluronic acid gel for volume restoration and contouring of the buttocks: 24-month efficacy and safety. *Aesthetic Plast Surg.* 2014;38:404–412.

8. Bartus C, William Hanke C, Daro-Kaftan E. A decade of experience with injectable poly-L-lactic acid: a focus on safety. *Dermatol Surg.* 2013;39:698–705.

9. Hart D, Fabi S, White W, Fitzgerald R, Goldman M. Current concepts in the use of PLLA: clinical synergy noted with combined use of MFUS and PLLA on the face, neck and décolletage. *Plast Reconstr Surg.* 2015;136:180S.

10. Machado Filho C, Santos T, Rodrigues A, Cunha MG. Poly-L-lactic acid: a biostimulating agent. *Surg Cosmet Dermatol.* 2013;5(4):345–350.

11. Mazzuco R, Sadick N. The use of poly-L-lactic acid in the gluteal area. *Dermatol Surg.* 2016;42:3.

12. Vanaman M, Fabi S. Décolletage: regional approach with injectable fillers. *Plast Reconstr Surg.* 2015;136:276S.

# 26

# Earlobe rejuvenation

Laurel Naversen Geraghty

## Summary and Key Features

- The earlobe is a site of adornment and a reflection of beauty across world cultures.
- With increasing interest in facial and neck rejuvenation, the earlobes have emerged as a site of cosmetic concern.
- Like other sun-exposed areas of skin, the earlobes may exhibit signs of age, including pigmentary changes and increased laxity, loss of volume, and elongation (ptosis).
- Volume loss of the earlobes can be corrected safely and effectively using injectable fillers.
- The quality of the earlobe skin can be improved with laser and other energy-based devices.

## Introduction

With a growing interest in minimally invasive cosmetic procedures, a new anatomic site is gaining increasing attention: the earlobes. Like sun-exposed areas of the face, chest, neck, and hands, the ears can show significant signs of aging. These may include wrinkling, dyspigmentation, and elongation (ptosis) due to chronic exposure to ultraviolet light, loss of elastic fibers and collagen, and natural aging. Such changes can be exacerbated by the use of heavy earrings. Earlobe restoration is indicated in patients with ptosis or other signs of lobule aging; those who have undergone cosmetic procedures on the face and neck and desire similarly youthful earlobes; and those with piercing holes that have stretched or are suboptimally placed, such that the lobule cannot adequately support earrings. Soft tissue augmentation using injectable fillers can safely restore volume and minimize sagging and wrinkling. Lasers and other energy-based treatments can improve skin dyspigmentation and the overall quality of the earlobe skin.

### Pearl 1

Earlobes can exhibit signs of aging and can become elongated as a result of gravity, photoaging, and the pull of heavy earrings.

### Pearl 2

With volume loss, the earlobes can become thin and wrinkled and can lose the ability to adequately support earrings.

## Anatomy and classification of earlobes

The earlobe is composed of tough areolar and adipose tissue and can have a natural shape that is round, flat, or triangular. Lobules are generally smooth but occasionally exhibit creases. Creased or crumpled earlobes can suggest an underlying genetic disorder, such as Beckwith-Wiedemann syndrome or congenital contractural arachnodactyly, respectively. Diagonal earlobe creases extending from the lateral cheek toward the inferior helix have been reported as a risk factor for myocardial infarction and ischemic heart disease. However, earlobes lack the firmness and elasticity of the rest of the pinna and can become creased and elongated with age, even in the absence of heart disease.

Elongated earlobes increase a person's perceived age and negatively impact her perceived attractiveness, according to a study by Forte et al.[1] Pendulous earlobes, which do not adhere to the lateral cheek, are most likely to elongate and become asymmetric with time (Fig. 26.1). These are inherited in autosomal dominant fashion. Nonpendulous earlobes attach to the lateral cheek, are less likely to elongate with age, and are inherited in a recessive pattern (see Fig. 26.1).

The earlobe is commonly measured from the intertragal notch to the subaurale (Fig. 26.2). Ptosis has been defined as an elongated free caudal segment (otobasion inferius to the subaurale), whereas pseudoptosis refers to elongation of the attached cephalic segment (intertragal notch to otobasion inferius) (see Fig. 26.2). In 1972 Loeb observed the natural range of the cephalic segment to be 1 to 2.5 cm and advocated for surgical correction when this segment (psuedoptosis) exceeds 2.0 cm.[2] A more recent study describes pseudoptosis as cephalic segment length exceeding 1.5 cm. Mowlavi (2003) reported increased incidence of earlobe ptosis and pseudoptosis following facelift surgery, highlighting the need to address signs of earlobe aging at the time of facial rejuvenation.

Using another means of evaluating the ear, in a randomized, prospective study of 547 men and women aged 20

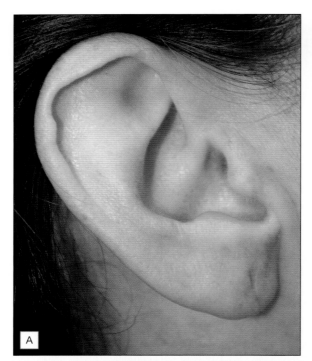

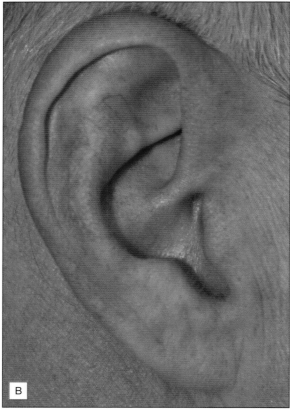

**Figure 26.1** Anatomic shape of earlobes: (A) unattached and (B) attached.

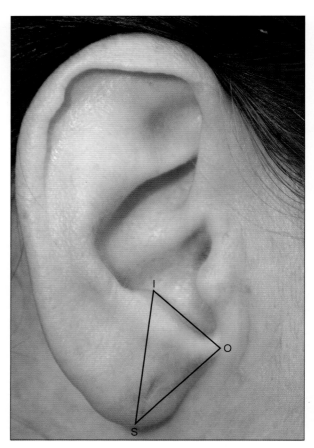

**Figure 26.2** The anatomic landmarks of the *I*, *O*, and *S* are labeled. Earlobe height parameters are defined with respect to the attached cephalic segment (*I* to *O segment*) and the free caudal segment to *S* segment). *I*, Intertragal notch; *O*, otobasion inferius; *S*, subaurale.

to 80 years, Azaria et al. measured earlobe length using a line of balance through the long axis of the ear (intertragic notch to caudal tip) (Fig. 26.3).[3] The authors demonstrated that the left earlobe is shorter than the right, on average (1.97 cm vs. 2.01 cm; mean difference 0.4 mm). Earlobe size and symmetry varied by race (individuals of African descent had the shortest earlobes, and Ashkenazi and Sephardic Jews had relatively long left earlobes), and earlobe length increased slightly with heavier body weight among women. Earlobe length increased by 30% to 35% between the youngest and oldest age groups, but no significant change was noted in women aged 40 years and older. Prior to treatment, it is beneficial to discuss ear size and any natural asymmetry with the patient and offer anticipatory guidance about earlobe changes based on age and body habitus.

## Fillers for earlobe rejuvenation

Soft tissue augmentation using fillers is a safe, effective, and increasingly popular means of restoring volume to

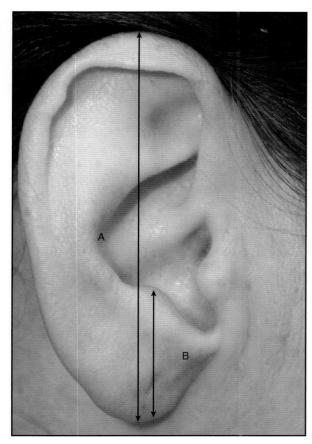

**Figure 26.3** Measurement technique of earlobes: line of balance (*line A*) and earlobe length (*line B*).

the earlobes. Hyaluronic acid fillers include Restylane, Restylane Silk, and Perlane (Galderma, Fort Worth, Texas) and Juvéderm, Juvéderm Ultra, and Juvéderm Voluma (Allergan Inc., Ivrine, California). Longer-lasting fillers, such as calcium hydroxylapatite (Radiesse, Merz Aesthetics, San Mateo, California) and poly-L-lactic acid (Sculptra, Galderma, Fort Worth, Texas), could also be attempted, although their use for earlobe rejuvenation has not been reported in the literature.

The earlobe is a small anatomic site but can require 0.3 to 1.0 mL or more to correct volume loss. A 27-gauge 0.5-inch (1.25-cm) needle is large enough to allow the product to flow quickly into the tissue and with less resistance relative to smaller needles. However, a 30-gauge needle or other size could also be used. Topical anesthesia or ice can be applied prior to injections, but this is often unnecessary, particularly with hyaluronic acid formulations containing anesthesia. After cleansing the area with antiseptic, the practitioner may grasp the earlobe firmly between the thumb and index finger and direct the needle into the mid-dermis at a 30- to 45-degree angle. Serial injections can be used to deliver small aliquots of filler; some authors have proposed making injections in a circular pattern around the hole of a pierced ear. This method helps to tighten the diameter of the piercing while allowing filler to be massaged outward to fill the entire lobule, ultimately providing better support for earrings (Fig. 26.4). With a threading or tunneling technique, the needle may be inserted into the inferior pole of the lobule, and a depot of filler is injected as the needle is withdrawn (Fig. 26.5). Firm pressure can be applied for 1 minute afterward to help to reduce the risk of bruising and edema, and the lobule may be gently massaged to distribute the product.

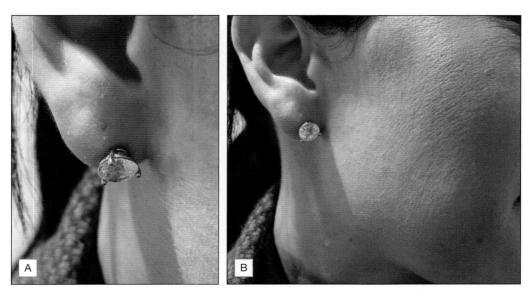

**Figure 26.4** The earlobe of a young woman before (A) and after (B) injections using Juvéderm Voluma (Allergan Inc., Irvine, California). Note how the earring is better supported by the lobule and oriented anteriorly (rather than downward) in the after photo.

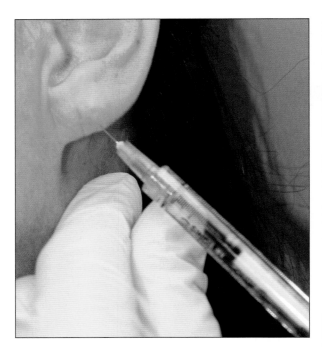

**Figure 26.5** Injection technique using Restylane (Galderma, Fort Worth, Texas) to restore volume from the inferior aspect of the earlobe in a patient who has previously had earlobe repair surgery.

### Pearl 3

Fillers can be delivered by making serial injections of small aliquots into the earlobe, or by placing a depot of filler through the inferior pole of the lobule. Either method can restore volume and allow the lobule to better support earrings.

As with soft tissue augmentation of other sites, there is a risk of bruising, swelling, and erythema following injections. Because of the earlobe's rich vascularity, the lobule can appear red and edematous for a prolonged period. Patients can resume wearing earrings immediately after the procedure, and the earlobe can be reassessed after 2 weeks to consider the need for more product. Hyaluronic acid filler has been noted to last longer in the earlobes relative to the face, but repeat injections are needed to maintain results.

### Conclusion

As more patients elect to undergo cosmetic treatments for the face and neck, earlobe restoration is garnering increasing attention. Research on soft tissue rejuvenation of this anatomic site remains in its nascent stages. However, empiric use of injectable fillers can safely and effectively improve the appearance of elongated or wrinkled ears, can help to support earrings in lobules with excess laxity or

poorly placed piercing holes, and can prevent a discordant appearance between the ears and a rejuvenated face and neck. Laser and other energy-based treatments can further improve the quality of the earlobe skin.

### Pearl 4

As with any injection of filler, there is a risk of bruising, edema, and erythema that may be more pronounced on the earlobe due to its rich vascularity. Repeat injections are needed to maintain results.

Little has been written on treatments for earlobe photoaging, but wrinkling and discoloration are common in this site among patients who are middle-aged and older. The skin of the earlobes responds well to laser and light devices used for retexturing and for treating dyschromia. Q-switched lasers and intense pulsed-light (IPL) treatments are among the therapies that can be effective for sun-induced earlobe dyspigmentation, whereas nonablative and ablative fractional lasers can help to improve earlobe texture.

### Pearl 5

The use of hyaluronic acid fillers for earlobe rejuvenation is safe, effective, and well-tolerated.

### References

1. Forte AJ, Andrew TW, Colasante C, Persing JA. Perception of age, attractiveness, and tiredness after isolated and combined facial subunit aging. *Aesthetic Plast Surg.* 2015;39:856–869.
2. Loeb R. Earlobe tailoring during facial rhytidoplasties. *Plast Reconstr Surg.* 1972;49:485–488.
3. Azaria R, Adler N, Silfen R, Regev D, Hauben DJ. Morphometry of the adult human earlobe: a study of 547 subjects and clinical application. *Plast Reconstr Surg.* 2003;111(7):2398–2402.

### Further reading

Christoffersen M, Frikke-Schmidt R, Schnohr P, Jensen GB, Nordestgaard BG, Tybjærg-Hansen A. Visible age-related signs and risk of ischemic heart disease in the general population. *Circulation* 2014;129:990–998.

De Oliveria Monteiro E. Hyaluronic acid for restoring earlobe volume. *Skin Med.* 2006;5(6):293–294.

Farkas LG. Anthropometry of the normal and defective ear. *Clin Plast Surg.* 1990;17:213.

Friedlander AH, López-López J, Velasco-Oretga E. Diagonal ear lobe crease and atherosclerosis: a review of the medical literature and dental implications. *Med Oral Patol Oral Cir Bucal.* 2012;17(1):e153–e159.

Hotta T. Earlobe rejuvenation. *Plast Surg Nurs.* 2011;31(1):39–40.

Jemec BI. Earlobe augmentation. *Aesthetic Plast Surg.* 1986;10:35–36.

Mowlavi A, Meldrum G, Kalkanis J, Wilhelmi BJ, Russell RC, Zook EG. Surgical design and algorithm for correction of earlobe ptosis and pseudoptosis deformity. *Plast Reconstr Surg.* 2005;115(1):290–295.

Mowlavi A, Meldrum D, Wilhelmi B, Zook EG. Incidence of earlobe ptosis and pseudoptosis in patients seeking facial rejuvenation surgery and effects of aging. *Plast Reconstr Surg.* 2004;113(2):712–717.

Mowlavi A, Meldrum DG, Wilhelmi BJ, Zook EG. Effect of face lift on earlobe ptosis and pseudoptosis. *Plast Reconstr Surg.* 2004;114(4):988–991.

Murray CA, Zloty D, Warshawski L. The evolution of soft tissue fillers in clinical practice. *Dermatol Clin.* 2005;23:343–363.

Saedi N, Kaminer MS, Dover JS. Earlobe rejuvenation. *Soft Tissue Augmentation: Procedures in Cosmetic Dermatology.* ed 3. Elsevier, 2012;166–169.

# 27

# Tower technique of filler injection

Gerhard Sattler, Sonja Sattler, Birgit Woerle

## Summary and Key Features

- Previous injection techniques for facial rejuvenation aimed at simply "filling" lines and furrows.

- Volume loss has become an important hallmark of the aging face, thanks to greater knowledge and understanding of how we age.

- New techniques focus on providing structural support and are performed vertically, rather than horizontally.

- The tower technique features 90-degree injections with gradually tapering product deposition as the needle is withdrawn, like placing flat washers in each anatomic level.

- In the vertical supraperiosteal depot technique, small aliquots of filling agent are deposited on the periosteum for maximum support.

- Softer hyaluronic acid formulations are recommended for more superficial injections, whereas more robust and cohesive products may be chosen for deeper implantation.

## Introduction

In the early 1980s, when soft tissue augmentation began its meteoric rise to become one of the most important procedures in cosmetic dermatology, bovine collagen was the only product available, and treatment focused solely on filling lines and furrows that marked the onset and progression of the aging face. Intradermal injections were performed superficially in the epidermal–dermal junction, whereas more stabilized preparations were recommended for "deeper" injections into the dermis. After piercing the surface of the skin, the needle was positioned parallel to the skin; examples of horizontal injections include the multiple puncture or linear threading technique, either singularly or in a fanlike manner.

Further developments in soft tissue augmentation—among them the recognition of the importance of volume loss—have led to a better understanding of what is needed to rejuvenate and restore the individual potential beauty of an aged or "mature" human face. As new materials

have become available and greater anatomic knowledge is gained, clinicians now have a better opportunity to restore volume lost through the aging process using innovative, vertical injection techniques that aim to provide optimal structural support to perform a predictable long-lasting correction of a focal aesthetic deficit.

## Anatomic considerations

Initial treatment approaches for volume restoration did not focus on the existing facial anatomy. As a result, dynamic muscular activity led to pronounced compression of all soft tissues, negatively affecting the superficial appearance of the surface of the skin resulting in a possible overcorrection. With the transition to more vertical injection techniques, augmentation results have become more predictable. However, it has become increasingly obvious that precise knowledge and understanding of the subcutaneous facial anatomy are prerequisites for successful volume restoration in facial rejuvenation.

The facial skin and subcutaneous tissue (referred to as the soft tissue "flap") comprise a dense, superficial formation of connective tissue that makes up the dermis and epidermis, a honeycomb weblike subdermal structure of connective tissue embedded in fat lobules, and muscle, which traverses the soft tissue flap (Fig. 27.1). Anatomic studies show that the immediate subdermal layer contains a large connective tissue network made up of small fat lobules with many septa, whereas the deeper subdermal layer features large fat lobules with only a few septa. Dynamic musculature presents in sometimes overlapping, multiple layers and may even form entire complexes—as in the brow area where the frontalis, corrugator, and orbicularis muscles merge into one complex with the ability to move medially, proximally, and distally (F. Anderhuber, personal communication).

The analysis of the anatomic composition of the connective tissue is of greatest interest in volume augmentation. The soft tissue flap is attached to the underlying bony structure via connective tissue bands called retinacula or *real* retaining ligaments (Fig. 27.2), which show no or very limited elasticity. So-called *false* retaining ligaments—the most important of which include the nasolabial fold, the zygomatic ligament, and the maxillary-buccal ligament (Fig. 27.3)—add to the character of the flap surface. Although false retaining ligaments have no bony attachment, they

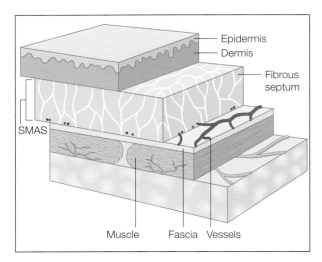

**Figure 27.1** Facial skin and subcutaneous tissue.

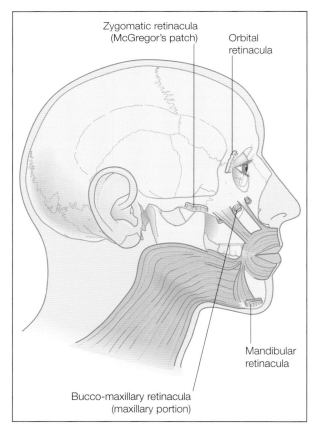

**Figure 27.2** Real retaining ligaments.

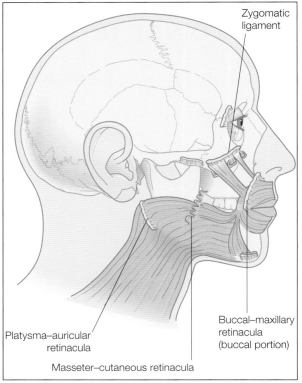

**Figure 27.3** False retaining ligaments.

act in a fence-like manner, compressing dynamic muscular activity and influencing the appearance, shape, and correction of the skin surface.

A brief description of the soft tissue anatomy of the human face is not complete without a discussion of the fat compartments, which are located around and below the eye, in the cheek, and in the perioral region (Fig. 27.4). The suborbicularis oculi fat (SOOF) and retro-orbicularis oculi fat (ROOF) pads are the dominant features of the periorbital region. As the most proximal entity in the midfacial region with the least coverage of musculature structures, the SOOF pad plays a key role in the process of facial aging of the midface and has a direct impact on the clinical presence of the medial and lateral infraorbital hollow. Another important, shape-relevant structure in the submalar area is induced by an indented groove from the medial orbital hollow to the lateral lower midface caused by the zygomatic ligament.

The strongest real retaining ligament in the lower third of the face is the mandibular ligament, which is located at the anterior aspect of the mandible lateral to the chin and anterior to the jowls at the caudal end of the marionette line or so-called prejowl sulcus. Posterior of the marionette line, there is a clinical impression of a descending fat pad of the superficial medial cheek

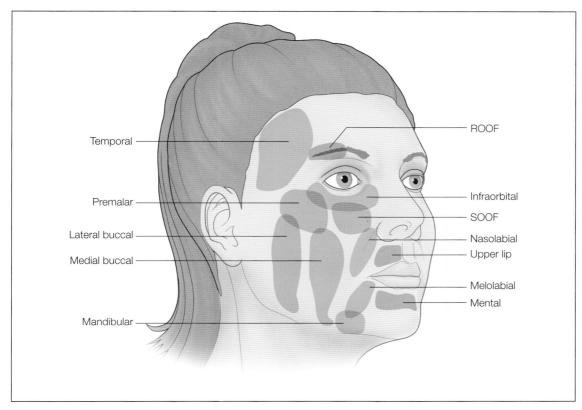

Temporal

Premalar

Lateral buccal

Medial buccal

Mandibular

ROOF

Infraorbital

SOOF

Nasolabial

Upper lip

Melolabial

Mental

**Figure 27.4** Fat compartments of the face. *SOOF,* Suborbicularis oculi fat; *ROOF,* retro-orbicularis oculi fat.

fat that is commonly described as "sagging." Because the superficial cheek fat layer is very cohesive due to the high quantity of connective tissue and therefore does not have the propensity to descend, it is more likely that real retaining ligaments like the mandibular ligament are causing areas of soft tissue atrophy due to surrounding dynamic muscles leading to an effective continuous soft tissue stress by pressure and tension.

This would suggest that age-related elastosis is not the dominant factor in facial aging, but instead the retaining ligaments would promote soft tissue atrophy and are the main cause for the development and existence of wrinkles.

## Biological characteristics of filler materials

Autologous fat or other biodegradable materials, such as hyaluronic acid (HA), calcium hydroxylapatite (CaHA), or poly-L-lactic acid (PLLA), are currently the most frequently used agents in volume replacement soft tissue augmentation. All agents differ with respect to interaction with the recipient site and therapeutic effect in the tissue. In this respect, the main characteristics of interest include overall duration of effect, neocollagenesis, and water retention.

## Autologous fat

Although autologous fat is usually harvested from a tumescent donor site, the hydrated fat tissue will dehydrate after injection at the recipient site. Owing to the microanatomic structure of fat tissue, injections must be performed using 18-gauge cannulas, or larger. After transplant, neofibrogenesis and neocollagenesis occur; no significant additional water retention can be observed.

## Hyaluronic acid

Multiple formulations of HA are currently available for different purposes in soft tissue augmentation. For volume replacement, preparations with concentrations of 20 to 24 mg/mL are produced. Aside from the primary effect of volume contribution through implantation of the physical material, HA leads to marked water retention generated by osmosis; this additional accumulation of fluid due to the binding capacity of the filler leads to a biological change in the atrophied subcutaneous tissues, wherein the rehydration at the site of injection is followed by a secondary redistribution of subcutaneous fluids. Theoretically, shrunken and atrophied fat lobules—from severely diminished blood supply during the aging process—will reinflate (F. Anderhuber, personal communication). In 2007 Wang et al.[1] found that degradation depends on the stabilization of HA; highly stabilized products can produce a secondary neocollagenesis.

## Calcium hydroxylapatite

CaHA is a long-lasting, biodegradable filler that can also accumulate water but only to approximately 10% of the amount that HA is capable. The persistence of its augmentative effect is due to the mass of filler material injected, which, as it degrades only slowly, affords long-term correction, also due to neofibrogenesis.

## Poly-L-lactic acid

PLLA induces neofibrogenesis and leads to a reinforcement of connective tissue fibers that have undergone the process of elastosis. The interaction between tissue and filler material spurs the production of new collagen fibers by fibroblasts without any relevant fluid retention.

## New concepts in injection techniques

Soft tissue volume correction of the mature face has to respect a regenerative treatment of all levels of tissue that are involved in the aging process. Accordingly, correction of soft tissue volume deficiencies needs to address the underlying structural support at all levels and compartments, as well as the surface defects, respecting anatomic identities and their influence on dynamic three- and four-dimensional aspects. Vertical injections, such as the tower technique (TT) and the vertical supraperiosteal depot technique (VSDT), offer the best control for an exact and predictable soft tissue augmentation approach.

## The tower technique

TT—to be used with HA fillers alone—is a novel method of soft tissue augmentation that reintroduces structural support that has been lost through lipodystrophy and bone resorption. Horizontal layers of tissue (fascia, connective tissue, muscle, fat, and dermis) are attached to each other with a limited lateral flexibility. The TT deposits small amounts of HA in the tissue planes, like multiple flat washers between each layer (Fig. 27.5). By injecting filler vertically (90 degrees to the base of the injection site) and gradually tapering product deposition as the needle is withdrawn, the clinician is able to build towers or columns of HA that serve as scaffolds for the overlying soft tissue structures, thus creating a deep base of support that extends through the entire subcutis.

The clinician gathers up the area to be injected between the thumb and second finger of the nondominant hand. A 24- to 27-gauge, half-inch (1.25-cm) needle is inserted perpendicular to the skin at the desired depth based on the anatomic location (Table 27.1). After reassuring that the needle has not been placed in a vessel, the plunger is

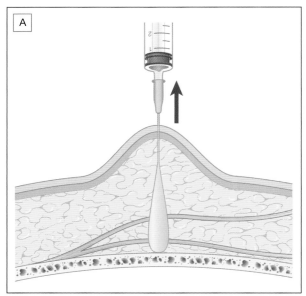

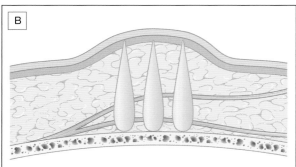

**Figure 27.5** The Tower Technique: The vertically directed injection technique uses a retrograde application of filler material starting from the supraperiosteal level and while withdrawing the needle, small amounts of filler is applied. This can be performed as a singular manoever (A) or as a geometrical arrangement (B).

**Table 27.1**   Injection depth based on anatomic location

| Treatment area | Depth |
| --- | --- |
| Lateral brow | Periosteum |
| Infraorbital hollow | Periosteum |
| Cheek | Deep subcutis |
| Zygomatic ligament | Deep subcutis |
| Nasolabial folds | Deep subcutis |
| Inferior marionnette lines | Periosteum |
| Superior marionnette lines | Deep subcutis |
| Prejowl sulcus | Periosteum |
| Chin | Periosteum |

pressed with light pressure, so HA is slowly injected as the needle is withdrawn vertically, using ever-decreasing amounts of product to create a pyramid-like support with a larger volume of HA deposited at the base and a gradual tapering of product deposition (see Fig. 27.5A). The towers are usually placed in a line along the fold or groove, with each injection approximately 0.5 to 1 cm apart (see Fig. 27.5B).

The columns are self-supporting, floating in the soft tissue plane without any additional support required, although the technique is best used in areas with underlying bony landmarks, a thick subcutis, or a thicker overlying dermis. As such, the TT is recommended to fill nasolabial folds and marionette lines, revolumize the chin and prejowl sulcus, and add volume to the lateral brow and cheek. Thin-skinned areas, such as the periorbital area, are unlikely to tolerate a more superficial placement of HA; it is best to avoid placement in the superficial dermis to avoid the Tyndall effect. Other areas that may be less amenable include the glabella, nasal dorsum, and the lips, although it is possible to use submuscular injections into the white part of the upper or lower lip for more controlled augmentation.

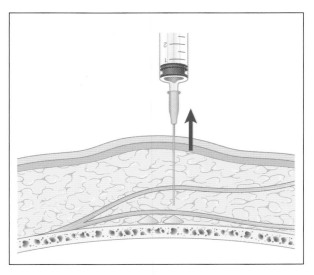

**Figure 27.6** The vertical supraperiosteal depot technique (VSDT).

| Pearl 1 |
| --- |
| Vertical injections in the real mandibular retaining ligaments will elongate the ligaments, thus creating a continuous jawline. |

## Vertical supraperiosteal depot technique

In comparison to the TT, the VSDT features vertical injections directly on the bone, or more precisely, on the periosteum (Fig. 27.6). As in the TT, the clinician grasps the area to be injected between thumb and forefinger of the nondominant hand for maximum penetration and pierces the skin at the thinnest entry point with a 27-gauge half-inch needle, using a 90-degree angle. After repositioning the cannula at the level of the bone and advancing slowly below the soft tissues, the augmenting agent can be deposited in aliquots of 0.02 to 0.1 mL at each injection point, depending on the depth of the defect, with a distance of up to 5 mm between injection sites.

Because of the bony support, only a minimal amount of filler is needed to have a pronounced correction on the surface of the skin ("sweet spot"), as can be observed in the area of the orbital hollow over the medial part of the orbital rim (Fig. 27.7) or the zygomatic bone. Using small amounts of filling agent reduces the incidence of overcorrection and risk of associated side effects. Other areas that may benefit from the VSDT include

the upper orbital rim just below the brow, the dorsal area of the nose, the mandibular bone, and the entire forehead.

## Injection tips and posttreatment recommendations

In areas without sufficient underlying firm anatomy, as in the cheek and perioral region, both techniques can be used with the additional intraoral placement of the contralateral indicator finger for an "in-oral" support, as well as for control and correct placement of the filler material. To achieve the desired results, HA fillers should be placed below the dynamic musculature, particularly in the perioral region for the volumetric correction of the nasolabial fold, marionette lines, and the upper and lower lips. Softer HA gels are recommended for more superficial use, whereas the more robust or cohesive products can be chosen for deeper volumizing implantations.

Careful and cautious manual massage of the treated sites after augmentation will help distribute the filler material evenly and allow the clinician to gauge the extent of correction and check for untreated areas. After treatment, the patient should be advised to apply continuous light pressure for 10 to 15 minutes in the area of the treatment. However, the minimal injection points and limited subcutaneous movement of the needle keep the level of discomfort low and reduce the risk of bruising or other damage caused by tissue trauma.

Three-dimensional augmentation using vertical injection techniques and biodegradable or semibiodegradable agents is a long-term commitment with multiple treatment sessions required to optimize and sustain the

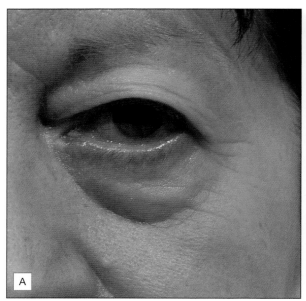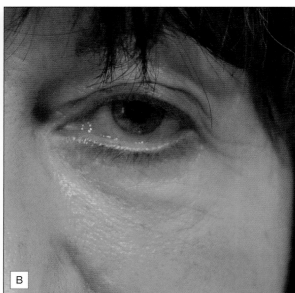

**Figure 27.7** Infraorbital hollow before and after treatment with hyaluronic acid (HA) and the vertical supraperiosteal depot technique (VSDT). (A) 60 year old female showing a severe condition of infra orbital hollowness, marked tear trough deformity with atrophy of the sub orbicular-occular fat pocket (SOOF) and pronounced condition of the lateral palpebral groove. (B) 1 year post after a single treatment by using highly stabilized HA filler injected with a vertical injection technique. Along the orbital rim, 7 injections of a total of 0,3 cc were performed. In the mid-pupillar line in the area of the SOOF, 0,7 cc of HA was injected slowly into the fatpad and then massaged very carefully.

cosmetic result. In the first year, two to four treatments may be necessary; after complete restoration and patient satisfaction have been achieved, one follow-up treatment per year is usually all that is needed to maintain the result, which will eventually become permanent. Combination therapy with botulinum toxin markedly supports the effect of augmentation procedures.

The most common injection-related side effects include bruising and swelling. Severe bruising can be avoided by persistent compression. More severe bleeding can lead to an extensive hematoma lasting for up to 2 months, which can be troublesome for the patient. Postinjection swelling is common, particularly after treatment with HA fillers. A dramatically swollen appearance is often alarming. Using lower total volumes and advising patients to sleep with the head elevated will do much to alleviate the incidence of edema.

**Pearl 2**

Postinjection hematomas or deep bruising lasting 1 to 2 weeks can be avoided or diminished by focused manual compression for more than 10 min.

**Pearl 3**

The use of blunt cannulas can reduce or even eliminate bruising and may be considered in patients with immediate appointments or other work-related functions following treatment.

**Pearl 4**

High volumes up to 5 mL of a 20 mg/mL HA filler per session should not be exceeded.

Serious complications in facial augmentation are extremely rare when the correct filler materials are used. However, the theoretical possibility of an intravascular injection exists and happens more often than one would like. If HA has been used as the augmenting agent, immediate injection of hyaluronidase directly into the vessel or in the area of the thrombotic situation is advised. Similarly, biofilm-like inflammatory reactions to HA fillers may lead to a firm swelling and tissue reaction, as well as a moderate rise in tissue temperature. Treatment includes focal injection of hyaluronidase in the area of swelling, and the addition of antiinflammatory and antibiotic therapy administered accordingly.

## CASE STUDY 1

A 58-year-old woman requests aesthetic improvement around and below her eyes to alleviate what she feels is a "tired" look. A shy woman, she has contemplated facial rejuvenation for a long time but has been too embarrassed to ask. She refuses a major surgical procedure, such as a facelift, but is interested in something less invasive to improve her outward appearance. Examination shows a marked blepharochalasis of the upper lids and severe loss of volume in the lower eyelid and midface areas. Furthermore, the patient exhibits clearly visible horizontal forehead lines and glabellar fold, lipohypertrophy of the lower eyelids, a deep and pronounced nasolabial fold, and severe marionette lines. Multiple, hypertrophic nevi on both cheeks are evident.

Treatment begins with 4 mL HA (Juvéderm Voluma) injected into each side of the midface region using the vertical supra-periosteal depot injection technique, with another 2 mL injected using the TT into the nasolabial fold and marionette lines. Superficial rhytides in those areas are treated with a lighter HA product (Juvéderm Ultra II). A total of 50 U botulinum toxin type A (BoNT-A; BOTOX Cosmetic) is injected into the glabella,

both eyebrows, the lateral canthal rhytides, midforehead, and the chin. Approximately 1 month later the patient returns for an additional 1 mL of HA (Juvéderm Voluma) into each side of the residual existing zygomatic ligaments using the TT. After another month the treating clinician performs a bilateral upper eyelid blepharoplasty and removal of four nevi in both cheeks and right upper lip, under local anesthesia. The stitches are removed after 5 days. The following month, the patient receives another touch-up of 2 mL HA (Juvéderm Voluma) in the cheeks, zygomatic ligaments, nasolabial folds, and marionette lines, along with treatment of superficial wrinkles using 1 mL of lower-viscosity HA (Juvéderm Ultra II). Botulinum toxin follows, with another 50 U in the glabella, eyebrows, lateral canthal rhytides, midforehead, and chin. Two injections of 0.3 mL hyaluronidase, spaced 1 month apart, are required in the very superficial aspect of each tear trough and zygomatic ligament. The patient receives a total of five treatment sessions in 5 months, with follow-up 1 year later (Fig. 27.8).

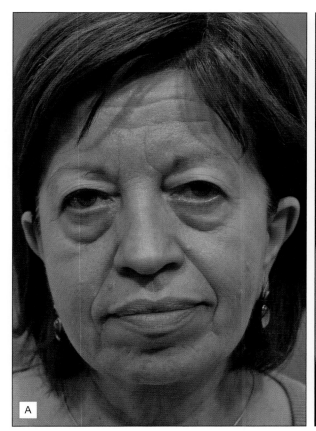 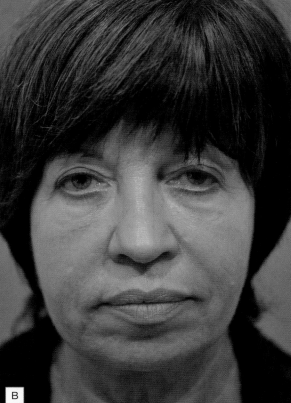

**Figure 27.8** Patient before (A) and at 1-year follow-up (B) after a total of five treatments between May and October 2010.

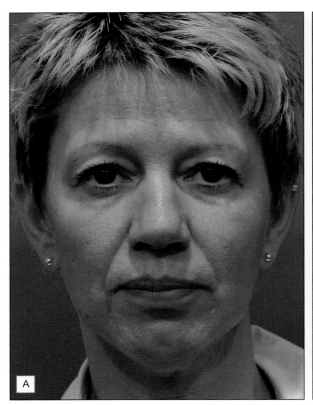
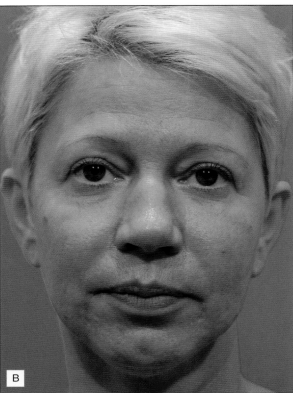

**Figure 27.9** Woman before (A) and after (B) treatment with botulinum toxin (glabella, brows, canthal rhytides, chin), hyaluronic acid (HA) augmentation (cheek, nasolabial folds, marionette lines), and upper lid blepharoplasty.

### CASE STUDY 2

A 41-year-old female who considers herself "an early ager" wants to improve her appearance and receives a total of four injectable treatments: three treatments of 50 U per session of BoNT-A (Xeomin) in the area of the glabella, brows, lateral canthal rhytides, and the chin; and soft tissue augmentation of the cheek with 4 mL of high-viscosity HA (Belotero Intense; VSDT), plus an additional 8 mL of lower-viscosity HA (Belotero Basic) to fill the nasolabial folds and marionette lines using the TT. To complete her rejuvenation, the patient undergoes an upper blepharoplasty under local anesthetic (Fig. 27.9).

### Pearl 5

In severe cases, treatment regimens encompass a multistep approach, with a preferred injection interval of 2 to 4 months.

### Conclusion

Soft tissue augmentation nowadays has changed from a fairly simple, superficial wrinkle treatment to an extensive facial restoration process with a high potential for

### CASE STUDY 3

A 62-year-old male has the impression that his outward appearance looks too "hard" and does not reflect his romantic emotionality. He requests a softer, more attractive look (Fig. 27.10). He receives a total of five treatment sessions performed at intervals of approximately 2 months. Invasive procedures include surgeries (an upper blepharoplasty, a subcision of the submental fold, and multiple nevi excisions), and ablative carbon dioxide laser resurfacing of his lower eyelids (Fraxel repair). The TT and VSDT are used to augment his face with different formulations of HA (Restylane, Perlane, and SubQ) to a total of 14 mL in the cheeks, nasolabial folds, lower eyelid margins, and marionette lines. In addition, BoNT-A (Xeomin) is administered three times, 50 U per session, in the glabella, forehead, brows, lateral canthal rhytides, and chin.

superior results. Modern filling agents capable of creating volume can be combined with innovative vertical injection techniques layered between soft tissue or deposited in aliquots directly on the periosteum to provide exceptional support and pronounced, long-lasting correction that excisional facelift surgery will never be able to generate.

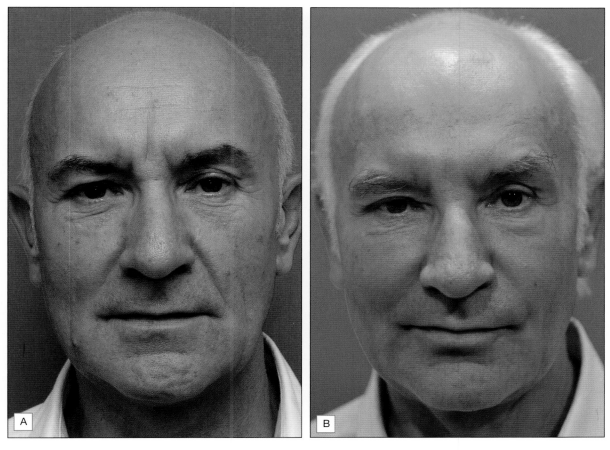

**Figure 27.10** Male patient before (A) and after (B) five treatment sessions including surgery, laser resurfacing, and soft tissue augmentation using the tower and vertical supraperiosteal depot techniques.

## Reference

1. Wang F, Garza LA, Kang S, et al. In vivo stimulation of de novo collagen production caused by cross-linked hyaluronic acid dermal filler injections in photodamaged human skin. *Arch Dermatol.* 2007;143(2):155–163.

## Further reading

Bartus CL, Sattler G, Hanke CW. The tower technique: a novel technique for the injection of hyaluronic acid fillers. *J Drugs Dermatol.* 2011;10:1277–1280.

Coleman SR, Grover R. The anatomy of the aging face: volume loss and changes in 3-dimensional topography. *Aesthet Surg J.* 2006;26(1S):S4–S9.

Donofrio LM. Fat distribution: a morphologic study of the aging face. *Dermatol Surg.* 2000;26:1107–1112.

Rohrich RJ, Pessa JE. The retaining system of the face: histologic evaluation of the septal boundaries of the subcutaneous fat compartments. *Plast Reconstr Surg.* 2008;121:1804–1809.

Sattler G, Gout U. *Illustrated Guide to Injectable Fillers.* Hanover Park, IL: Quintessence Publishing Group; 2015. ISBN 978-1-85097-251-8.

Sattler G, Sommer B. *Bildatlas der Ästhetischen Augmentationsverfahren mit Fillern.* Marburg: KVM Dr Kolster Verlags-GmbH; 2010.

Sattler G, Sommer B, Kolster BC. *Filler in der Ästhetischen Medizin (Patientenratgeber).* Marburg: KVM Dr Kolster Verlags-GmbH; 2010.

Shaw RB Jr, Katzel EB, Koltz PF, et al. Aging of the facial skeleton: aesthetic implications and rejuvenation strategies. *Plast Reconstr Surg.* 2011;127:374–383.

# 28

# Vascular compromise

## Katie Beleznay, Derek Jones

### Summary and Key Features

- Soft tissue fillers are generally very well tolerated. However, serious vascular complications, including blindness, can occur.
- When filler is injected into blood vessels, ischemic or embolic phenomena may result.
- It is important to understand the depth and location of vessels in high-risk sites, such as the glabella and nasal region.
- Strategies to prevent vascular compromise are critical and include using a reversible hyaluronic acid filler, injecting slowly and with minimal pressure, and using a cannula.
- A treatment protocol should be instituted urgently at the first sign of vascular compromise. The goal of treatment is rapid restoration of perfusion.

## Introduction

The use of soft tissue fillers continues to grow in popularity, in part, due to their favorable side-effect profile. However, serious complications can occur. The most feared and potentially serious complications are vascular in nature. It is critical for injecting physicians to have a firm knowledge of the vascular anatomy and to understand key prevention and management strategies.

Vascular complications occur when filler is injected into blood vessels, resulting in ischemic or embolic phenomena. Skin necrosis occurs when the blood supply to the skin is compromised. Typically the first indication of vascular compromise of the skin is painless blanching. This can be subtle and may go unnoticed. Over the following days, progression to a painful, violaceous, reticulated patch may occur (Fig. 28.1). Necrosis and subsequent scarring may develop.

Blindness results from retrograde embolization of filler into the ocular vessels. Visual complications after filler injection may present with immediate unilateral vision loss, ocular pain, headache, nausea, or vomiting. In addition, central nervous system complications, including infarction and hemiplegia, have been seen in association with blindness. In a recent review of the world literature there were 98 cases of blindness reported after filler injection. Autologous fat was the most common filler type to cause this complication, at 48% of the cases. Hyaluronic acid (HA) was the cause in 24% of cases. The most high-risk site was the glabella, followed by the nasal region, nasolabial fold, and forehead, but virtually every anatomic location on the face where filler is injected is at risk for vascular compromise (Fig. 28.2).

## Anatomy

It is important to understand the depth and location of vessels in high-risk sites. In the glabella and forehead the two major arteries are the supratrochlear artery, which is found along the medial canthal vertical line, and the supraorbital artery, which is more lateral in the region of the medial iris (Fig. 28.3). Both of these arteries start out deep and become more superficial approximately 15 to 20 mm above the supraorbital rim as they travel superiorly on the forehead. As such, injections within 2 cm of the supraorbital rim should be superficial. However, injections more superiorly on the forehead should be deep in a supraperiosteal plane to decrease the risk of intravascular injection. In the nasal region there are many anastomotic vessels, and as such filler is most safely placed in the avascular deep supraperiosteal plane. If the patient has had prior surgical procedures to the nose, filler injections should only be performed with extreme caution. The most high-risk blood vessel for compromise in the medial cheek, nasolabial fold, and medial periorbital area is the angular artery. The angular artery has variable patterns after it branches off the facial artery and can be located more superficially in the subcutaneous layer, so it is imperative to be cautious when injecting this region. With the rich vascular supply of the face and multiple anastomoses, it is very important to understand the location of vessels and appropriate depth of injection. If a needle enters a blood vessel and enough pressure is applied to the plunger when injecting filler, the arterial pressure can be overcome and filler can travel retrograde to the ocular vessels causing blindness.

## Prevention

Strategies to prevent vascular compromise are critical because we do not have well-documented successful

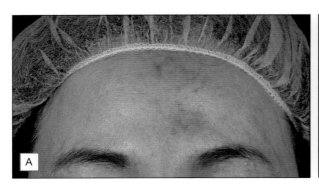
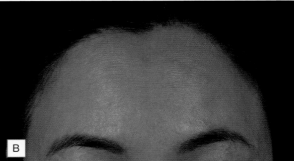

**Figure 28.1** Mottled erythema to forehead, 5 days post injection **(A)**. Resolution of vascular compromise with no sequelae, 2.5 months post injection **(B)**.

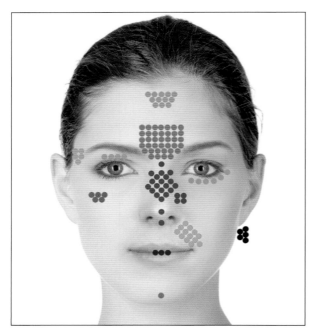

**Figure 28.2** The coloured dots are the location of injection for each case of blindness from filler. The five black dots represent cases in which the location was not specified and listed as "face." *With permission from Beleznay K, Carruthers J, Humphrey S, Jones D. Avoiding and treating blindness from fillers: a review of the world literature.* Dermatol Surg. *2015;41:1097–1117.*

*When injecting autologous fat, many experts recommend using larger 16- to 18-gauge blunt cannulas because small sharp needles and cannulas are more likely to perforate blood vessels. The syringe size should be limited to 1 mL and no more than 0.1 mL of autologous fat should be injected with each pass of the cannula.

treatments, particularly when it comes to ocular complications. First and foremost, having a firm understanding of the facial vascular anatomy and proper depth and plane of injection is important, particularly in high-risk sites, such as the glabella, nasolabial fold, and nose. Choosing a reversible HA filler allows for treatment with hyaluronidase and potential reversal of vascular occlusion if used early. Injecting slowly and using a small-gauge needle or cannula are other strategies to implement. Key prevention strategies are highlighted in Box 28.1.

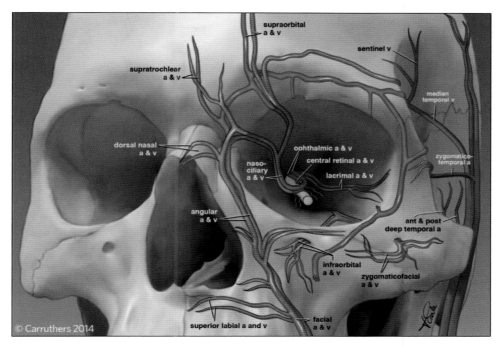

**Figure 28.3** Vascular anatomy of the upper face. *a, Artery; v, vein. Copyright Jean D. Carruthers, MD, 2014.*

## Treatment

Despite implementing prevention strategies, the risk of vascular compromise remains. Treatment should be instituted immediately at the first sign of vascular compromise. However, it is important to recognize that treatment recommendations are not based on a large body of evidence. Injecting physicians should have a treatment protocol in place to be implemented if vascular complications are suspected. The goal of treatment is rapid restoration of perfusion. Key management strategies for vascular compromise with skin sequelae (Box 28.2) and ocular complications (Box 28.3) are reviewed.

If blanching occurs while injecting filler, immediately discontinue the injection. If the complication occurs with an HA filler, hyaluronidase is recommended. Hyaluronidase works to break down and hydrolyze HA. Hyaluronidase has also been shown to have edema-reducing benefits and theoretically can reduce occluded vessel pressure. Animal studies have shown that occlusion after HA injection can be reversed when the hyaluronidase is injected within 4 hours after the occlusion. However, later injection may help to decompress the vessel and aid in healing. Different formulations are available for hyaluronidase, which makes it difficult to establish standardized dosing. Variable doses have been reported from 10 to 30 U per $2 \times 2$ cm$^2$ area along the artery and its branches up to 1500 IU. Further treatments that should be initiated include warm compresses and vigorous massage. Other reported therapies include topical nitroglycerin paste, aspirin, oral prednisone, hyperbaric oxygen, and low-molecular-weight heparin. A thorough individual assessment and treatment plan with close follow-up should be initiated for each patient to optimize outcomes. If necrosis does occur, diligent wound care is critical, and long-term scar management should be addressed.

---

**Box 28.2**
**Treatment of vascular compromise with skin sequelae**

- If blanching occurs, stop the injection immediately.
- Inject hyaluronidase if an HA filler was used.
- Apply warm compresses every 10 min for the first few hours.
- Vigorous massage.
- Consider topical nitroglycerin paste 2%. Can be applied as frequently as every 1–2 h initially.
- Consider aspirin, 325 mg under tongue immediately and 81 mg daily thereafter.
- Consider oral prednisone 20–40 mg daily for 3-5 days.
- In certain cases, consider such therapies as hyperbaric oxygen and low-molecular-weight heparin.
- Follow patient daily until improvement. Provide them with clear care instructions and contact information.

> **Box 28.3**
> **Treatment of vascular compromise with ocular complications**
>
> - If vision changes, ocular pain, headache, nausea, or vomiting occur while injecting filler, stop the injection at once. Immediately contact an ophthalmologist colleague and urgently transfer the patient directly there.
> - Consider treating the injection site and surrounding area with hyaluronidase in the case of an HA filler.
> - Consider retrobulbar injection of 300–600 units (2–4 mL) of hyaluronidase if an HA filler was used.
> - Mechanisms to reduce intraocular pressure should be considered, such as ocular massage, anterior chamber paracentesis, intravenous mannitol, and acetazolamide.

Management of blindness following filler injection is more challenging because there are few reported successful treatments and most commonly vision loss is permanent. In addition, there is a strict timeline because after approximately 90 minutes the damage secondary to the retinal ischemia is more likely to be irreversible.

First and foremost, if the patient complains of ocular pain, vision changes, headache, or nausea, the injection should be stopped at once. The patient should be immediately transferred to an ophthalmologist or oculoplastics colleague. Large volumes of hyaluronidase should be injected at the location of filler injection and surrounding areas if an HA filler was used. It has been shown that hyaluronidase can diffuse through the blood vessel walls without needing to be directly injected into the vessel. If vision loss occurs after an HA filler, retrobulbar injection of hyaluronidase has been proposed as a potential vision-saving treatment. The treatment, as described in the literature, involves an injection of 300 to 600 units of hyaluronidase into the retrobulbar space. The first step is to anesthetize the lateral lower eyelid. A 25-gauge needle is then advanced at this location until it is at least 1 inch in depth. Two to 4 mL of hyaluronidase are injected in the inferolateral orbit (video of retrobulbar injection). Other therapies that have been tried include treatments that will decrease intraocular pressure, including anterior chamber decompression, mannitol, and acetazolamide. Further strategies include hyperbaric oxygen, systemic and local intraarterial fibrinolysis, and oral corticosteroids; however, these treatments have not been proven consistently successful.

Injecting physicians should help to educate their ophthalmic and oculoplastic colleagues about this rare complication and build relationships with them, so if an event occurs they will be ready to help and understand the rationale and the urgency. Further discussion among experts relating their experiences with this complication and management strategies can help to build consensus that will improve patient safety.

## Conclusion

With the increased use of soft tissue augmentation for revolumization, it is imperative to be aware of the risk of devastating vascular complications. To minimize any adverse events, a thorough understanding of facial anatomy and proper injection technique is critical. Key prevention strategies, such as injecting small amounts under low pressure, using smaller needles or cannulas, and injecting slowly, should be implemented. Despite proper technique, the possibility of vascular occlusion and embolization of filler into ocular vessels remains. As such, injectors should have a treatment protocol in place, which should include immediate transfer to an ophthalmologist in the case of ocular complications, and injection of high doses of hyaluronidase if an HA filler was used. Immediate and ongoing care ensures optimal outcomes and decreases the risk of permanent complications.

## Further reading

Alam M, Gladstone H, Kramer EM, et al. ASDS guidelines of care: injectable fillers. *Dermatol Surg*. 2008;34(Suppl 1): S115–S148.

Beleznay K, Carruthers J, Humphrey S, Jones D. Avoiding and treating blindness from fillers: a review of the world literature. *Dermatol Surg*. 2015;41:1097–1117.

Beleznay K, Humphrey S, Carruthers J, Carruthers A. Vascular compromise from soft tissue augmentation: experience with 12 cases and recommendations for optimal outcomes. *J Clin Aesthet Dermatol*. 2014;7:37–43.

Carruthers JD, Fagien S, Rohrich RJ, Weinkle S, Carruthers A. Blindness caused by cosmetic filler injection: a review of cause and therapy. *Plast Reconstr Surg*. 2014;134: 1197–1201.

Coleman SR. Avoidance of arterial occlusion from injection of soft tissue fillers. *Aesthetic Surg J*. 2002;22:555–557.

Dayan S, Arkins JP, Mathison CC. Management of impending necrosis associated with soft tissue filler injections. *J Drugs Dermatol*. 2011;10:1007–1012.

DeLorenzi C. Complications of injectable fillers, Part 2: vascular complications. *Aesthetic Surg J*. 2014;34:584–600.

DeLorenzi C. Complications of injectable fillers, Part I. *Aesthetic Surg J*. 2013;3:561–575.

FDA Safety Communication. *Unintentional Injection of Soft Tissue Filler into Blood Vessels in the Face*. <http://www.fda.gov/medicaldevices/safety/alertsandnotices/ucm448255.htm>. 2015.

Flowers FP, Breza TS. Surgical anatomy of the head and neck. In: Bolognia JL, Jorizzo JL, Schaffer JV, eds. *Dermatology*, ed 3, Philadelphia, China: Elsevier; 2012:2235–2236.

Funt D, Pavicic T. Dermal fillers in aesthetics: an overview of adverse events and treatment approaches. *Clin Cosmet Investig Dermatol*. 2013;6:295–316.

Jones D, Tezel A, Borell M. In-vitro resistance to degradation of HA by ovine testicular hyaluronidase. *Dermatol Surg*. 2010;36(s1):804–809.

Kleintjes WG. Forehead anatomy: arterial variations and venous link of the midline forehead flap. *J Plast Reconstr Aesthet Surg*. 2007;60:593–606.

Larrabee WF, Makielski KH, Henderson JL. *Surgical Anatomy of the Face*. ed 2. Philadelphia, PA: Lippincott Williams & Wilkins; 2004:97–101.

Lazzeri D, Agostini T, Figus M, Nardi M, Pantaloni M, Lazzeri S. Blindness following cosmetic injections of the face. *Plast Reconstr Surg*. 2012;129:994–1012.

Rzany B, DeLorenzi C. Understanding, avoiding, and managing severe filler complications. *Plast Reconstr Surg*. 2015;136;196S–203S.

Saban Y, Andretto Amodeo C, Bouaziz D, Polselli R. Nasal arterial vasculature. Medical and surgical applications. *Arch Facial Plast Surg*. 2012;14:429–436.

Yoshimura K, Coleman SR. Complications of fat grafting how they occur and how to find, avoid, and treat them. *Clin Plast Surg*. 2015;42:383–388.

# 29

# Complications of temporary fillers

Joanna G. Bolton, Sabrina Guillen Fabi

## Summary and Key Features

- Soft tissue augmentation with temporary fillers continues to be among the most commonly performed cosmetic procedures.
- There are a variety of temporary dermal fillers with an ever-increasing number coming to market. As more fillers become available, it is imperative that the aesthetic physician who injects dermal fillers has proper training in their use and understands the differences between them.
- Though generally safe, complications can occur with temporary fillers; physicians need to recognize and manage these complications when they present.
- Such periprocedural adverse events as bruising, swelling, and pain are extremely common and usually resolve in less than 7 days.
- Proper injection technique is crucial to minimize visible and/or symptomatic papules and nodules.
- To minimize the risk of infection and biofilm formation, one should consider a skin preparation using chlorhexidine and/or isopropyl alcohol.
- The cause of granulomatous reaction is multifactorial and may be due to a true foreign body reaction to the particulate or gelatinous filler or to the emergence of a biofilm.
- Early institution of antibiotics, often for a prolonged period, is vital when a patient presents with inflammatory papules and nodules.
- Early recognition of impending necrosis after injection is critical; treatment with hyaluronidase, topical nitroglycerin, and massage may be required.
- Judicious use of injectables requires an appreciation of normal facial anatomy and the changes that occur with the aging process.
- Virtually every anatomic location where filler is injected on the face is at risk for blindness because of the anastomotic nature of the facial vasculature and the end artery morphology of the retinal circulation.
- There is an alarming trend of nonaesthetic physicians and midlevel, nonphysician providers using these products; one may expect to see potential complications in the office.

## Introduction

Soft tissue fillers are used to fill wrinkles and folds, to add volume lost during senescence, to sculpt facial structure, and to correct defects, such as scars and facial lipoatrophy. Soft tissue augmentation using temporary fillers continues to be among the most commonly performed cosmetic procedures. The increasing demand is due to a population demanding facial rejuvenation with less invasive approaches, fast actualization of results, and minimal morbidity. In 2014 approximately 5.5 million injections of temporary filler agents were performed worldwide, representing a significant increase over previous years. Given their favorable safety profiles, effectiveness, and versatility and the availability of multiple filler options, it is expected that the popularity of these products will continue to increase. Despite their impressive safety record, as the number of patients seeking treatment with fillers increases, so do the reports of complications and adverse events. In particular, there has been an alarming trend of increasing numbers of untrained or poorly trained physicians and nonphysicians using these products; therefore one must be prepared to see complications in our offices even if we were not the injector.

Materials approved for soft tissue augmentation can be divided into biodegradable, semibiodegradable, and nonbiodegradable products. These classifications correlate with their duration of effect as being temporary (approximately 6 to 12 months), semipermanent (duration of 18 months or more), or permanent (Box 29.1). As more fillers become available, it is imperative to understand the differences between them, the complications that can occur from each, and how best to avoid and treat them when they do occur.

### Pearl 1

It is imperative that physicians are familiar with the potential complications and management that may result from use of current fillers. As the number of augmentations increases worldwide and with the advent of new filler agents, there is an expected likelihood of increase in complications.

Potential complications associated with temporary soft tissue fillers can be categorized by the time of onset (Box 29.2). In general, adverse events can be subdivided into

---

**Box 29.1**
**Historical and currently available dermal fillers**

- Temporary
  - Bovine collagen (Zyderm, Zyplast)—no longer available.
  - Porcine collagen (Fibrel, Evolence)—no longer available.
  - Human-derived collagen (CosmoDerm, CosmoPlast)—no longer available.
  - Hyaluronic acid (Restylane, Restylane Lyft, Restylane Silk, Juvéderm, Voluma, Volbella, Volift, Belotero Hydro, Belotero Soft, Belotero Intense, Belotero Volume, Belotero Balance, Emervel Touch, Emervel Classic, Emervel Lips, Emervel Deep, Emervel Volume, Elevess/Hydrelle, Captique, Hylaform, Prevelle Silk).
  - Calcium hydroxylapatite (Radiesse).
  - Autologous fat.
- Semipermanent
  - Poly-L-lactic acid (Sculptra).
  - Autologous fibroblasts (Fibrocell).
- Permanent
  - Collagen + polymethylmethacrylate (Artecoll/Artefill/Bellafill).
  - Silicone (Adato SIL-OL 5000, NY; Silikon 1000).
  - Hydroxyethylmethacrylate/ethylmethacrylate fragments and hyaluronic acid (Dermalive).
  - Polyacrylamide hydrogel (Aquamid).

---

**Box 29.2**
**Onset of adverse events**

**Acute (occurring up to 1 week after treatment)**
Injection site reactions.
Nodules.
Infection.
Hypersensitivity.
Tissue necrosis.
Blindness.

**Delayed (occurring from weeks to years after treatment)**
Infection.
Biofilm formation.
Granuloma formation.

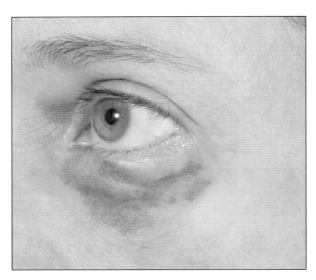

**Figure 29.1** Severe periocular ecchymosis 7 days following injection of hyaluronic acid deep into the supraperiosteal fat pads.

is exceedingly low. Delayed reactions are related to the product itself or the interaction between the filler and the host response. They are usually manifested by persistent erythema, swelling, nodules, and indurations developing months to years after. The nature of these reactions and their treatment will be summarized in this chapter.

## Injection site reactions

The most common adverse events associated with fillers are local injection site reactions, manifested by tenderness, erythema, and edema. They are typically mild, localized, and transient, resolving within 4 to 7 days. A study by Brandt et al. evaluating the efficacy and safety of biphasic hyaluronic acid Restylane and Perlane in the lower face revealed that the majority of patients treated with both small and large gel-particle hyaluronic acid experienced at least one injection site reaction. The reported events in decreasing order of occurrence consisted of bruising, tenderness, swelling, and redness. In another study comparing hyaluronic acid (Restylane) with collagen (Zyplast) for the treatment of nasolabial folds in contralateral sides, injection site reactions occurred at 93.5% and 90.6% of the hyaluronic acid and collagen treated sites, respectively. The bruising can be severe, especially in patients who have taken antiplatelet agents, such as aspirin or nonsteroidal antiinflammatory agents, as shown in Fig. 29.1.

acute and delayed reactions. Acute, or early, reactions are procedural or related to injection technique. They are usually transient and are manifested by erythema, edema, ecchymosis, pruritus, and pain in the first week after injection. Although blindness and hearing impairment are catastrophic potential acute complications, the risk

**Pearl 2**

Most patients will develop a local injection site reaction: erythema, edema, or ecchymosis. They are usually transient and resolve in the first week after injection. Make patients aware of this before injecting them.

## Pain

Pain during injection is often one of the commonly reported adverse events associated with filler agents. Pain is often attributable to hydrostatic dissection of tissue during injection, as well as the discomfort of numerous needle punctures during the implantation of the product. Certain anatomic sites, such as the lips and perioral region, are more sensitive as a result of increased sensory innervation of these sites. A number of techniques may be used to minimize the pain associated with injections. These include the use of topical anesthetics, local anesthetics ("numbing dots"), application of ice before and after injection, and vibratory distraction. Some clinicians also use infraorbital and mental nerve blocks. Placement of small aliquots of lidocaine along a few points of the gingival sulcus has also been found to be beneficial in minimizing pain associated with injections of the lips. A number of fillers have now packaged the filler syringe premixed with lidocaine.

### Pearl 3

Pretreatment of the site with a topical mixture of betacaine, lidocaine, and tetracaine 30 minutes prior to treatment and the use ice pretreatment can minimize pain associated with injections.

## Edema and ecchymosis

Some of the most common postprocedural adverse events are bruising and swelling secondary to local trauma from the injection (see Fig. 29.1). Reviewing all medications and supplements with the patient can minimize the degree of edema and ecchymosis. Avoidance of agents that inhibit coagulation is recommended, including aspirin (unless taking for "therapeutic" indications) and nonsteroidal antiinflammatory medications, as well as supplements, such as garlic and *ginkgo biloba*, that have an inhibitory effect on platelets. Other supplements, such as vitamin E, niacin (vitamin B3), fish oil, glucosamine, ginger, ginseng, green tea, chamomile, and celery root, can inhibit coagulation pathways and further increase bleeding and bruising. It is recommended to withhold these supplements at least 5 days prior to treatment.

### Pearl 4

Avoiding anticoagulants that are not medically necessary and a thorough pretreatment review of all supplements will minimize posttreatment ecchymosis and edema. Therapeutic aspirin or other anticoagulants, such as warfarin, clopidogrel, or dabigatran, should not be discontinued because the risk outweighs the benefit.

Bruising can often be minimized by choosing the injectable filler least likely to cause this problem, as well as minimizing the number of injection points and using a smaller-gauge needle when possible. Collagen-based fillers were less likely to cause ecchymosis secondary to their inherent platelet-aggregating properties. However, they are not available at the time of this writing. Conversely, it has been suggested that hyaluronic acid fillers have an anticoagulant effect and can cause more swelling and bruising because they are structurally similar to heparin.

During the injection, signs of bleeding must be carefully monitored. Immediate pressure and posttreatment cold packs should be applied to these areas. Some injectors incorporate blunt-tipped cannulas in certain treatment areas, which, theoretically, have a lower chance of traumatizing blood vessels and negate the need for multiple injection points. Nonetheless, bruising is still often a reality in many filler patients.

When bruising occurs there are a few things that can be used to minimize the degree and duration of the ecchymosis. Some advocate supplements, such as bromelain and homeopathic arnica, in reducing posttreatment ecchymosis. Bromelain has been shown to decrease vascular permeability in animal models by lowering the levels of bradykinin, thereby potentially resulting in less edema, pain, and inflammation. Helenalin, an extract of arnica, has been shown to possess antiinflammatory effects and inhibits platelet function in vitro. Patients may also start arnica before the procedure.

Clinical studies of both these compounds have provided conflicting results, with some revealing a decrease in posttreatment bruising, whereas others show no statistical difference. A comprehensive review by Waldorf et al. concluded there are insufficient data to routinely support use of arnica and bromelain to prevent and/or treat postprocedure ecchymosis and edema. Their review included published clinical trials using oral and topical arnica and oral bromelain. No studies on topical bromelain were found. Based upon the authors' review of the literature, the beneficial effects of arnica and bromelain, if observed, were best demonstrated when administered preoperatively and continued 1 to 4 days postoperatively. Further investigations are recommended to substantiate their efficacy and safety.

Aside from these "natural" remedies, some physicians choose to minimize posttreatment ecchymosis by using their vascular laser at subpurpuric treatment settings (lower fluences; pulse durations of 3 to 6 ms). Settings we have found useful with the pulsed dye laser (PDL) (Vbeam Perfecta, Syneron Candela) are 10 mm spot, 6.0 to 8.5 J/$cm^2$, 6 ms pulse duration with dynamic cooling (40/30) for 1 to 2 passes or stacking 2 pulses. When the bruise is dark purple, stacking pulses is not recommended out of concern for bulk heating. With milder bruising, pulses may be stacked with a 2- to 3-second delay in between. PDL can be used immediately upon discovering an ecchymosis (same day as filler treatment) or within the first few days after filler injection, as long as the bruising is still purple in color (due to the presence of deoxyhemoglobin). After the bruise starts to fade to green (biliverdin), then to orange-yellow (bilirubin), PDL is no longer effective due to the absence of the target chromophore. PDL may be used in most skin types, although longer pulse durations and lower fluences are generally preferred with darker skin tones.

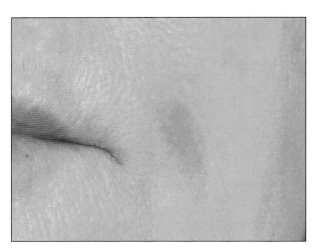

**Figure 29.2** The Tyndall effect is shown following injection of the hyaluronic acid Restylane intradermally in the superior modiolus.

Adverse effects of PDL may include transient erythema and mild edema. Importantly, patients must understand that PDL treatment will accelerate the resolution of a bruise but will not make it instantly disappear.

## Nodules and papules

Inappropriate placement of fillers may result in the development of subcutaneous nodules and papules. The majority of these are manifested as palpable and/or visible bumps under the skin. Injecting too superficially can lead to lumps of visible product or bluish bumps under the skin explained by the Tyndall effect with hyaluronic acid fillers (Fig. 29.2). Such reactions can for the most part be prevented by use of correct technique. Treatment of visible papules can often be accomplished by firm digital pressure, by aspiration, or by incision and drainage. When persistent papules and nodules are due to the use of a hyaluronic acid filler, the enzyme hyaluronidase can be used to treat them. Vanaman et al. provide a concise review of expert recommendations for hyaluronidase dosing and indications.

| Pearl 5 |
| --- |
| When using hyaluronidase derived from an ovine or bovine source for nonemergent complications, such as overcorrection, superficial implantation, or inflammatory reactions, skin testing is considered optional but is recommended because there have been reports of sensitivity to the animal-derived enzyme. For emergent complications, such as vascular occlusion, hyaluronidase manufactured from a human recombinant source (Hylenex, Halozyme Therapeutics, Inc.) is the safest product to use because immediate, larger volumes are typically required, and a pretest is of less concern. Bedside availability of epinephrine is advisable with the use of any hyaluronidase when there is no pretest. |

Historically, the incidence of injection site nodules from temporary fillers appears to be higher in patients receiving poly-L-lactic acid (PLLA; Sculptra), particularly in the human immunodeficiency virus (HIV)-infected population. In early clinical studies conducted in Europe, nodules at the site of injection that were asymptomatic, palpable, but generally not visible were described in approximately 30% to 50% of patients, and without treatment they tended to persist for months to years. Subsequent studies in the United States reported a lower incidence of PLLA papules and nodules, occurring in approximately 6% to 13% of patients. In a more recent study comparing PLLA with collagen for the correction of nasolabial fold rhytides in non-HIV-infected patients, papules less than 5 mm in diameter occurred in 8.6% of patients receiving PLLA and 3.4% of those receiving collagen. Nodules greater than 5 mm diameter occurred in 6.9% of subjects receiving PLLA and 6.0% of subjects receiving collagen. The literature now reveals most of the early problems encountered with PLLA resulted from suboptimal methodology, in part from inadequate on-label reconstitution with 5 mL of sterile water for injection (SWFI), short powder hydration times, and subsequent injection of highly concentrated product.

Therefore, in recent years, Narins and others have recommended changes in the protocol for product reconstitution, hydration, and administration that have helped limit this potential complication. Current consensus recommendations state that PLLA should be reconstituted ≥24 hours prior to injection with approximately 7 to 8 mL of SWFI or bacteriostatic water, with 1 to 2 mL of lidocaine added at the time of injection. Dilution in this volume range leads to even PLLA distribution, easier injection, with reduced risk of needle blockage, and decreased incidence of papules and nodules. Product placement in the appropriate deep injection planes will also help minimize nodules. Fig. 29.3 shows a visible periocular papule following too-superficial placement of PLLA using an older dilution technique. For injection of the cheek, preauricular area, nasolabial folds, and lower face, injection should be into the deeper subcutaneous plane. For treatment of the temples, PLLA should be injected beneath the temporalis fascia, and for injection of the zygoma, maxilla, and mandibular regions, depot injection in the subperiosteal plane is desired. Care should be taken not to inject the precipitate at the end of the syringe. Following implantation, vigorous massage of the treatment area with instructions for the patient to massage at home is recommended. The posttreatment "rule of 5s" is easy for the patients to remember: massage 5 times per day, for 5 minutes, for 5 days. However, data supporting posttreatment massage are limited and may be of less concern with the updated consensus recommendations for reconstitution and administration.

Even with recent alterations in protocol to minimize this complication, papules and nodules may still occur, as illustrated by a case report of a woman who developed numerous nodules 3 years after PLLA injections. This

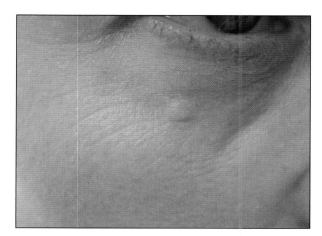

**Figure 29.3** An obvious small noninflamed papule in the periocular region following injection of PLLA. An older, more concentrated dilution technique was used and the product placed too superficially. This nodule was subsequently excised and showed particles of PLLA and no inflammation.

may be more likely due to a delayed foreign body reaction or a reaction to a latent infectious process rather than to product placement. It is important to note that the incidence of nodules is greater in areas where PLLA is able to aggregate in the muscle, which include highly mobile or dynamic areas, such as the perioral and periocular regions, as well as the hands and neck because of the proximity between the platysma and the skin; therefore differences in regional thickness of skin should be considered when injecting PLLA. Diligence is needed when injecting these sites, and treatment should not be performed by novice injectors.

A retrospective chart review of 4702 Juvéderm Voluma (HA-V) treatments revealed 23 patients (0.5%) developed delayed-onset nodules, with a median time from injection to reaction of 4 months. The most common nodule locations were the melomental folds and the midface. Nine of the 23 (39%) had an identifiable immunologic trigger, such as flulike illness, dental procedure, or trauma before the nodule onset. In their study Beleznay et al. noted a median time to resolution of 6 weeks. First-line therapies to consider include watchful waiting, intralesional triamcinolone or hyaluronidase, and oral prednisone.

Although triggering events from infectious agents or trauma likely play a role in nodule development after HA-V injection, evidence suggests that hyaluronic acid on its own plays a role in activating the immune system. In particular, when there is a higher proportion of low-molecular-weight (LMW) (<1 mDa) hyaluronic acid and a minority of high-molecular-weight (HMW) (≥1 mDa) hyaluronic acid, as is the case with HA-V. Published data suggest that HMW hyaluronic acid is mostly antiinflammatory, whereas LMW hyaluronic acid is proinflammatory and triggers the immune system. The addition of LMW hyaluronic acid chains significantly improves the efficiency

of hyaluronic acid cross-linking, resulting in a highly cohesive gel with longer duration and ability for greater lift. However, it is believed that when HA-V is injected into a predisposed individual, an overactive immune response may ensue, contributing to delayed nodules. Hyaluronic acid fragments of low-to-intermediate size have been shown to activate macrophages and dendritic cells and deliver costimulatory signals to T cells via their primary cell surface receptor, CD44, or TLR4.

Beleznay et al. acknowledge that although HA-V has a higher proportion of LMW hyaluronic acid, it is not known whether this proportion on its own is more inflammatory compared with other products. It is known that during inflammation there is an increased breakdown of HA. Theoretically it is possible that 3 to 5 months after injection, there is an increased breakdown of hyaluronic acid, exposing LMW hyaluronic acid fragments, which coincides with the time most inflammatory nodules are observed. Thus the short-chain composition of HA-V may serve to highlight the active immunologic properties of hyaluronic acids previously thought to be structurally inert. Additional research is needed to evaluate this mechanism further; however, the proposed etiology of delayed nodules does fit with the successful management that has been observed in practice. Interestingly, the authors noted the majority of patients who developed delayed-onset nodules, and were subsequently retreated with HA-V, did not experience repeated episodes.

> **Pearl 6**
>
> Calcium hydroxylapatite (Radiesse) injected too superficially can result in visible white nodules. These can usually be treated by puncturing the nodules with a no. 11 blade or needle and then expressing the contents. As a result of the thin skin in the tear trough, a higher incidence of nodule formation may occur when treating the nasojugal sulcus.

## Inflammation (hypersensitivity reactions)

With the exception of autologous fat, all soft tissue augmentation agents are composed of foreign body material. As a result, varying degrees of immune system reactivity can occur. It is important to be able to recognize inflammatory reactions and manage them.

Prior to the introduction of hyaluronic acids in 2004, the most common agent for soft tissue augmentation was bovine collagen in the form of Zyderm 1, Zyderm 2, and Zyplast. Given its animal source, it could be immunogenic, resulting in allergic reactions. Two separate skin tests were recommended to test for sensitivity because 3% of the population may develop a delayed hypersensitivity response. In other studies it has been reported that the incidence of foreign body reactions is approximately 1.3%. Allergic reactions to bovine collagen may be treated with topical, intralesional, or a brief course of systemic corticosteroids, or other topical immunomodulators, such as tacrolimus.

To avoid the risk of hypersensitive adverse reactions to bovine collagen, human-based collagen was then generated for injection. Obtained from human donor tissues, CosmoDerm and CosmoPlast were the most frequently used agents within this class. There are very few cases of true hypersensitivity reactions to human-derived collagen fillers. However, one must be aware that it may still rarely be possible. There are some physicians who favor collagen products and some patients who still request it for their augmentation; however, it was not available at the time of this publication.

Hyaluronic acid is one of the components of the extracellular matrix of the dermis and has no organ or species specificity. When introduced to the market, non-animal stabilized hyaluronic acid (NASHA) compounds were thought to have been considered to be nonimmunogenic. Indeed, in spite of its frequent use for cosmetic reasons, there are very few descriptions of hypersensitivity reactions secondary to injections of hyaluronic acid. A case of circulating antibodies against hyaluronic acid in patients after several injections was reported; however, these findings could not be confirmed by other investigators. In a randomized clinical trial using Restylane and Perlane, researchers failed to detect clinical or laboratory evidence for elicitation of humoral (type I hypersensitivity) or cell-mediated (delayed type IV hypersensitivity) immunity to NASHA in the majority of patients treated. At most, it is estimated by some experts that one in every 10,000 individuals undergoing augmentation with these materials reports a clinical hypersensitivity reaction. Many now feel, based on their clinical course and response to treatment, that a number of these reported hypersensitivity reactions are likely due to an infectious process.

Severe systemic hypersensitivity reactions secondary to injections of hyaluronic acid fillers are even more rare than local side effects. A case was reported in 2009 of a patient who developed acute facial angioedema, accompanied by generalized urticarial lesions, pruritus, and fever 3 weeks after implantation of 1 mL of NASHA (Restylane) in her nasolabial folds. The patient subsequently developed palpable purpura on the trunk and extremities with a biopsy consistent with leukocytoclastic vasculitis. Whether this was a true immunologic reaction in this specific case is questionable; however, it is important to be conscious that there may be coincidental or idiosyncratic reactions with the use of dermal fillers.

In cases where there have been reports of clinical hypersensitivity reactions, it is postulated that the reactions were caused by residual proteins or impurities resulting from the manufacturing process, rather than by the hyaluronic acid itself. There were two sources for industrial production of the hyaluronic acid used as agents for soft tissue augmentation: an animal hyaluronic acid produced from rooster combs (Hylaform) and a non-animal stabilized hyaluronic acid produced by bacterial fermentation from specific strains of streptococci (Restylane family, Juvéderm family, and Belotero). Some studies have shown that LMW fragments obtained from different preparations of hyaluronic acid stimulated the synthesis of interleukin-12 and tumor necrosis factor alpha in monocytes and that these findings might explain the rare reports of delayed hypersensitivity reactions in patients treated with hyaluronic acid injections. Others have postulated that when the cross-linked hyaluronic acid is broken down, the components used to stabilize the hyaluronic acid molecules might lead to inflammation or precipitate an immunologic response. In early European use of NASHA, delayed hypersensitivity reactions were reported at relatively low incidences, 0.15% to 0.42%. Since then, manufacturing processes have become even more stringent, subsequently reducing the protein load by sixfold and virtually eliminating the incidence of implant-site hypersensitivity reactions.

Though the incidence is low, there have been case reports of localized and generalized hypersensitivity reactions, immune-mediated granuloma formation, and sarcoidosis-like disease following injection with temporary soft tissue fillers. A rare but dramatic type of reaction that was reported in 2005 was an angioedema-type hypersensitivity to 1 mL of Restylane following injection into the upper lip. One hour after injection, the patient developed an angioedema-type swelling of the upper lip without systemic complaints. The patient was treated with intramuscular corticosteroids, with stabilization of swelling occurring 2 hours later, and was subsequently treated with an oral steroid taper with complete resolution of edema within 5 days.

---

**Pearl 7**

The documented incidence of allergic reactions to NASHA gel remains extremely low. However, with the surge in popularity of these fillers, this risk may increase. It is incumbent upon physicians to discuss with patients not only the benefits but also the risks of a potential for an allergic response.

---

## Infection

As with any procedure in which there is a breach in the structural integrity of the skin, infection after injection of temporary soft tissue fillers can occur. Potential infectious etiologies may be bacterial, fungal, or viral in nature. It is possible that trauma from injection may trigger recurrent herpetic lesions. Therefore, in patients with a history of herpes outbreaks, prophylactic antiviral treatment is recommended if the filler is to be used for the purpose of lip augmentation; alternatively avoid the site of the herpetic outbreak. Delay filling if an active herpes lesion is present near the area of augmentation.

To minimize the risk of infection, one should consider a more formal sterile surgical preparation using chlorhexidine. Commonly recovered bacterial microorganisms associated with injections of dermal fillers include *Staphylococcus* and *Streptococcus*. Patients with a lesion clinically suspicious for an infection often present with a single or multiple tender erythematous and/or fluctuant nodules. This may be accompanied by systemic symptoms, such as fever and fatigue. When an infection is suspected, the lesion should be cultured or biopsied, and the specimens sent for bacterial, fungal, and acid-fast stains. Empiric treatment with an antibiotic, such as clarithromycin or minocycline, should be initiated until the more specific culture results become available.

When a lesion that may be infectious in nature appears at the site of injection more than 2 weeks post procedure, it may be suggestive of an atypical infection, such as a *Mycobacterium* organism. There have been reports of an outbreak of *M. chelonae* infection after soft tissue augmentation with a hyaluronic acid-based filler. It is not clear whether the injected material was contaminated with the mycobacteria during the manufacturing process or whether the patient was inoculated during the injection procedure. Contamination of the filler agent is of concern because there have been individuals who used non-US Food and Drug Administration (FDA)-approved products and have illegally imported products outside of approved US distributors. With the expansion of nonphysicians and untrained personnel performing aesthetic procedures and with the possibility of non-FDA-approved agents or even counterfeit products being used, it is possible that we may see an increase in these types of complications.

## Biofilms

A biofilm is a quiescent infection by bacteria, introduced at the time of injection, resulting in the formation of a structured community of microorganisms adherent to an inert surface and encapsulated by a protective self-developed polymeric matrix. Biofilms are extremely difficult to eradicate because they are often resistant to the immune system and conventional anti-infectives. The most common biofilm-forming microorganisms responsible for approximately two-thirds of infections with foreign material are *Staphylococcus aureus*, *Staphylococcus epidermidis*, *Pseudomonas aeruginosa*, and *Enterococcus* species. Biofilms may also be composed of fungal elements, such as *Candida*. Biofilm formation is a crucial step in the pathogenesis of many subacute and chronic bacterial infections. They have been problematic to many fields of medicine, ranging from orthopedic devices to heart valves, indwelling catheters, and stents. Active clinical infections have flared weeks, months, and even years after the initial surgery. It is now acknowledged that biofilms are a concern when using temporary fillers for soft tissue augmentation.

Biofilm reactions have been reported more frequently when a permanent nondegradable gel, such as silicone or polyacrylamide gel, is injected; however, they can also occur with the use of temporary filler agents. Following filler injections, there may be both acute and delayed onset of erythematous papules and nodules. Some of

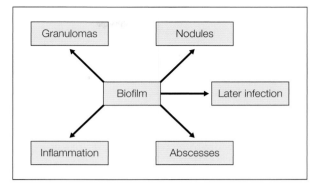

**Figure 29.4** Potential complications from biofilms.

these reactions have been reported years after injection of the product. Often culture of these lesions will lead to negative results because standard culturing techniques are not sensitive enough to detect these types of infections, leading some to incorrectly refer to them as "sterile abscesses." It is important to understand how a biofilm can be responsible for many filler side effects, particularly those that present as early- or late-onset "angry red bumps." Biofilms can result in a clinical picture of an inflammatory response, a local infection including an abscess or cellulitis, a systemic infection with sepsis, a granulomatous response with a foreign body granuloma, or a nodule (Fig. 29.4). It has been noted that subsequent trauma or injection at sites of previous filler placement can activate biofilms, with the possible induction of a "granulomatous or an infectious response."

Any inflammatory nodule should first be treated as an infection. The first treatment of choice for most papules and nodules, whether they are red and/or painful, should be an antibiotic, such as clarithromycin or minocycline, for 2 to 6 weeks, in lieu of initial treatment with intralesional corticosteroid or 5-flourouracil injections. If these lesions are treated initially with steroids, intralesionally or systemically, it can make the inflammation much worse by further activating the biofilm and prolonging the infectious process. Intralesional steroid injections should be used only if the patient is already taking an antibiotic. If the substance injected is a long-lasting particulate filler, excision must be considered if antibiotics and steroids are not successful (Box 29.3).

### Pearl 8

The first treatment of choice for most papules and nodules, whether they are red and/or painful, should be an antibiotic, such as clarithromycin or minocycline, for 2 to 6 weeks. Avoid the use of steroids as a first-line agent for treatment of these lesions because they can worsen the situation.

Because biofilm-associated infections are difficult to treat, it is extremely important to use a sterile reliable

> **Box 29.3**
> **Algorithm for the treatment of inflammatory nodules**
>
> - Incision and drainage to expel as much of the substance as possible.
> - Send for culture.
> - Oral antibiotics for at least 2 to 6 weeks. May need multiple agents if no response, or intravenous antibiotics if severe.
> - Avoid initial use of intralesional steroids. Use only if the patient is already on an antibiotic regimen.
> - Inject hyaluronidase if caused by hyaluronic acid-based filler.
> - Excision or débridement of the nodule if no response and long-term persistence.

antiseptic protocol for skin cleansing prior to injection, so as to prevent early colonization. High-risk patients, such as immunocompromised patients and diabetics, who are more prone to infection, need special attention. Patients with chronic sinusitis and chronic dental problems may have a greater tendency to develop an infection after a filler is injected in the periorbital area or central face. It is commonly recommended to avoid filler implantation until 2 weeks after any dental work has been performed, or wait 4 weeks after filler placement to perform dental work.

Biofilm bacteria show much greater resistance to antibiotics than do their free-living counterparts. One potential reason for this increased resistance is the penetration barrier that biofilms may present to antimicrobials. In addition, bacterial biofilms have several antimicrobial resistance mechanisms. Investigations have identified genes that may be specifically involved in increased antibiotic resistance of biofilm cells. It has been shown that bacteria in biofilms have enhanced penicillin resistance as a result of a dual strategy: impaired penetration of the biofilm through its matrix and rapid efflux of the antibiotic. Other molecular studies have cast light on new facts about the virulence factors of biofilms. The biofilm matrix has been shown to include a variety of structural components, including DNA, polysaccharides, and proteins. This finding has stimulated interest in developing substances that enzymatically disrupt these elements, leading to a breakdown of the biofilm. Others have been investigating the role of photodynamic therapy to disrupt biofilms. Research continues to ascertain the mechanics of pathogenic biofilms, which could lead to the development of new drugs to combat them.

> **Pearl 9**
>
> Biofilms may account for many of today's delayed-onset complications, including granulomas, nodules, inflammation, and abscesses. Prolonged antibiotic use may be necessary even when cultures do not reveal a definitive organism.

## Granulomas

Although it happens infrequently, local and regional delayed and recurrent granulomatous reactions, manifested as persistent nodules, may complicate nonpermanent dermal filler injections. Because all synthetic fillers act as foreign bodies, the host response ranges from a few macrophages to an intense foreign-body reaction with fibrosis, depending on the filler. A fibrotic response by the patient is often the desired basis of volumization for such products as PLLA and calcium hydroxylapatite (Radiesse). These granulomas are usually secondary to an inflammatory response to a specific product, and there is speculation that the composition and the size of the filler agent can be associated with the risk of developing this type of reaction. It is not yet fully understood why these granulomas develop years after injection.

Because collagen is usually resorbed in approximately 3 to 4 months, the risks of delayed or persistent granulomas are quite low. Rare examples of palisading granulomas resembling granuloma annulare and disseminated and recurrent sarcoid-like granulomatous panniculitis have been reported in the past, following bovine collagen injections. Hyaluronic acid products have been rarely associated with granuloma formation, as evidenced by delayed erythema and either painful or nontender swollen nodules. Whether this reaction is due to an inherent continuous foreign-body reaction or to a biofilm is up for debate. Many problems that were previously assumed to be foreign body granulomas or allergic reactions on the basis of negative bacterial cultures are now thought to be due to biofilms. As stated previously, evidence has pointed to bacterial contamination at the time of device implantation as a potential etiology of these granulomatous responses.

Nevertheless, there have been reports of true granulomatous reactions to Restylane. In a specific case a patient received a hyaluronic acid product in the vermilion border and subsequently developed discrete nodules initially associated with eczematous changes in the overlying skin 6 weeks after injection. Histologic analysis revealed the presence of a sharply demarcated nodule in the subcutaneous fat that was consistent with a granulomatous foreign body reaction to the filler. These granulomas have been shown at times to respond to intralesional steroids and calcineurin inhibitors. In cases of hyaluronic acid-related granulomatous foreign body reactions that do not respond to initial treatment with topical antiinflammatory medications, hyaluronidase may be used to resolve the problem.

There have been reports of histologically confirmed foreign body granulomas to PLLA, as well at the sites of injection. The granulomatous reaction to PLLA particles may persist for at least 18 months after injection. Bacteria have been searched for to find the etiology of this reaction, but no microorganisms were detected by DNA analysis of the granulomatous reaction in a series of cases. There has been a concern of a vigorous granulomatous response to PLLA in patients who have had immune reconstitution, in which a previously immunodeficient patient became relatively immunocompetent while being treated for HIV. The hypothesis is that these patients may develop an overactive response to infectious or foreign substances. One paper reported three cases with significant visible deformity as a result of foreign body-induced giant cell granulomatous reactions following skin augmentation. These reactions were attributed to the aberrant reactivity of the recipient to the material. Treatment with intralesional steroids and 5% imiquimod cream resulted in no visible clinical improvement, and excision was required to remove the largest of nodules. Severe systemic adverse effects secondary to PLLA injections are extremely rare, with only one case being described as an anaphylactic reaction necessitating treatment interruption. As noted previously, with appropriate deposition technique and adequate dilution, late-onset foreign body granulomas are reported to be rare, with overall incidence in studies as low as 0.1%. Nevertheless, patients and physicians must be aware of this potential side effect.

Injectable calcium hydroxylapatite tends to be associated with a high incidence of nodules when this agent had been injected into the lips. However, these nodules do not appear to be inflammatory in nature. Histologically, microspheres of calcium hydroxylapatite stimulate almost no foreign body reaction, and only a few macrophages are seen around the injected material. Migration of this product from the original site of injection to a distant location has been described with this filler and it should be avoided for augmentation of the lips.

## Necrosis

Necrosis of the skin is a rare but severe complication following injection of temporary fillers. Judicious use of the fillers with proper placement and selection of products and recognition of this serious complication is vital. There have been reports of all filler agents leading to necrosis of the skin. Some experts have seen an increase in the incidence of necrosis following injections, possibly paralleling the rise in treatments. There is a growing concern regarding the varied experience level and training backgrounds of those who are treating the expanding market. Regardless, if you inject enough fillers, it is likely you are going to have some type of vascular incident at some point. It is important to be prepared with firm knowledge and appropriate products for quick intervention to mitigate the damage.

Necrosis can result from inadvertent placement of filler within the lumen of a vessel or from compression of blood vessels if excess product is used—both of which can lead to obstruction of blood flow and poor tissue oxygenation with resulting tissue necrosis. This often presents with a mottled pattern of violaceous, or dusky, discoloration of the overlying skin that was treated. If not recognized and ameliorated this can progress to further discoloration, pain, and ulceration with resultant scarring of the skin upon healing. The areas at greatest risk for injection necrosis and complications are in the glabellar region corresponding to the supratrochlear artery and its small-caliber branches that supply this watershed region with minimal collateral circulation. This complication can also occur along the course of the facial artery, angular artery, lateral nasal artery, or their branches. An appreciation of normal facial anatomy, with consideration given to location and course of major arteries and differences between regional properties and thickness, is of importance to minimize this complication. Both Belezany and Carruthers et al. have published articles detailing the facial vascular anatomy.

A number of precautions can be taken to avoid necrosis. Aspiration before injecting, injecting slowly in a retrograde manner, and keeping the needle constantly mobile are all advised. If your patient complains of pain out of proportion to normal discomfort, stop the injection immediately and reassess. Although customary to perform, controversy exists concerning the need for aspiration before injection with hyaluronic acid fillers because it may not be possible to get flashback into a syringe through fine needles with thick gels. A 2015 study of found that withdrawal of the hyaluronic acid syringe plunger, using slow or fast techniques, with no visible blood in the syringe does not eliminate the possibility of intravascular placement of the syringe needle. Selection of appropriate agents that are small in particle size and are intended for superficial use is also imperative in helping to minimize this complication. Also avoid injection in the immediate vicinity of large named facial vessels. Some experts have adopted the use of blunt-tipped cannulas, which reduce but do not eliminate the risk of intravascular entry.

Impending necrosis presents in one of three patterns: immediate, early (within 24 to 48 hours), or delayed. Several protocols exist for managing this complication. Treatment is dependent on the time of onset. First, recognition of vascular compromise is evident by blanching followed by a dusky or purple discoloration of the area. Upon recognition of this, injection should be immediately discontinued. Applying warm compresses and massaging the area will facilitate vasodilation and blood flow. Approximately 0.5 inch (12 mm) of 2% nitroglycerin paste should be massaged onto the affected area, which will often result in revascularization as manifested by a pink hue within a few minutes. Sildenafil citrate (Viagra, Pfizer, Inc.) or any similar drug may be considered to increase blood flow. Hyaluronidase, which enzymatically degrades hyaluronic acid, is recommended if the above treatments are ineffective. Anaphylaxis has been reported after retrobulbar injection but not after subcutaneous administration. Because hyaluronidase is one of the active components of bee venom, its administration in patients with a history of allergy to bee stings should be performed cautiously. Skin testing for hypersensitivity is recommended prior to administration of two hyaluronidase formulations: bovine-derived Amphadase (Amphastar Pharmaceuticals, Inc., Rancho Cucamonga, California) and sheep-derived Vitrase (ISTA Pharmaceutical, Irvine,

California). However, a consensus report on the treatment of filler-induced necrosis did not find it necessary to conduct a skin test prior to administration of hyaluronidase in these urgent situations; rather the physician should be prepared to treat the patient for hypersensitivity or anaphylaxis, should it occur.

Hyaluronidase has been shown to reduce edema, which could minimize occluding vessel pressure. Therefore hyaluronidase is of benefit in the management of impending necrosis even if not using a hyaluronic-based filler. In more severe or unresponsive cases of necrosis, Schanz et al. described their success using deep subcutaneous injections of LMW heparin into the affected area. Finally, a course of oral steroids may decrease inflammation and improve blood flow to the area. Fortunately in many cases the skin necrosis remodels and the resultant damage is less than expected. Should contour irregularities persist, fillers may be placed to correct depressed areas followed by a fractionated laser to smoothen the surface and stimulate collagen formation.

---

### Pearl 10

Necrosis is a serious complication, and, albeit rare, all physicians need to have a treatment protocol in place to effectively manage this. Injections of hyaluronidase may help to minimize impending necrosis from all types of fillers.

---

## Blindness

Although exceedingly rare, blindness is perhaps the most feared and catastrophic complication of filler injection. Belezany's 2015 review of world literature revealed 98 cases of vision changes following fillers, ranging from mild impairment to complete vision loss. The most common symptoms were immediate vision loss and pain. Autologous fat (47.9%) was the most common filler associated with ocular complications, followed by hyaluronic acid (23.5%). Autologous fat had a higher risk of permanent blindness, with an ultimate ocular outcome at 80.9% compared with hyaluronic acid at 39.1%. This could reflect use of larger volumes, larger syringes, and higher extrusion pressures with fat injections. The injection sites that were high risk for ocular symptoms were the glabella (38.8%), nasal region (25.5%), nasolabial fold (13.3%), and forehead (12.2%); however, virtually every anatomic location where filler is injected on the face is at risk for blindness due to vascular anastomoses and the ability of filler material to travel in retrograde fashion.

Blindness from autologous fat injection has been universally irreversible, whereas vision loss from hyaluronic acid has been partially reversed in some cases. The goal of treatment after impending blindness is suspected is rapid restoration of perfusion to the eye. Carruthers et al. have presented techniques for retrobulbar and peribulbar injection of hyaluronidase to attempt reversal of vision loss. It has been shown that damage secondary to retinal ischemia becomes irreversible after 90 minutes; however, many experts feel this overestimates the time one has to

---

### Box 29.4
### Key prevention and management strategies to avoid blindness

- Prevention
  - Know location and depth of facial vessels.
  - Inject slowly and with minimal pressure.
  - Inject in small increments (0.1 mL aliquots).
  - Move the needle tip while injecting to prevent large deposit in one location.
  - Aspirate prior to injection (efficacy controversial but recommended, especially with PLLA).
  - Use a small-diameter needle (necessitates slower injection).
  - Smaller syringes are preferred to larger ones to control volume.
  - Use caution if prior surgical procedure in area (i.e., rhinoplasty, face lift).
  - Consider using a cannula to reduce the chance of entering a blood vessel (i.e., highly vascularized areas such as tear trough).
- Management
  - If ocular pain or vision changes, stop injecting at once.
  - Immediately contact an ophthalmologist or oculoplastic surgeon and transfer the patient directly there.
  - Consider treating the injected area and surrounding tissue with hyaluronidase.
  - Consider retrobulbar injection of 300 to 600 units (2 to 4 mL) of hyaluronidase, regardless of which filler is used.
  - Consider reduction of intraocular pressure (i.e., ocular massage, intravenous mannitol).
  - Monitor the patient's neurologic status and order relevant imaging studies (high prevalence of central nervous system [CNS] complications accompany blindness).

Adapted from Beleznay K, Carruthers JD, Humphrey S, Jones D. Avoiding and treating blindness from fillers: a review of the world literature. *Dermatol Surg.* 2015;41:1097–1117.

---

perform sight-saving intervention. Beleznay et al. proposed key prevention and management strategies (Box 29.4). Ideally, with careful injection technique, iatrogenic blindness from filler is preventable and should never occur, but this complication is more likely with the increasing use of fillers by those less familiar with facial vascular anatomy.

## Conclusion

Soft tissue augmentation with temporary fillers continues to be among one of the most commonly performed cosmetic procedures. Performed with good care and by experienced physicians, it is a highly effective, extremely well-tolerated procedure. As both the number of patients seeking injections and the types of fillers expands, it is imperative that physicians have the proper training and are familiar with their potential complications and treatment. Though complication rates are generally low with these classes of agents, they can still occur even in the best of hands; therefore early recognition and management of them are imperative. To ensure the best possible outcomes while minimizing avoidable adverse events, a thorough understanding of facial anatomy, as well as proper product selection and injection techniques, is required.

## Further reading

Alam M, Dover JS. Management of complications and sequelae with temporary injectable fillers. *Plast Reconstr Surg.* 2007;120:S98–S105.

Alsaad S, Fabi SG, Goldman MP. Granulomatous reaction to hyaluronic acid: a case series and review of the literature. *Dermatol Surg.* 2012;38(2):271–276.

Beer K. Avoiding complications with fillers. *Dermatologist.* 2014;22(11):20–21.

Beleznay K, Carruthers JD, Carruthers A, Mummert ME, Humphrey S. Delayed-onset nodules secondary to a smooth cohesive 20 mg/mL hyaluronic acid filler: cause and management. *Dermatol Surg.* 2015;41:929–939.

Beleznay K, Carruthers JD, Humphrey S, Jones D. Avoiding and treating blindness from fillers: a review of the world literature. *Dermatol Surg.* 2015;41:1097–1117.

Berlin, AL, Cohen, JL. Improving bruising after facial filler injections. *Dermatologist.* 2016;24(1):20–21.

Brandt F, Bassichis B, Bassichis M, O'Connell C, Lin X. Safety and effectiveness of small and large gel-particle hyaluronic acid in the correction of perioral wrinkles. *Drugs Dermatol.* 2011;10:982–987.

Carey W, Weinkle S. Retraction of the plunger on a syringe of hyaluronic acid before injection: are we safe? *Dermatol Surg.* 2015;41:S340–S346.

Carruthers J, Fagien S, Dolman P. Retro or peribulbar injection techniques to reverse visual loss after filler injections. *Dermatol Surg.* 2015;41:S354–S357.

Christensen L. Normal and pathologic tissue reactions to soft tissue gel fillers. *Dermatol Surg.* 2007;33(suppl 2):S168–S175.

Christensen L. Host tissue interaction, fate, and risks of degradable and nondegradable gel fillers. *Dermatol Surg.* 2009;35(suppl 2):S1612–S1619.

Cohen JL. Understanding, avoiding, and managing dermal filler complications. *Dermatol Surg.* 2008;34(suppl 1):92–99.

Cohen JL, Biesman BS, Dayan SH, et al. Treatment of hyaluronic acid filler-induced impending necrosis with hyaluronidase: consensus recommendations. *Aesthet Surg J.* 2015;35(7):844–849.

Coleman SR. Cross-linked hyaluronic acid fillers. *Plast Reconstr Surg.* 2006;117:661–665.

Dayan SH, Arkins JP, Brindise R. Soft tissue fillers and biofilms. *Facial Plast Surg.* 2011;27(1):23–28.

Dover JS, Rubin MG, Bhatia AC. Review of the efficacy, durability, and safety data of two nonanimal stabilized hyaluronic acid fillers from a prospective, randomized, comparative, multicenter study. *Dermatol Surg.* 2009;35(suppl 1):S322–S331.

Glashofer MG, Cohen JL. Complications from soft-tissue augmentation of the face: a guide to understanding, avoiding, and managing periprocedural issues. In: Jones D, ed. *Injectable Fillers, Principles and Practice.* Oxford: Wiley-Blackwell; 2010:121–139.

Grunebaum LD, Allemann I, Dayan S, Mandy S, Baumann L. The risk of alar necrosis associated with dermal filler injection. *Dermatol Surg.* 2009;35(suppl 2):S1635–S1640.

Hamilton DG, Gauthier N, Robertson BF. Late-onset, recurrent facial nodules associated with injection of poly-L-lactic acid. *Dermatol Surg.* 2008;34:123–126.

Hamilton RG, Strobos J, Adkinson NF. Immunogenicity studies of cosmetically administered nonanimal-stabilized hyaluronic acid particles. *Dermatol Surg.* 2007;33(suppl 2):S176–S185.

Hirsch RJ, Cohen JL. Surgical insights: challenge: correcting superficially placed hyaluronic acid. *Skin Aging.* 2007;15:36–38.

Hirsch RJ, Cohen JL, Carruthers JD. Successful management of an unusual presentation of impending necrosis following a hyaluronic acid injection embolus and a proposed algorithm for management with hyaluronidase. *Dermatol Surg.* 2007;33:357–360.

Ho D, Jagdeo J, Waldorf HA. Is there a role for arnica and bromelain in prevention of post-procedure ecchymosis or edema? A systematic review of the literature. *Dermatol Surg.* 2016;42:445–463.

Lam SM. Periorbital and midfacial volume enhancement with cannula. *J Am Med Assoc Fac Plast Surg.* 2016;18(1):71–72.

Landau M. Hyaluronidase caveats in treating filler complications. *Dermatol Surg.* 2015;41:S347–S353.

Lee A, Grummer SE, Kriegel D, Marmur E. Hyaluronidase. *Dermatol Surg.* 2010;36:1071–1077.

Lee WR, Kim SJ, Park JH, et al. Bee venom reduces atherosclerotic lesion formation via anti-inflammatory mechanism. *Am J Chin Med.* 2010;38:1077–1092.

Lemperle G, Rullan PP, Gauthier-Hazan N. Avoiding and treating dermal filler complications. *Plast Reconstr Surg.* 2006;118(suppl 3):S92–S107.

Leonhardt JM, Lawrence N, Narins RS. Angioedema acute hypersensitivity reaction to injectable hyaluronic acid. *Dermatol Surg.* 2005;31:577–579.

Lowe NJ, Maxwell CA, Patnaik R. Adverse reactions to dermal fillers: review. *Dermatol Surg.* 2005;31:1626–1633.

Monheit GD, Rohrich RJ. The nature of long-term fillers and the risk of complications. *Dermatol Surg.* 2009;35(suppl 2):S1598–S1604.

Mummert ME. Immunologic roles of hyaluronan. *Immunol Res.* 2005;31:189–206.

Narins RS. Minimizing adverse events associated with poly-L-lactic acid injection. *Dermatol Surg.* 2008;34(suppl 1):S100–S104.

Narins RS, Coleman WP, Glogau RG. Recommendations and treatment options for nodules and other filler complications. *Dermatol Surg.* 2009;35:1667–1671.

Narins RS, Jewell M, Rubin M, Cohen J, Strobos J. Clinical conference: management of rare events following dermal fillers—focal necrosis and angry red bumps. *Dermatol Surg.* 2006;32:426–434.

Percival SL, Emanuel C, Cutting KF, Williams DW. Microbiology of the skin and the role of biofilms in infection. *Int Wound J.* 2011;9(1):14–32.

Requena L, Requena C, Christensen L, Zimmermann US, Kutzner H, Cerroni L. Adverse reactions to injectable soft tissue fillers. *J Am Acad Dermatol.* 2011;64:1–34.

Resko AE, Sadick NS, Magro CM, Farber J. Late-onset subcutaneous nodules after poly-L-lactic acid injection. *Dermatol Surg.* 2009;35:380–384.

Rzany B, DeLorenzi C. Understanding, avoiding and managing severe filler complications. *Plast Reconstr Surg.* 2015;136:S196–S203.

Vanaman M, Fabi SG, Carruthers J. Complications in the cosmetic dermatology patient: a review and our experience (Part 1). *Dermatol Surg.* 2016;42:1–11.

Vleggaar D, Fitzgerald R, Lorenc P, et al. Consensus recommendations on the use of injectable poly-L-lactic acid for facial and nonfacial volumization. *J Drugs Dermatol.* 2014;13(suppl 4):S44–S51.

# 30

# Complications of permanent fillers

Shilpi Khetarpal, Jeffrey S. Dover

## Summary and Key Features

- Permanent fillers comprise mostly synthetic materials that cause collagen deposition via fibroplasia as their mechanism of action.
- Permanent fillers are better at facial volumizing and deep structural augmentation than at "line filling."
- Silicones, polyalkylimides, polyacrylamides, polymethylmethacrylate, and acrylic hydrogels are the most common permanent fillers worldwide.
- All cosmetic fillers, whether temporary or permanent, may induce adverse reactions.
- Permanent filler complications may be due to the injection itself, injector-dependent variables, or host tissue and filler interactions.
- Permanent filler complications are difficult to treat because the product will not dissipate but rather remains in vivo.
- Foreign body and late-onset granulomas are the most challenging permanent filler complications to treat.
- Late-onset granulomas can be caused by biofilms from bacteria introduced at the time of injection.
- Effective treatments of granulomas must target bacterial etiologies and host immune response mechanisms.
- Invasive and scarring treatments, such as surgery, should be reserved and used after more conservative treatments have failed.

## Introduction

Injectable facial fillers have become a cornerstone of aesthetic medicine during the past several decades. Although soft tissue augmentation using industrial-grade silicones can be traced to the early 20th century, widespread adoption of injectable fillers began in the 1980s with the advent of bovine collagen. Since the 1990s soft tissue augmentation to fill lines and volumize or recontour the face has surged to become the second most popular nonsurgical aesthetic procedure in North America, with more than 2.2 million soft tissue filler procedures performed in 2013.

Based on the axiom that an aged facial appearance is due in some part to dermal, subcutaneous, and osseous atrophy that naturally occurs over time, injectable facial fillers offer the ability to replace lost volume and restore youthful proportions, providing a foundation for facial rejuvenation.

As with certain other nonsurgical aesthetic modalities, facial filling is a product-driven procedure. Beyond an adroit injection technique, judicious use of the appropriate product in the proper location is a prerequisite to success. To know the art of injection, one must know the products, and the products vary significantly. In 2010 more than 200 fillers from more than 60 manufacturers worldwide were available for tissue augmentation. Although some share characteristics that may predict a similar clinical response or comparable side effect profile, inappropriate substitution with a dissimilar product, particularly by an inexperienced provider, invites complications and ultimately patient dissatisfaction and compromises patient safety.

Although there is no universally accepted classification for soft tissue fillers, they can be classified based on their origin—natural animal, synthetic, or natural synthetic. Fillers may be further divided based on their longevity: temporary, semipermanent, or permanent. Temporary fillers are typically biologically derived products that are eventually broken down in vivo after a period of a few months to a few years. This category includes collagens and hyaluronic acids (HAs), the most predominant fillers worldwide. In contrast, permanent fillers comprise mostly synthetic materials that have an in vivo, biodynamic mechanism of action, causing collagen deposition via fibroplasia. They are composed of nonabsorbable, permanent material. For this reason, permanent fillers are better at facial volumizing and deep structural augmentation than at "line filling," which is better accomplished with temporary fillers. It is important to note that "permanence" refers to a lack of degradation of the in vivo material over time rather than to a "permanent" cosmetic result. Once placed, permanent fillers remain in the skin and subcutaneous tissues indefinitely. Permanent aesthetic results are seldom possible owing to continued tissue volume loss, bone resorption, and other factors associated with the aging face. Nevertheless, duration of correction is more extensive than with temporary fillers. As such, permanent fillers are less "forgiving." Experience and precise technique are required to achieve favorable outcomes.

## Liquid injectable silicone

Silicone is one of the oldest and longest-lasting injectable fillers. Liquid injectable silicone (LIS) received US Food and Drug Administration (FDA) approval in 1959 for intraocular use as a retinal stabilizing agent during vitreous surgery. Its off-label use as a filler is controversial due to potential long-term complications. The FDA-approved medical-grade silicone oils that are recommended for cosmetic use include Silkon-1000 (Alcon, Fort Worth, Texas) and Adatosil-5000 (Bausch & Lomb, Rochester, New York). Although injectable silicone has been effectively used for more than 50 years, its use remains controversial owing to the historical widespread reports of complications, most of which are confounded with unknown or impure products labeled as "silicone" and purified silicones injected by improper techniques. When critically evaluating silicone, the distinction must be made between modern products intended for injection (LIS) in contrast to adulterated or impure products lumped under the "silicone" label that is manufactured outside the United States. LIS demonstrates a unique aptness for the correction of specific cutaneous and subcutaneous atrophies owing to its versatility, permanence, excellent cost–benefit profile, and natural texture in vivo. Furthermore, evidence continues to mount demonstrating that modern silicone oils approved by the FDA for injection into the human body may be successfully used off-label when injected according to strict protocol, which includes using the microdroplet serial puncture technique with limited quantities per session and adequately spaced treatment sessions. In contrast, adulterated and impure silicone products, even when labeled "medical-grade," are rife with complications.

## Polyalkylimide gel

Bio-Alcamid (Polymekon, Italy) was first launched in 2000 and has been used in more than 20 countries. It does not require skin allergy testing prior to use (Protopapa, Sita, Caporale, Cammarota, 2003). Its use was originally as an "endoprosthesis" for the treatment of pectus excavatum and postoperative defects and aesthetic use in the lips, cheeks, and nasolabial folds (Fig. 30.1). It contains a nonbiodegradable, nontoxic, nonimmunogenic synthetic polyalkylimide cross-linked polymer suspended in water. Although it is approved in Europe, it is not currently approved by the US FDA. Bio-Alcamid contains a ratio of 3% alkylimide polymer to 97% sterile water. The product is a gel that is injected as a large bolus subcutaneously. After injection, the polyalkylimide gel is completely covered by a thin collagen capsule (0.02 mm) that isolates it from host tissues, making it a type of endogenous prosthesis (Formigli & Protopapa, 2004). It has been successful and safe in treating human immuno-deficiency virus (HIV)-associated facial lipoatrophy and showed persistent correction at 18 months. There have been reported cases of product migration and infection that occurred 12 months after injection (Karim, Hage, Rozelaar, Lange & Raaijmakers, 2006).

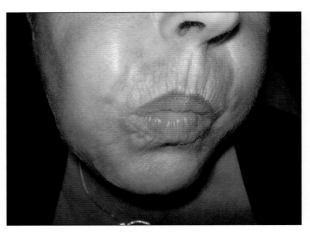

**Figure 30.1** Granuloma of the nasolabial fold 4 years after injection of Bio-Alcamid.

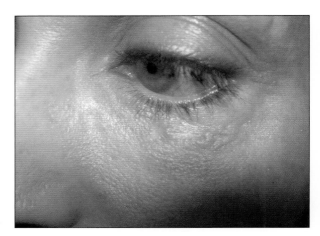

**Figure 30.2** Aquamid granuloma.

## Polyacrylamide gels

Polyacrylamide hydrogels contain a nondegradable, non-toxic, nonimmunogenic synthetic polyacrylamide cross-linked polymer suspended in water that belong to the family of acryl derivatives. Polyacrylamide products are available in Europe and Asia; however, none are currently available for use in the United States.

Aquamid (Contura International, Denmark) contains a 2.5% cross-linked polyacrylamide gel in 97.5% sterile water. It has been in use in Europe and worldwide since 2001, primarily for augmentation of nasolabial folds and lips, facial contouring, and correction of HIV facial lipoatrophy (Fig. 30.2). On histology, Aquamid appears as a multivacuolated nonbirefringent material with a surrounding layer of thin fibrous connective tissue, macrophages, multinucleated giant cells, and lymphocytes.

Amazingel (NanFeng Medical Science and Technology Development Co. Ltd, Shijiazhuang, People's Republic of China) is a product manufactured in China and available throughout Asia. Although it is readily available for purchase through internet distributors, it has not been extensively studied in the Western medical literature. There have been reports of Amazingel used for breast augmentation, lip enhancement, and correction of facial scarring. Late-onset complications have been reported including induration, nodules, hematoma, inflammation, and infection and resolved after removing the product (Do & Shim, 2012).

## Polymethylmethacrylate

Polymethylmethacrylate (PMMA) is a nonresorbable, biocompatible material first synthesized in the early 1900s and used for varied medical purposes, including intraocular implants and bone cements. It was first engineered for soft tissue augmentation in the early 1980s in an attempt to provide a safe implant, with the theory that such a synthetic material might induce long-lasting tissue fibroplasia, in contrast to the temporary volume displacement seen with collagens. Currently available PMMA products are biphasic and suspended in either bovine collagen (Artefill, Suneva Medical, San Diego, California) or carboxyglutamate (Metacril, private lab, Rio de Janeiro, Brazil).

Arteplast was the first-generation commercial PMMA product with less than 20 µm microspheres suspended in a gelatin carrier. It was used in Germany through the early 1990s but was found to have a high incidence of granuloma formation within the first 18 months of implantation. Such complications were likely due to an inconsistent particle size and the presence of surface impurities found with processing methods.

Artecoll (Rofil Medical International, Breda, The Netherlands) (Fig. 30.3) was then introduced in 1992 as a second-generation product with an improved processing and washing method that reduced impurities. Significantly, the carrier was also reformulated, and the PMMA was suspended as a 20% product in 80% bovine collagen with 0.3% lidocaine for improved comfort. The PMMA particles were larger at 30 µm, leading to lower rates of foreign body reaction. Because of the bovine collagen component, Artecoll requires allergy testing prior to injection. As such, Artecoll is considered a biphasic implant, inducing augmentation through displacement with an early collagen component and later through a fibroplastic component caused by PMMA. In 1998 Artecoll was approved in Canada, and processing methods were further improved to reduce particle size variability, resulting in fewer incidences of late-granuloma formation compared with Arteplast. Histology of skin biopsy specimens from areas treated with Artecoll show round, sharply circumscribed, translucent, nonbirefringent particles, epithelioid histiocytes, multinucleated giant cells, lymphocytes, and occasional eosinophils surrounding the microspheres.

Artefill, now known as Bellafill, the third-generation iteration of PMMA was further improved by enhancing the uniformity of the PMMA particle size (30 to 50 µm) and by eliminating nanoparticles that had plagued earlier

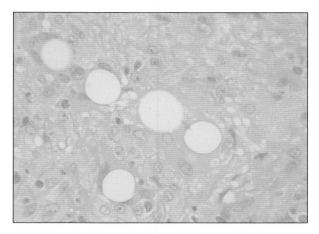

**Figure 30.3** Artecoll.

formulations. The collagen matrix was also improved, and Artefill was approved by the FDA in 2006 for use in the nasolabial folds based on safety studies performed earlier in the United States with Artecoll. Bellafill was approved for moderate-to-severe, atrophic, distensible facial acne scars on the cheeks in 2014. Importantly, Bellafill is the only permanent filler currently approved by the FDA for aesthetic use.

## Acrylic hydrogel plus hyaluronic acid

Dermalive and Dermadeep (Dermatech, Paris, France) are biphasic permanent fillers composed of a mixture of 40% hydroxyethylmethacrylate and ethylmethacrylate particles and 60% biodegradable, fluid cross-linked, bacterially derived HA (Fig. 30.4). The acrylic particles are hydrophobic and irregularly shaped in a polygonal fashion. Dermalive contains acrylic particles 45 to 65 µm in diameter, whereas Dermadeep contains particles 80 to 110 µm in diameter. Both products are intended for injection in the deep dermis and subcutaneous regions, with the Dermadeep product indicated for deep subcutaneous injection only. Both products were CE-approved and available in Europe in 1998 but were withdrawn several years ago, owing to the high incidence of complications. Neither product has ever been FDA-approved for use in the United States. Histology of acrylic hydrogels in tissue reveals pseudocystic structures of different sizes and shapes containing polygonal, pink, translucent, nonbirefringent foreign bodies with a surrounding granulomatous reaction of epithelioid histiocytes, multinucleated giant cells, some lymphocytes, and occasional eosinophils surround the microstructures.

## Treatment sites

Although appropriate indications and uses are beyond the scope of this chapter, it is worthwhile to note that permanent fillers have been extensively used throughout the face and body, and complications in each area have been reported. Documented facial complications have occurred in the eyelids, eyebrows, glabella, temples, cheeks, nose, nasolabial folds, labiomental folds, lips, and prejowl sulci. Traumatic surgical scars and atrophic acne scars have also been treated with permanent fillers and have been noted to have complications. Nonfacial complications have been reported in the chest, breasts, penis, and buttocks, particularly when large amounts of product were injected in single sessions.

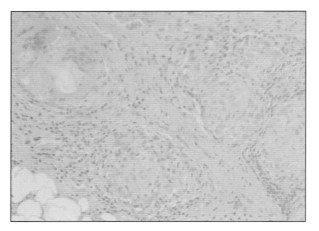

**Figure 30.4** Dermalive.

## Complications

Most permanent fillers are found outside North America, including Europe, Asia, and South America. They are less common in Canada and uncommon in the United States, primarily because of the stringent FDA approval requirements. Those submitted for approval to the FDA must undergo a rigorous clinical trials process prior to approval. The upside of such a process with respect to patient safety is that many complications are identified prior to widespread use. Such is the case for Bellafill, the only permanent filler currently approved in the United States. Outside the United States, standards are less stringent. Europe requires all products used in the European Union to have a CE certificate. However, such a certificate ensures only the technically correct manufacturing of the preparation and is not a guarantee of biological safety. Because clinical trials are not held before product approval, identification of filler complications must be performed retrospectively and gathered through anecdotal evidence. This system allows the widespread use of most permanent filler products prior to the assurance of safety, and therefore the largest numbers of reports of permanent filler complications originate in Europe.

All cosmetic fillers, regardless of their longevity, can have adverse reactions (Table 30.1). Complications can be divided into early (0 to 14 days), late (14 days to 1 year), and delayed (beyond 1 year) reactions. Early reactions include erythema, pain, edema, bruising, and bleeding.

**Table 30.1** Selected permanent fillers by category and composition

| Category | Branded product | Composition |
|---|---|---|
| Liquid injectable silicone | Silikon-1000 | Purified polydimethylsiloxane polymer |
| | Adatosil-5000 | Purified polydimethylsiloxane polymer |
| Other "silicones" | Adulterated and unknown products | Variable and often unknown |
| Polyalkylimide gels (hydrophilic) | Bio-Alcamid | 3% or 4% polyalkylimide gel in 97% or 96% sterile water |
| Polyacrylamide gels (hydrophilic) | Amazingel | Polyacrylamide gel in sterile water |
| | Aquamid | 2.5% polyacrylamide gel in 97.5% sterile water |
| Polymethylmethacrylate (hydrophobic) | Arteplast (first generation) | 30–42 µm PMMA microspheres in a gelatin carrier |
| | Artecoll (second generation) | 30–50 µm PMMA microspheres in a bovine collagen carrier |
| | Artefill (third generation) | 30–50 µm PMMA microspheres in a bovine collagen carrier |
| | Metacril | PMMA in carboxyglutamate |
| Acrylic hydrogel (hydroxyethyl-methacrylate/ethylmethacrylate) (hydrophobic) | Dermalive | 45–65 µm polygonal fragments acrylic hydrogel (40%) in HA (60%) |
| | Dermadeep | 80–110 µm polygonal fragments acrylic hydrogel (40%) in HA (60%) |

*HA*, Hyaluronic acid; *PMMA*, polymethylmethacrylate.

Such reactions are inherently due to the invasive nature of the injection itself, are usually mild to moderate, and are typically self-limited to the first 14 days. However, they may be exacerbated by poor technique.

---

**Pearl 1**

Select patients carefully when considering permanent fillers. The best candidate is a patient who has extensive prior experience with temporary fillers and who desires longstanding correction.

---

Other early and late complications that may occur with both temporary and permanent fillers are due to injector variables. Inexperience and poor technique increase the risk of complications, such as discoloration, vascular occlusion, embolism, cutaneous necrosis, undercorrection or overcorrection, asymmetry, contour irregularity, textural irregularity, and migration. Complications, when seen with short-term resorbable and even long-term resorbable fillers, will eventually resolve as the product is resorbed. However, complications from the use of a permanent filler as the augmenting agent will then no longer dissipate but rather remain in vivo and serve as a continued source of complication.

---

**Pearl 2**

Thorough injector training is crucial with permanent fillers. Extensive injector experience with temporary fillers is essential prior to injections with permanent fillers.

---

However, the most vexing complications occur because of poorly understood phenomena that result from host tissue interactions with the injected product in addition to bacterial interference. This may be related either to the product itself or to the biological interaction of the product and host response to a foreign body, or foreign antigen in residence on the foreign body. Inflammation, infection, biofilm formation, foreign body granulomas, and late-onset granulomas may all occur with both temporary and permanent fillers, but they occur disproportionately with permanent ones. These complications can occur any time after product placement but are skewed toward the late and delayed periods with permanent products. With permanent fillers increasing dramatically during the past decade, both in number of fillers and in number of patients treated, delayed adverse events are now more commonly seen. Furthermore, they are increasingly recognized as the most challenging aspects of permanent tissue augmentation, owing to their tenacity and resistance to treatment. The characteristic of duration that makes a permanent product seemingly advantageous with respect to good results is also the one that engenders the least desirable group of complications. However, not all complications are created equally, and the following adverse reactions are exacerbated owing to the permanent nature of the product.

---

**Pearl 3**

Avoid using permanent fillers, or for that matter any filler in patients with active concomitant infectious or inflammatory processes.

---

*Overcorrection* is an injector-dependent iatrogenic complication that is particularly troublesome with permanent fillers and may occur with any of the permanent fillers (see Table 30.1). Overcorrection may be due to both too much product placed in a particular area, as well as an underestimation of the degree of fibroplasia that will occur over time. With bovine collagens in the 1980s and 1990s, slight overcorrection was intentional at the time of treatment because a significant degree of the immediate correction achieved in the office would dissipate over the next few days. Gross volume displacement was the mechanism for achieving results with collagen alone, and further augmentation by fibroplasia was not expected. However, such a strategy does translate well into the realm of permanent fillers because these depend heavily on augmentation by fibroplasia over time in addition to immediate volume displacement. To apply the overcorrection strategy of collagens to the permanent fillers is to invite disaster because products that work by inducing collagenous deposition will continue to effect augmentation over several weeks to months afterwards. That is, tissue will be augmented beyond the immediate gross displacement due to product volume. For this reason, most permanent fillers should be placed in smaller amounts over multiple sessions spaced several weeks to months apart to allow adequate time for tissue augmentation to occur between sessions.

*Asymmetry* may occur with all permanent fillers by a similar mechanism (delayed fibroplastic augmentation), and care should be taken to ensure equal amounts of product are symmetrically placed. Such a strategy is elementary but may sometimes prove challenging when working with permanent filler products that do not show an immediate volume correction. Cognizance of how much product is being placed as one proceeds through the injection is important, and the amount injected in each site or region should be recorded. Allowing adequate time between injection sessions is also important to avoid placing too much product in a particular area.

*Contour and textural irregularities* may also occur with all of the permanent fillers and are due either to placement of the filler product too superficially (textural irregularity) or to placement of too much product too superficially (contour irregularities). As a rule, permanent fillers are best for deep placement and should rarely be placed more superficial than the deep reticular dermis. Most should be placed in the subcutaneous layer or deeper. Moreover, the particulate nature of some permanent fillers, such as PMMA and the acrylic hydrogels, does not allow for the smooth, soft, and pliable texture desirable for superficial placement. However, LIS is soft and pliable but may still lead to textural and contour irregularities when placed superficially. Fibroplastic fillers are essentially best used as deep fillers rather than superficial ones to avoid these complications. Caution should also be taken when injecting permanent fillers into areas with overlying thin skin.

---

**Pearl 4**

Fill only the appropriate defects. Some treatment areas, such as lips, have a higher rate of complications with permanent fillers. The lips are a notoriously unforgiving site for textural and contour irregularities, owing to their anatomic characteristics—a thin cutaneous and mucosal layer overlying a region particularly sensitive to volume changes. All but the most experienced of injectors should avoid permanent fillers in the lips.

---

**Pearl 5**

With permanent fillers, fill at the appropriate tissue level. Place the product in the subcutaneous tissue and avoid placement of permanent fillers in the superficial and mid-dermis.

---

*Migration* of product along tissue planes to sites distant from injection is a concern with all permanent fillers when large volumes are injected. Injection of large boluses of silicone in a single site or single session is known to increase the risk of product tracking along tissue planes to distant body sites. Indeed, historically adulterants have been intentionally added to silicone oils in an effort to prevent LIS migration, causing further complications owing to a host response to the adulterants. With LIS, using the microdroplet serial puncture technique prevents migration from occurring. The total surface area and resulting surface tension of a given volume of LIS are greatly increased when divided into multiple microdroplets. The increased surface tension holds the microdroplet in place. As fibrosis occurs in the ensuing weeks following LIS microdroplet deposition, a collagenous capsule is created around the microdroplet. The collagenous capsule results in further containment of the microdroplet and prevents migration to other tissue sites. LIS injected in large boluses demonstrates the physical properties of an oil and may track along the planes of least resistance, whereas microdroplets of LIS remain in place long enough for slow collagenous anchoring to occur. Moreover, the increased surface area of multiple microdroplets results in an increased total volume of collagen deposition and a subsequent improved clinical response. These principles may be extended to other permanent fillers as well to help to avoid migration.

---

**Pearl 6**

Use the appropriate technique. With liquid injectable silicone (LIS), a microdroplet serial puncture technique spaced over several sessions is necessary for success.

---

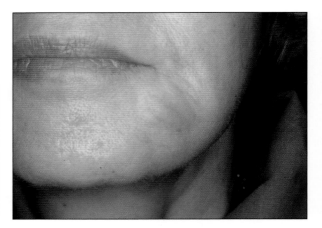

**Figure 30.5** Silicone granuloma (foreign body granuloma).

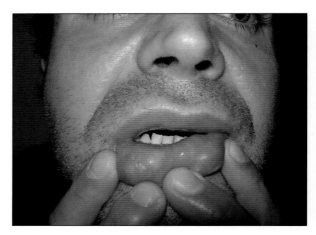

**Figure 30.6** Lower lip granuloma 6 months after injection of Aquamid.

Complications are due to the host response to a foreign body or product and host tissue interactions. Inflammation, foreign body granulomas (**Figs. 30.5** and **30.6**), and late-onset granulomas (**Fig. 30.7**) may be due to the host immune response independent of infection, in which case the filler serves as the foreign body. However, they may also be due to bacterial biofilm formation, in which case both the filler and biofilm colony serve as a foreign body nidus for pathologic inflammation. Such complications have been seen but are poorly understood. Only in the past decade have theories regarding the etiology of such complications begun to coalesce, and, although biofilms are now viewed as the likely culprit, more research is needed to fully understand all mechanisms involved.

Although an exhaustive discussion of bacterial biofilms is beyond this chapter, this phenomenon is increasingly recognized as a possible etiology of permanent filler complications, including inflammation, recurrent infection, and granulomas. Bacterial biofilms are durable subclinical

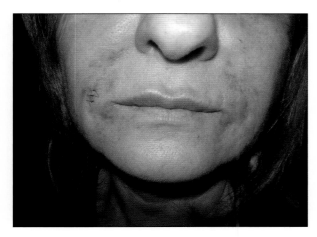

**Figure 30.7** Delayed-onset granuloma 2.5 years after injection with Dermalive.

infections on the surface of a foreign body or prosthesis. They are living colonies that adhere to the foreign body surface, in this case a microdroplet or bolus of permanent filler, and are self-encapsulated by a protective matrix to help to avoid a host response. This protective capsule also helps the biofilm to avoid penetration and destruction by antibiotics. Bacteria in biofilms may remain quiescent for months or years, then reactivate to a free planktonic state to cause inflammatory and infectious sequelae. Importantly, biofilm colonization may remain subclinical because bacteria in the biofilm state are resistant to culture, likely explaining the "sterile" abscesses seen at times with permanent fillers. The irregularities of particulate fillers (PMMA and acrylic hydrogels) may support biofilms, but they may also be found on the smooth surfaces of LIS microdroplets and any other permanent substrate. Biofilms may occur with temporary fillers as well, although they are less significant owing to the lack of substrate permanence. Bacteria that cause biofilms are likely introduced during injection through the skin or mucosa, and, although the normal flora encountered during injection can never be completely eliminated, some authors have begun to advocate adopting a sterile approach when injecting permanent fillers, in contrast to the clean approach that is used for temporary fillers, with the idea that the chance for introduction of bacteria and subsequent biofilm formation may be reduced. Biofilms may play a more important causative role in hydrophilic gels in contrast to hydrophobic fillers. Christensen and colleagues found in polymer nonbiodegradable gels the major cause of foreign body granuloma was likely biofilm formation, which they found in all specimens of patients treated with Aquamid. Such a distinction has strategic implications for treatment, as biofilm causation on hydrophilic products may respond very well to antibiotic treatment. In contrast, hydrophobic fillers with microspheres may not be associated with biofilms and may respond better to steroid treatment. Luitgart Wiest has collected data on 52 patients with foreign body granulomas after Artecoll or Dermalive.

Neither biofilms nor bacteria could be detected in any patient with electron microscopy (Luitgart G. Wiest, personal communication).

*Inflammation* manifesting as tissue erythema and swelling has been reported as a complication during both the late and delayed periods. It has been reported with both LIS and PMMA products but appears particularly prevalent with the polyalkylimide gels, polyacrylamide gels, and acrylic hydrogels.

*Foreign body granulomas* and *late-onset granulomas* are the most challenging complications to treat and are the archetypal permanent filler complications. Both are manifestations of the host's natural immunologic response to a foreign body. Indeed, injecting a foreign body into the host, even a biocompatible, nontoxic, inert one as the permanent fillers are, naturally elicits a granulomatous foreign body response, characterized by the appearance of macrophages and foreign body giant cells that arrive to both phagocytose the foreign material and deposit a fibroplastic collagenous response in an effort to "wall-off" or neutralize it. This is, after all, the main mechanism of action for fibroplastic tissue augmentation. Ideally, the foreign body granulomatous reaction creates a controlled fibrous area around the surface of the implanted filler, and augmentation proceeds in a controlled, limited, and predictable manner. However, if the fibroplastic response does not cease, either because of an ongoing interaction with the foreign product itself or because of the synergistic presence of bacteria, possibly present in a bacterial biofilm, the fibroplastic response will manifest as a foreign body granulomatous complication. Late-onset granulomas result from the same phenomena but typically occur at least 1 year after injection. These may be explained by continued host–filler interactions because there is evidence that the "permanent" microparticles and gels can be further modified by the host immune response even years after injection. Alterations to the surface of Dermalive particles have been documented by electron microscopy (EM) at 2 years, suggesting the product is altered in some fashion over time. This may be due to incomplete polymerization, in which low-molecular-weight oligomers are left in the copolymer after final processing, or ongoing hydrolization. However, most late-onset granulomas are likely explained by bacteria being introduced during injection having the opportunity to establish a biofilm around the injected product, and the biofilm having been reactivated or triggered to cause a host response, either by distant inflammation or infection or by further mechanical insult (Box 30.1).

## Evaluation methods

Histopathology, scanning EM, high-frequency ultrasound, bacterial culture, polymerase chain reaction (PCR), and fluorescent in situ hybridization (FISH) have all been used to evaluate granulomatous and infectious complications due to permanent fillers. Two questions naturally arise when a granulomatous complication ensues: (1) What product was placed? (2) Is the area infected?

> ### Box 30.1
> #### Reported possible triggers of granulomas
>
> - Injecting different types of fillers in the same location
> - Systemic infections
> - Sinusitis
> - Pharyngitis
> - Bronchitis
> - Pleurisy
> - Enteritis
> - Pyelonephritis
> - Flu-like syndrome
> - Autoimmune thyroiditis
> - Acupuncture
> - Hyperthyroidism
> - Ulcerative colitis
> - Crohn disease
> - Pemphigus
> - Sarcoidosis
> - Breast cancer
> - Psychologic shock
> - Facial trauma
> - Facelift operation
> - Dental focus of infection
> - Periodontal disease/inflammation

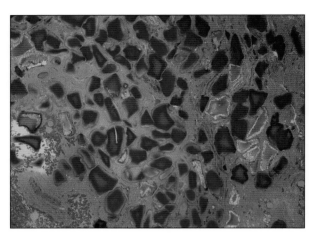

**Figure 30.8** Histology of Dermalive particles 4 years after injection, showing incomplete polymerization.

The first question is best addressed through histopathology rather than history. Histopathological study of the lesions is the "gold standard" technique to identify the responsible filler. With modern products, the particles of each filler have specific microscopic characteristics that allow identification (Fig. 30.8). EM may be used if histopathological studies prove inconclusive or further research is warranted (Fig. 30.9). High-frequency ultrasound has also been reported to identify and quantify the presence of filler in vivo, as well as to detect inflammation, granulomas, and the presence of different fillers in the same area. Nevertheless, evaluation of the exact offending agent may prove difficult when a patient presents with a history of injection with an "unknown" product or an illicitly injected one. A history of "silicone" injections most often eludes detection. Although silicone may be detected on histopathology, the clinician has no method of testing whether or not adulterants were also present in the injected material. Nonpurified and unknown products are often lumped under "silicone" injections by patient history, and these should be distinguished from modern purified products meant for human soft tissue augmentation and appropriately injected.

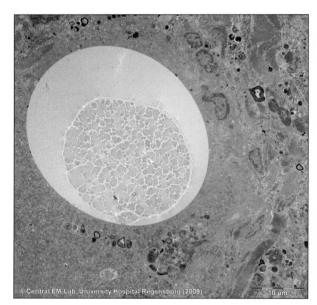

**Figure 30.9** Electron microscopic photograph of an Artecoll microsphere surrounded by a multinucleated giant cell. *Courtesy Dr Josef Schroeder, Central EM-Unit, Department of Pathology, University Hospital Regensburg, Germany.*

### Pearl 7

In the case of granulomas, identify the agent used and treat according to the properties of the filler. Detection of infection may be accomplished through routine bacterial cultures of tissue samples or exudate, but granulomas will often be negative on culture. This should not allay the concern for latent bacterial infection because biofilms may be present in the face of negative cultures. In such cases, PCR may also be used to detect bacterial presence but has also reportedly been negative in the setting of a suspected infection. FISH analysis may also help to detect bacterial presence in the setting of a negative Gram stain and bacterial culture.

## Treatment

Treatment of transient, self-limited filler complications due to injection, including erythema, bleeding, bruising, edema, pain, and herpes simplex virus activation, has been well documented in the literature. However, treatment of permanent filler complications in the second and third categories (Table 30.2) presents a greater challenge. Several treatment methods have been reported in the literature, including topical products, systemic medications,

**Table 30.2** Filler complications

| Cause | Complication | Temporary filler | Permanent filler |
|---|---|---|---|
| Due to injection:<br>• Inherent in invasive procedures<br>• Usually mild to moderate<br>• May be exacerbated by poor technique | Erythema | ++ | ++ |
| | Bleeding | ++ | ++ |
| | Bruising | ++ | ++ |
| | Edema | ++ | ++ |
| | Pain | ++ | ++ |
| | HSV activation | ++ | ++ |
| Due to procedural technique:<br>• Iatrogenic<br>• Operator-dependent | Discoloration | ++ | ++ |
| | Vascular occlusion | ++ | ++ |
| | Embolism | ++ | ++ |
| | Cutaneous necrosis | ++ | ++ |
| | Undercorrection | ++ | ++ |
| | Overcorrection | ++ | ++ |
| | Asymmetry | ++ | ++ |
| | Contour irregularity | + | ++ |
| | Textural irregularity | + | ++ |
| | Migration | + | ++ |
| Due to product/tissue interactions and/or biofilm formation | Inflammation | ++ | ++ |
| | Infection | ++ | ++ |
| | Extrusion | + | ++ |
| | Biofilm formation | + | ++ |
| | Foreign body granuloma | + | ++ |
| | Late-onset granuloma | +/− | +++ |

HSV, Herpes simplex virus.
Gray shading signifies reactions that take on extra significance due to permanent nature of filler.

minimally invasive procedures and modalities, and surgical excision. Treatment options are dependent upon the specific product and patient reaction, and should be individualized. One tenet is to avoid surgical excisions that will result in scarring until all other treatment options have been exhausted.

Treatment of complications in the second category, those due to procedural technique, becomes more challenging when the product placed is permanent because there is generally no reversing agent as is seen with hyaluronidase for HA products. *Discoloration* may be treated with the appropriate laser for the target chromophore if one exists. However, discoloration is often due to a Tyndall effect, and no target chromophore

exists. Destruction with a carbon dioxide laser has been reported to be effective. *Vascular occlusion, embolism,* and *cutaneous necrosis* should be managed aggressively immediately upon recognition with vasodilating agents, such as nitroglycerin paste. If the filler contains an HA component (Dermalive, Dermadeep), hyaluronidase may help to dissolve a portion of the product. *Undercorrection* is simply treated in subsequent sessions. However, *overcorrection, asymmetry, contour irregularities,* and *texture irregularities* require the permanent filler to be reduced or removed in some fashion. *Needle aspiration, liposuction, extrusion* after incision with an angled blade or Nokor needle, and *surgical removal* have all been reported as effective with permanent fillers. Alternatively,

**Box 30.2**
**Anecdotal treatments of granulomas**

- Triamcinolone intralesional + cryotherapy
- 5-Fluorouracil intralesional
- Bleomycin (1.5 IU/mL) intralesional
- Prednisone (1 mg/kg/day) oral
- Prednisone (60 mg/day) oral + ibuprofen (1800 mg/day)
- Cortivazol (3.75 mg/1.5 mL) intralesional
- Amoxicillin (1.5-3 g twice daily) oral (Christensen)
- Ciprofloxacin (500 mg to 1 g twice daily) oral (Christensen)
- Minocycline (2 × 100 mg/day) oral
- Minocycline (2 × 250 mg/day) + prednisolone (4 mg/day) oral
- Cyclosporine (5 mg/kg/day) oral
- Allopurinol (200-600 mg/day) oral
- Imiquimod (Aldara) cream 5% topical
- Tacrolimus cream 0.5% topical
- Laser 532 nm and 1064 nm
- Intense pulsed light

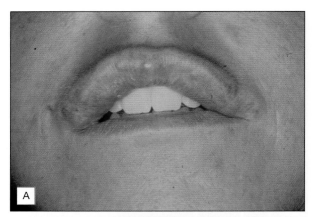

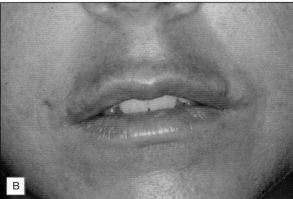

**Figure 30.10 A,** Dermalive granuloma. **B,** With improvement after treatment with intralesional 5-fluorouracil and steroids.

an injected steroid may cause tissue atrophy and help counter slight irregularities, as is done with hypertrophic scarring. However, one must take caution not to create a "doughnut" effect, with residual central prominence and surrounding atrophy. *Migration* is better avoided than treated, but surgical removal and liposuction are strategies for gross debulking of filler products in this situation.

Treatment of complications in the third category, which includes inflammation, infection, extrusion, and granuloma formation, is best geared toward the host immune response and infectious agents or ultimately by product reduction and removal (Box 30.2). Treatment is difficult, and no one single method has reliably proven effective. Immuno-modulators strike at the biologic mechanisms underlying the granulomatous response. Topical immunomodulating treatments, such as imiquimod, have been reported effective for granulomas, likely through dampening of the local host immune response. Injected immunomodulating medications, such as corticosteroids and 5-fluorouracil (5-FU), can also be effective for localized inflammation and granulomas (Fig. 30.10A and B). Oral steroids work by systemic, nonspecific immunomodulation and may be required for severe reactions over short to medium durations. Systemic biologic medications, such as etanercept and infliximab, have also been successful in altering the systemic immune response and decreasing granuloma activation and formation. There have been few reported cases using allopurinol to treat delayed granulomas associated with PMMA. Allopurinol is a xanthine oxidase inhibitor that acts as a catalyst in the formation of superoxide. Allopurinol and its metabolite oxypurinol act as free radical scavengers. Free radicals play an important role in the pathogenesis of granulomatous diseases and reduction of their amounts could contribute to the mechanism of action leading to reduced granuloma formation in select patients.[1]

If product reduction or removal is necessary, minimally invasive techniques should be attempted first, including needle aspiration, extrusion after incision, and liposuction. Ultimately, laser destruction or surgical removal may be necessary, but these modalities should be reserved for cases that are particularly problematic or that have not responded to more conservative therapies. Cassuto et al. have described a minimally invasive, minimally scarring technique for laser-assisted evacuation of infectious lesions after hydrogels using a lithium triborate laser at 532 nm, as well as a method for intralesional treatment of granulomas caused by gels containing microparticles, with an 808 nm diode laser to facilitate product evacuation (Fig. 30.11A and B).

Particularly with respect to late-onset granulomas, oral and/or intralesional antibiotic therapy should be attempted prior to, or at least alongside, other treatment modalities because biofilms are likely the etiologic agent. Some authors feel that initial treatment with any agent

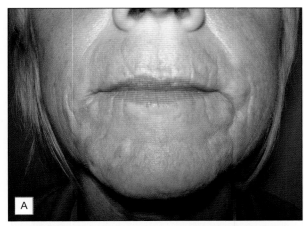

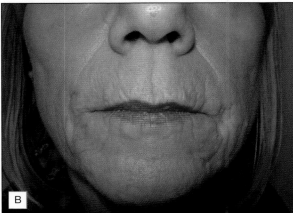

**Figure 30.11 A,** Late-onset granulomas. **B,** With improvement after treatment with the method described by Cassuto et al.

other than antibiotics may allow the biofilm colony to thrive, possibly setting up an opportunity for long-term and recurrent granulomatous sequelae. Ultimately, a multimodal treatment approach may be necessary. A suggested therapeutic ladder for late-onset granulomas includes treatment with antibiotics first and foremost, possibly along with an immunomodulating agent, such as a steroid. Failing that, escalating immunomodulating medications should then be used, followed by minimally invasive and ultimately surgically invasive treatments until a response is achieved.

### Pearl 8

Assume that late-onset granulomas are due in some part to bacterial biofilm colonization and direct therapy accordingly.

### Pearl 9

Use invasive and surgical options only after all other options have been exhausted.

### Pearl 10

Recurrent inflammation and granuloma formation may require chronic suppressive antibacterial therapy.

## Conclusions

All fillers are not created equal, and the aesthetic practitioner who wishes to treat the varied manifestations of facial aging and effectively guide patients to the desired outcome must know which ones will help to accomplish patient goals and which ones will not. Myriad "permanent" products are available, and most fall into particulate and nonparticulate categories. All may cause the full spectrum of filler complications. Permanent fillers share the same complications seen with temporary fillers, plus additional ones made more significant by their long-lasting nature. The most difficult complications, foreign body and late-onset granulomas, are increasingly recognized with permanent fillers and may be attributed to product–host interaction, as well as bacterial biofilm formation. A suggested therapeutic ladder includes antibiotic therapy, laser treatment with optic microfiber (as described by Cassuto et al.), immunomodulation, and possibly eventual surgical removal. Permanent fillers abound and will only increase over the next decade, as soft tissue augmentation has become the basis of an ever-expanding worldwide cosmetic industry. Even patients who do not have ready access to permanent fillers (such as in the United States) may easily find them abroad or illicitly for consumption. The modern aesthetic physician must recognize the products, the complications, and the treatment strategies, although there is more work to be done to elucidate underlying causes and best approaches for success.

## Reference

1. Park TH, Seo SW, Kim JK, Chang CH. Clinical experience with polymethylmethacrylate microsphere filler complications. *Aesthetic Plast Surg.* 2012;36(2):421–426.

## Further reading

Al-Qattan MM. Complications related to Artecoll injections for soft tissue augmentation of the hand: 3 case reports. *J Hand Surg Am.* 2011;36(6):994–997.

Carruthers J, Carruthers A, Humphrey S. Introduction to fillers. *Plast Reconstr Surg.* 2015;136(suppl 5):120–131.

Cassuto D, Marangoni O, de Santis G, Christensen L. Advanced laser techniques for filler-induced complications. *Dermatol Surg.* 2009;35(suppl 2):1689–1695.

Chrastil-LaTowsky B, Wesley NO, MacGregor JL, Kaminer MS, Arndt KA. Delayed inflammatory reaction to Bio-Alcamid polyacrylamide gel used for soft-tissue augmentation. *Arch Dermatol.* 2009;145(11):1309–1312.

Christensen L, Breiting V, Janssen M, Vuust J, Hogdall E. Adverse reactions to injectable soft tissue permanent fillers. *Aesthetic Plast Surg.* 2005;29(1):34–48.

Christensen LH. Host tissue interaction, fate, and risks of degradable and nondegradable gel fillers. *Dermatol Surg.* 2009;35(suppl 2):1612–1619.

Cohen SR, Rubin MG. Artefill. In: Sadick NS, ed. *Augmentation Fillers.* New York, NY: Cambridge University Press; 2010:53–67.

Do ER, Shim JS. Long term complications from breast augmentation by injected polyacrylamide hydrogel. *Arch Plast Surg.* 2012;39:267–269.

Epstein RE, Spencer JM. Correction of atrophic scars with artefill: an open-label pilot study. *J Drugs Dermatol.* 2010;9(9):1062–1064.

Formigli L, Zecchi S, Protopapa C, Caporale D, Cammarota N, Lotti TM. Bio-Alcamid: An Electron Microscopic Study after Skin Implantation. *Plas Reconstr Surg.* 2004;113(3):1104–1106.

Furmanczyk PS, Wolgamot GM, Argenyi ZB, Gilbert SC. Extensive granulomatous reaction occurring 15 years after DermaLive injection. *Dermatol Surg.* 2009;35(suppl 1):385–388.

Goldberg DJ. Bioalcamid. In: Sadick NS, ed. *Augmentation Fillers.* New York, NY: Cambridge University Press; 2010:113–116.

Grippaudo FR, Mattei M. The utility of high-frequency ultrasound in dermal fillers evaluation. *Ann Plast Surg.* 2011;67(5):469–473.

Jones DH. Semipermanent and permanent injectable fillers. *Dermatol Clin.* 2009;27(4):433–444.

Joseph JH, Eaton LL, Cohen BR. Current concepts in the use of bellafill. *Plast Reconstr Surg.* 2015;136(suppl 5):171–179.

Karim RB, Hage JJ, Van Rozelaar L, Lange CA, Raaijmakers J. Complications of Polyalkylimide 4% Injections (Bio-Alcamid): A report of 18 cases. *J Plast Reconstr Aesthet Surg.* 2006;59(12):1409–1414.

Khan I, Shokrollahi K, Bisarya K, Murison MS. A liposuction technique for extraction of Bio-Alcamid and other permanent fillers. *Aesthetic Surg J.* 2011;31(3):344–346.

Khetarpal S, Tomecki K, Billings SD. Foreign body granulomas from polymethylmethacrylate treated successfully with allopurinol. *Pract Dermatol.* 2014;10:35–36.

Lemperle G, Knapp TR, Sadick NS, Lemperle SM. ArteFill permanent injectable for soft tissue augmentation: I. Mechanism of action and injection techniques. *Aesthetic Plast Surg.* 2010;34(3):264–272.

Monheit GD, Rohrich RJ. The nature of long-term fillers and the risk of complications. *Dermatol Surg.* 2009;35(suppl 2):1598–1604.

Narins RS, Coleman WP 3rd, Rohrich R, et al. 12-Month controlled study in the United States of the safety and efficacy of a permanent 25% polyacrylamide hydrogel soft-tissue filler. *Dermatol Surg.* 2010;36(suppl 3):1819–1829.

Ono S, Ogawa R, Hyakusoku H. Complications after polyacrylamide hydrogel injection for soft-tissue augmentation. *Plast Reconstr Surg.* 2010;126(4):1349–1357.

Pacini S, Ruggiero M, Morucci G, Cammarota N, Protopapa C, Gulisano M. Bio-Alcamid: a novelty for reconstructive and cosmetic surgery. *Ital J Anat Embryol.* 2002;107(3):209–214.

Pallua N, Wolter TP. A 5-year assessment of safety and aesthetic results after facial soft-tissue augmentation with polyacrylamide hydrogel (Aquamid): a prospective multicenter study of 251 patients. *Plast Reconstr Surg.* 2010;125(6):1797–1804.

Prather CL, Jones DH. Liquid injectable silicone for soft tissue augmentation. *Dermatol Ther.* 2006;19(3):159–168.

Protopapa C, Sito G, Caporale D, Cammarota N. Bio-Alcamid in Drug-Induced Lipodystrophy. *J Cosmet Laser Ther.* 2003;5(3–4):226–230.

Rauso R, Freda N, Parlato V, Gherardini G, Amore R, Tartaro G. Polyacrylamide gel injection for treatment of human immunodeficiency virus-associated facial lipoatrophy: 18 months follow-up. *Dermatol Surg.* 2011;37(11):1584–1589.

Reisberger EM, Landthaler M, Wiest L, Schröder J, Stolz W. Foreign body granulomas caused by polymethylmethacrylate microspheres. *Arch Dermatol.* 2003;139(1):17–20.

Requena L, Requena C, Christensen L, Zimmermann US, Kutzner H, Cerroni L. Adverse reactions to injectable soft tissue fillers. *J Am Acad Dermatol.* 2011;64(1):1–34.

Rossner M, Rossner F, Bachmann F, Wiest L, Rzany B. Risk of severe adverse reactions to an injectable filler based on a fixed combination of hydroxyethylmethacrylate and ethylmethacrylate with hyaluronic acid. *Dermatol Surg.* 2009;35(suppl 1):367–374.

Sachdev M, Anantheswar Y, Ashok B, Hameed S, Pai SA. Facial granulomas secondary to injection of semi-permanent cosmetic dermal filler containing acrylic hydrogel particles. *J Cutan Aesthet Surg.* 2010;3(3):162–166.

Schelke LW, Van Den Elzen HJ, Erkamp PP, Neumann HA. Use of ultrasound to provide overall information on facial fillers and surrounding tissue. *Dermatol Surg.* 2010;36(suppl 3):1843–1851.

Schuller-Petrović S, Pavlović MD, Schuller SS, Schuller-Lukić B, Neuhold N. Early granulomatous foreign body reactions to a novel alginate dermal filler: the system's failure? *J Eur Acad Dermatol Venereol.* 2013;27:121–123. doi:10.1111/j.1468-3083.2011.04264.x.

Sclafani AP, Fagien S. Treatment of injectable soft tissue filler complications. *Dermatol Surg.* 2009;35(suppl 2):1672–1680.

Treacy PJ, Goldberg DJ. Use of a biopolymer polyalkylimide filler for facial lipodystrophy in HIV-positive patients underoging treatment with antiretroviral drugs. *Dermatol Surg.* 2006;32:804–808.

Wiest LG, Stolz W, Schroeder JA. Electron microscopic documentation of late changes in permanent fillers and clinical management of granulomas in affected patients. *Dermatol Surg.* 2009;35(suppl 2):1681–1688.

Wolter TP, Pallua N. Removal of the permanent filler polyacrylamide hydrogel (Aquamid) is possible and easy even after several years. *Plast Reconstr Surg.* 2010;126(3):138e–139e.

Yamauchi PS. Emerging permanent filler technologies: focus on aquamid. *Clin Cosmet Investig Dermatol.* 2014:7;261–266.

Zielke H, Wölber L, Wiest L, Rzany B. Risk profiles of different injectable fillers: results from the Injectable Filler Safety Study (IFS Study). *Dermatol Surg.* 2008;34(3):326–335.

# 31

# Reversers

## Gabriela Casabona, Jose Raul Montes, Paula Marchese

### Summary and Key Features

- Increasing popularity of soft tissue augmentation requires knowledge of reversal techniques.
- Adverse events due to filler injection can be totally or partially reversed depending on the filler type and timing.
- Biodegradable fillers are much more forgiving and more easily corrected.
- Hyaluronidase can be considered a treatment "eraser" for many complications arising from the injection of hyaluronic acid, and small doses can be effective.
- Vascular occlusion should be rapidly diagnosed and treated, especially if vision loss is involved, and large doses of hyaluronidase should be considered
- Late-onset inflammatory reactions may require more invasive techniques, particularly after complications due to nonbiodegradable filling agents.

## Introduction

Better and more profound knowledge of the anatomy involved in the aging process, in which volume restoration is one of the most important aspects, led to outstanding growth of the use of injectable products. According to statistics presented by American Society for Aesthetic Plastic Surgery (ASAPS) in 2015 the use of hyaluronic acid (HA) injection as a nonsurgical procedure grew 21% in United States.[1] As opposed to how it was performed in the past, when mainly nasolabial folds and lips were addressed, many other sites of injection are now being treated, such as nose, tear trough, and forehead, and more superficial techniques are now available ("blanching technique"). These changes in the use of injectables brought the need to a more deep knowledge on how to treat complications after injections. The products can be divided into two categories according to biodegradability: biodegradable (absorbable) or nonbiodegradable (permanent). In addition companies innovated cross-linking techniques with different HA concentrations for more versatile and long-lasting use of the products (Table 31.1).

Any of the listed products can lead to early or delayed complications, but only HAs can be really reverted with the use of hyaluronidase. Unlike biodegradable agents, particularly HAs, permanent fillers require more invasive techniques and can be more difficult to correct in the event of misplacement or serious adverse reactions.

## Why do we need reversers?

One of the reasons for a physician to use a reverser is an unwanted event after a filler injection. Looking from the perspective of the filler permanence, according to Table 31.1, only HA and collagen can be completely erased by two different enzymes: hyaluronidase and collagenase. However, if we look at all the adverse events after filler application, especially with nonabsorbable fillers, there are complications that can be partially reversed or at least treated with a variety of substances, lasers, or oral medicines without addressing the filler permanence, and those will be mentioned but not discussed in this chapter. This chapter will focus on the use of substances, procedures, or technology that can alter or change not only the permanence of filler itself but also change the elements involved in a specific adverse event.

## Filler complications and reversibility

Adverse effects following soft tissue augmentation are generally classified as early onset (up to 2 weeks after injection) or delayed onset (from 15 days to years after injections) (Box 31.1). Delayed-onset reactions are more commonly associated with nonabsorbable filling agents but have been more recently described with HA, calcium hydroxylapatite (CaHA), and poly-L-lactic acid (PLLA).

## Reversible adverse events and reversers (Figs. 31.1 to 31.5)

The early-onset adverse events are easier to treat and more common then the late-onset ones. According to reversibility classification (Box 31.1) HA and Collagen injection may be a clear advantage over other substances. The most common immediate complications are not related to the filler chosen but to the injection itself: bruising and swelling at the injection site. In review of the literature, we found

**Table 31.1** Products according to biodegradability, manufacturer, type of cross-link or vehicle, type of product and concentration, regulatory organs approval for United States, Canada, Europe, South America, and Central America

| Biodegradable products | | | | | |
|---|---|---|---|---|---|
| Product | Manufacturer | Cross-link tech/vehicle | Type product and concentration mg/mL | Approval by country | Biodegradability/ erasability |
| Juvéderme XC ultra | Allergan | Hylacross | HA-24 | All | Absorbable/ Erasable |
| Juvéderme XC ultra plus | Allergan | Hylacross | HA-24 | All | Absorbable/ Erasable |
| Restylane | Galderma | Nasha | HA-20 | All | Absorbable/ Erasable |
| Perlane | Galderma | Nasha | HA-20 | — | Absorbable/ Erasable |
| Radiesse | Merz | Carboximetilce-lullose 70% | Calcium hydroxylapatite 30% | All | Absorbable/ Nonerasable |
| Sculptra | Galderma/ Sinclair | Saline and Lidocaine | Poly-L-lactic acid (% depend on dilution) | All | Absorbable/ Nonerasable |
| Zyderm/Zyplast | Allergan | Collagen | Collagen bovine | All | Absorbable/ Erasable |
| Juvéderm voluma | Allergan | Vycross | HA-20 | All | Absorbable/ Erasable |
| Juvéderm volbella* | Allergan | Vycross | HA-15 | South America/Canada/ Europe | Absorbable/ Erasable |
| Juvéderm volift* | Allergan | Vycross | HA-17.5 | South, Central America/ Canada/Europe | Absorbable/ Erasable |
| Belotero balance | Merz | CPM | HA-22.5 | All | Absorbable/ Erasable |
| Beotero volume* | Merz | CPM | HA-26 | South, Central America/ Canada/ Europe | Absorbable/ Erasable |
| Belotero intense* | Merz | CPM | HA-25.5 | South, Central America/ Canada/Europe | Absorbable/ Erasable |
| Belotero soft* | Merz | CPM | HA-20 | South, Central America/ Canada/Europe | Absorbable/ Erasable |
| Emervel classic* | Galderma | OBT | HA-20 | South, Central America/ Canada/Europe | Absorbable/ Erasable |
| Emervel lips* | Galderma | OBT | HA-20 | South, Central America/ Canada/Europe | Absorbable/ Erasable |
| Emervel volume* | Galderma | OBT | HA-20 | South, Central America/ Canada/Europe | Absorbable/ Erasable |
| Restylane Silk/Vital | Galderma | NASHA | HA-20 | All | Absorbable/ Erasable |
| **Nonbiodegradable products (permanent)** | | | | | |
| Silikone 1000 | Alcon | — | Polymethylsiloxane | All (not aesthetic uses) | Nonabsorbable/ nonerasable |
| Belafill | Suneva Medical | Bovine collagen | PMMA + Bovine collagen | North America and Canada | Nonabsorbable/ nonerasable |

*CPM,* Cohesive polydensified matrix; *OBT,* optimal balance technology; *NASHA,* non-animal stabilized hyaluronic acid; *PMMA,* polimethylmetacrilate.
*Products not FDA approved.

<table>
<tr><td colspan="2">

**Box 31.1**
**Adverse events following soft tissue augmentation according to onset**

**1) Early onset (immediate to 15 days)**

Due to the procedure, not filler-related

- Bruising
- Swelling at site of injection
- Infection (viral or bacterial)

Due to filler behavior and placement technique

- Overcorrection
- Misplacement (palpable or visible implant)
- Hypersensitivity (type IV reaction)
- Angioedema (type I reaction)
- Vascular occlusion

**2) Late onset (from 15 days to years)**

Due to the procedure, not filler-related

- Chronic infection

Due to filler behavior and placement technique

- Skin discoloration (yellowish after CH )
- Migration of implants
- Nodules (product accumulation)
- Granulomas
- Recurrent edema
- Tindall effect
- Hypersensitivity (type IV reaction)
- Biofilm
- Hypertrophic scarring

</td></tr>
</table>

that pulsed dye laser (PDL) is the most effective technology used to help the clearance of a bruise and should start 1 to 2 days after the procedure, but YAG laser micropulsed can also be used. Infections are much less frequent, and herpes virus is the most common cause for physicians to be aware of the risk of an herpetic recurrence if there is a positive history. Adverse events related to injectable implants are more commonly due to inappropriate volume or too-superficial placement of the filling agent leading to palpable or visible material and textural changes (see Fig. 31.2A and B). Sometimes even nodules of product accumulation can be seen, especially with CaHA (see Fig. 31.5A and B), and can be easily treated with an injection of lidocaine 2% and saline 0.9% (1 : 1) and massage, as published by Voigts and Col (2010). Hypersensitivity and angioedema are very rare but can occur with all fillers composed of foreign body material. Anaphylaxis reaction symptoms are pruritus, erythema, urticarial lesions, angioedema, nausea, vomiting, breathlessness, dizziness, syncope, hypotension, or even cardiorespiratory arrest. The physician must be prepared to deal with anaphylaxis reactions. Epinephrine is the most important drug in this clinical emergency, maximally effective when injected promptly. H1-antihistamines are not drugs of choice in initial anaphylaxis treatment

because they do not relieve life-threatening respiratory symptoms or shock, although they decrease urticaria and itching. Diphenhydramine can be administered, and glucocorticoids remain in use for anaphylaxis because they potentially prevent biphasic anaphylaxis, reducing the risks of late symptoms. If symptoms are mild, oral prednisone can be prescribed, but more severe cases need intravenous methylprednisolone. It is important to have an oxygen cylinder and β2 agonist medication, such as salbutamol in the clinic in case of hypoxemia. After clinical stabilization the physician must decide whether the patient should be taken to the hospital or not.

Among all the adverse events related to filler placement, intravascular injection and its consequences can be devastating. Iatrogenic ophthalmic artery occlusion is characterized by severe ocular pain in the affected eye immediately after injection, but central retinal artery occlusion presents with only decreased vision without ocular pain. If there is any evidence of a visual problem or sudden ocular pain after dermal filler injection, prompt consultation with an ophthalmologist is recommended. Theoretically we have 90 minutes to reverse retinal ischemia and prevent tissue necrosis. Fagien and Carruthers has advocated that a large volume of retrobulbar hyaluronidase injection is the single most effective option to prevent retinal infarction after accidental hyaluronic filler embolization. Hyaluronidase 150 to 200 units/mL should be injected along the inferolateral orbit (see Fig. 31.3B). According to Cohen et al. when the occlusion involves skin, at least 200 U should be injected around the whole area of ischemia.[2] As mentioned previously, to reverse all immediate adverse events, timing is crucial, so we present an algorithm to treat and reverse each one. Every physician who performs filler injections needs to have in mind an algorithm for diagnosis and treatment of those catastrophic complications because timing is crucial to attempt reversal of permanent damage (see Figs. 31.1 and 31.3A and B).

Late-onset reactions are often the most difficult to treat. The ones related to injection procedures, such as skin discoloration, can be easily treated with lasers and intense pulsed light (IPL), as shown in Fig. 31.5, but chronic infections (e.g., mycobacterial due to preprocedure poor preparation) are difficult to treat and sometimes not completely reversed.

The most common complications of periocular filler injections with HA are Tyndall effect (blue light reflectance after HA superficially placed) and recurrent edema. The cause of recurrent inflammatory edema is not well known but, according to Beleznay (2015),[14] can be related to an immune response after viral or bacterial infection in other sites. Reversal of inflammatory edema requires oral oral steroids or just a small dose (4 to 28 U) (Table 31.2 and 31.3) of hyaluronidase, not to completely dissolve the product, but to reduce the amount of hyaluronan that may be triggering the immune response after a concomitant infection elsewhere or not (Figs. 31.5 to 31.7). Usually,

*Text continued on p. 222*

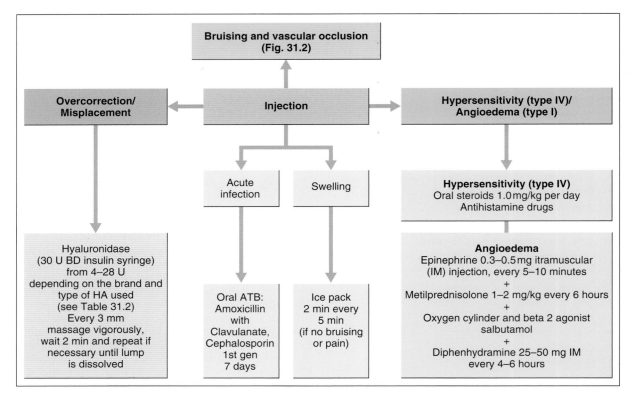

**Figure 31.1** Immediate-onset adverse events totally reversible.

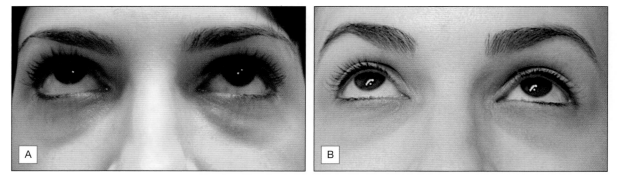

**Figure 31.2** (A) Patient after 6 months of HA filler for tear trough correction and (B) 15 days after 8 U hyaluronidase each side (4 U per lump).

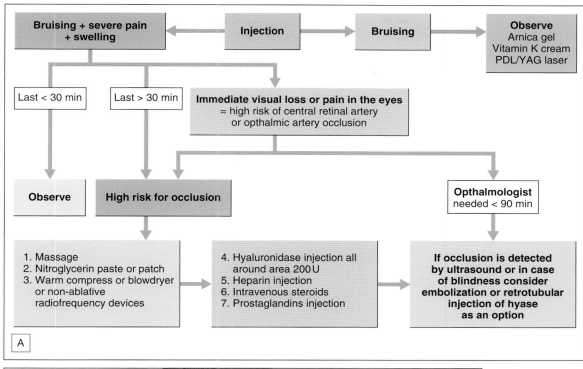

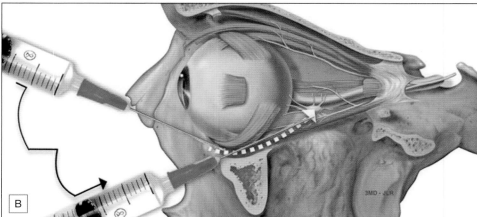

**Figure 31.3** (A) Vascular occlusion and bruising. (B) How to perform retrobulbar injection of hyaluronidase if occlusion of ophthalmic artery of retinal artery is suspected. *B*, modified. Original image attribution goes to Patrick J. Lynch http://commons.wikimedia.org/wiki/Category:Medical_illustrations_by_Patrick_Lynch

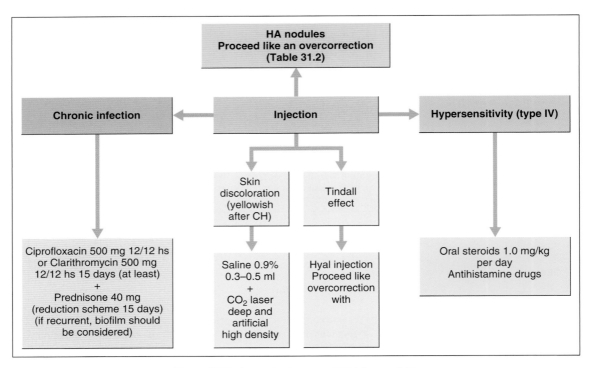

**Figure 31.4** Late-onset adverse events totally reversible.

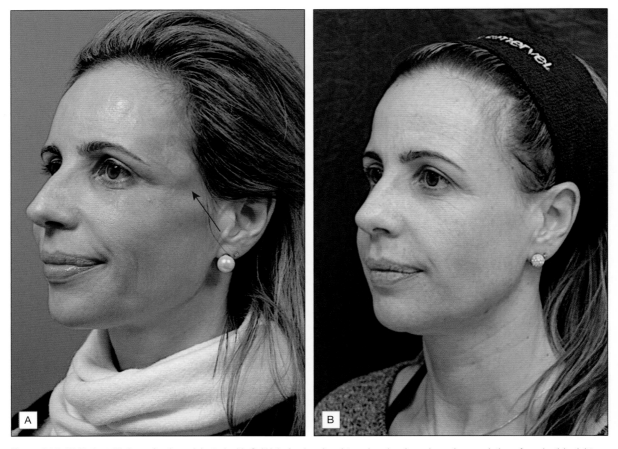

**Figure 31.5** (A) Patient 15 days after been injected with CaHA in forehead and temples showing a lump (accumulation of product) in right temple, and (B) (*arrow*). (C) After injection of 0.25 mL of lidocaine 2% and 0.25 mL of saline 0.9% using a 100 U BD insulin syringe and vigorous massage right after.

**Table 31.2** Brands, origin, manufacturer, availability by country, dilutions, and dose recommended for five different hyaluronidase products

| Product | Manufacturer | Available for use | Origin of hyaluronidase | Dose (mL) | Dilution | Amount to inject 4 U (using 30U BD syringe) (mL) |
|---|---|---|---|---|---|---|
| Hyaluronidase 2000 | Biometil Swiss, Sao Bento do Sul, SC, Brazil | Brazil | Purified bovine testicular | 2000 UI/5 | 5 mL of own diluent | 4 UI/0.01 |
| Vitrase | ISTA Pharmaceutical, Irvine, CA | USA, Canada | Purified ovine testicular* | 200 UI/1.2 | 1.2 mL already diluted | 4 UI/0.025 |
| Hylenex | Halozyme Therapeutics, San Diego, CA; marketed by Baxter Healthcare | USA, Canada | Recombinant human deoxyribonucleic acid (rDNA), hamster ovary cells | 150 UI | 1 mL saline 0.9% | 4 UI/0.025 |
| Hylase, Dessau | Riemser Pharma GmbH, Berlim Germany | USA, Canada and Europe | Purified bovine testicular | 150 UI | 1 mL saline 0.9% | 4 UI/0.025l |
| Reductonidasa | Mesoestetic Pharma Group, Barcelona, Spain | Europe | Purified bovine testicular | 1500 UI/10 | 10 mL saline 0.9% | 4 UI/0.025 |

*Preservative-free.

**Table 31.3** Dose recommended for five different hyaluronidase products according to each HA product tested at T0: units (UI) of hyaluronidase needed to clinically dissolve HA at time zero (immediately after HA injection)/T35: units (UI) of hyaluronidase needed to clinically dissolve HA 35 days after HA injection

| | Hyaluronidases (UI) | | | | | | | | | |
|---|---|---|---|---|---|---|---|---|---|---|
| | Reductonidasa (R)* | | Vitrase (V) | | Hylenex (Hx) | | Hylase (Hy) | | Biometil (B)* | |
| Volumes of fillers (mL) | T0 | T35 | T0 | T35 | T0 | T35 | T0 | T35 | T0 | T35 |
| Volbella 0.1* | 12 UI | 04 UI | 08 UI | 08 UI | 04 UI | 08 UI | 08 UI | 16 UI | 08 UI | 08 UI |
| Volbella 0.2* | 12 UI | 04 UI | 12 UI | 08 UI | 06 UI | 12 UI | 12 UI | 20 UI | 12 UI | 12 UI |
| Voluma 0.1 | 12 UI | 08 UI | 12 UI | 08 UI | 24 UI | 24 UI | 08 UI | 08 UI | 08 UI | 16 UI |
| Voluma 0.2 | 12 UI | 08 UI | 12 UI | 08 UI | 28 UI | 28 UI | 08 UI | 8 UI | 08 UI | 20 UI |
| Juvéderm Ultra Plus XC 0.1 | 4 UI | 04 UI | 06 UI | 06 UI | 04 UI | 20 UI | 04 UI | 08 UI | 04 UI | 04 UI |
| Juvéderm Ultra Plus XC 0.2 | 8 UI | 04 UI | 06 UI | 06 UI | 04 UI | 20 UI | 08 UI | 08 UI | 08 UI | 04 UI |
| Belotero balance 0.1 | 4 UI | 04 UI | 04 UI | 04 UI | 04 UI | 02 UI | 04 UI | 04 UI | 04 UI | 04 UI |
| Belotero balance 0.2 | 4 UI | 04 UI | 08 UI | 04 UI | 04 UI | 02 UI | 04 UI | 12 UI | 08 UI | 04 UI |
| Belotero volume 0.1* | 8 UI | 08 UI | 08 UI | 08 UI | 08 UI | 08 UI | 04 UI | 08 UI | 16 UI | 08 UI |
| Belotero volume 0.2* | 8 UI | 08 UI | 12 UI | 08 UI | 08 UI | 08 UI | 04 UI | 08 UI | 20 UI | 12 UI |

*Products not FDA-approved.

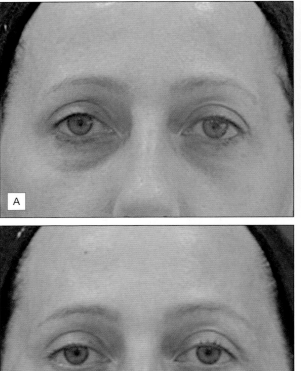

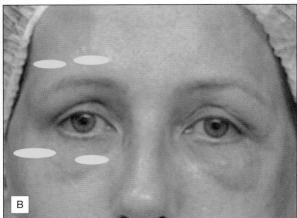

**Figure 31.6** (A) Patient preinjection. (B) Four months after injection of different densities of HA in forehead, temples, eyebrow, and malar areas, presented an inflammatory edema with pain. At first, treated with clarithromycin and oral steroids with mild response, and then hyaluronidase was injected during the course of antibiotics only at the points that had induration (*yellow dots*). (C) Two days after hyaluronidase there were a total response and the aesthetic effect could still be seen.

late-onset adverse events after HA injections may be totally reversed, whereas with other injectables, reversal is unpredictable.

## Hyaluronidase

Hyaluronidase is a naturally occurring enzyme (endo-β-N-acetyl-hexosaminidases) that degrades the substrate HA. Hyaluronidase breaks down HA by separating the 1,4-glucosa-minidic bond between C1 of the glucosamine moiety and C4 of the glucuronic acid. In its natural environment, hyaluronidase facilitates several important functions, ranging from fertility to bacterial pathogenesis. After injection, hyaluronidase immediately disperses in tissues, and rapid return to previous skin contour is achieved. The duration of hyaluronidase enzyme activity is dependent on location. Hyaluronidase acts immediately once in contact with its substrate, and the duration of activity is typically

24 to 48 hours in dermal tissues. However, it has an extended duration in ocular tissues that ranges from 60 to 112 hours. In contrast, the hyaluronidase enzyme is deactivated immediately when injected intravenously. It is hypothesized that the process is antibody-mediated; however, the true mechanism of deactivation is unknown. The US Food and Drug Administration (FDA) has approved hyaluronidase to break down and hydrolyze HA for the following three therapeutic indications:

1. Increase the absorption and dispersion of other injected drugs, particularly retrobulbar anesthetic block in ophthalmologic surgery (it reduces the viscosity of extracellular matrix, which facilitates the diffusion of the agent, enlarging the anesthetized area, and shortens diffusion time, increasing the permeability of tissues and enhancing the anesthesia effect).

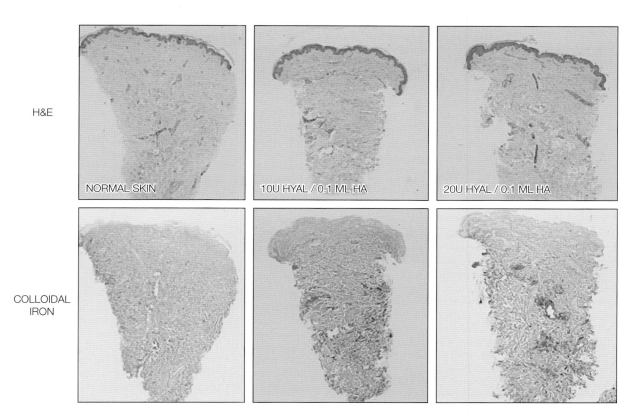

**Figure 31.7** Skin biopsy stained with colloidal iron to compare amount of hyaluronic acid in normal skin and after 10 and 20 U of hyaluronidase showing no natural HA difference.

**Table 31.4** Summary of data published on hyaluronidase doses and uses

| Author | Year | Dose (mL) (UNITS) | Repeat dose | Time for resolution | Recommendation |
|---|---|---|---|---|---|
| Soprarkar et al.[3]/Lambros[4] | 2004 | 75 U | UD | 24 h | Periocular overcorrection HA* |
| Soparkar et al.[3] | 2004 | 150–200 U/mL filler | UD | 1–2 h | Any adverse event |
| Brody[5] | 2005 | 15 U | 24 h | 24 h | Granulomatous reaction after HA* |
| Hirsch et al.[6] | 2006 | 150 U | UD | 72 h | Periocular misplacement HA* |
| Hirsch et al.[7] | 2007 | 30 U | 2 h | 13 days | Vascular occlusion nasolabial fold |
| Menon et al.[8] | 2010 | 1.5–3 U | 24 h | 24 h | Any adverse event |
| Cohen et al.[2] | 2015 | 200 U | 2 h | h–days | Vascular occlusion |

*HA- HYALURONIC ACID

2. Subcutaneous infusion of fluids (hypodermoclysis), used mostly in the elderly population for mild-to-moderate dehydration and in young infants or children in whom intravenous administration is not possible.
3. Adjunct for subcutaneous urography, improving the resorption of radiopaque agents.

Therapeutic off-label applications in dermatology have yielded variable success for the treatment of diabetic scleredema, scleroderma, and others. Hyaluronidase can be used after injection of HA fillers to correct asymmetry, overcorrection, the Tyndall effect, and vascular occlusion, and Table 31.4 show a summary of publications about its use.

## Available formulations

North American and Canadian commercial formulations of hyaluronidase include Vitrase, Hylenex, and Hylase Dessau. In most of the South American countries and Europe there are compounded hyaluronidases or they use the same ones used in the United States and Canada. In Brazil there is one extensively used, Hyaluronidase 2000 (Biometil Swiss, Sao Bento do Sul, SC, Brazil), which is prepared from purified bovine testicular hyaluronidase; in Europe there is one available, widely use, and produced in Germany, Hylase Dessau, and another produced in Spain, Reductonidase (see Table 31.2).

## Injection techniques and dosing

There is no consensus on dose or time comparing all hyaluronidases used in different countries. Most of the papers use US and Canadian hyaluronidase formulations. The dose will depend also on the type of HA product. Many different HA formulations are available, and each one has a different HA concentration and BDDE-based cross-linking 1,4 butanedioldiglycidyl ether (see Table 31.1). The degree of modification is one very important characteristic parameter that can affect the rheologic property, anti-degradation ability, and swelling property of modified HA hydrogel in the structural foundation. The modification type (pendent or cross-link modification) also affects the final properties of HA hydrogel. Cross-link modification is considered as the effective modification, which produces strong covalent bonds to retard the degradation and prolong duration of hydrogel. For that reason, an in vivo study on different hyaluronidase preparations and different HA products was performed by the author to try to quantify the amount of hyaluronidase and the time needed to dissolve clinical lumps (0.1 and 0.2 mL) of each HA product (Tables 31.2 and 31.3; immediately and a month after injection, respectively). According to the study five different hyaluronidases (Vitrase, Reductonidasa, Hylase, Hylenex, and Biometil) were studied to determine the minimum and maximum doses for each hyaluronidase and for each amount of different product. After statistical analysis, the study concluded that all five were effective in dissolving 0.1 to 0.2 mL of HA, and the dose varied from 4 to 28 U immediately and a month after injected HA. Dosages up to 150 U showed no compromise to the natural amount of HA of the skin (see Fig. 31.7), as Cavallini et al. reported that ovine hyaluronidase dosages below 14 U did not affect fibroblast viability.[9]

The dilution will depend on the hyaluronidase used, as in Table 31.2, and we suggest that the application should be performed with a 30 U BD insulin syringe. However, because all hyaluronidase formulations are very fluid, a 30- to 32-gauge needle can be used to diminish discomfort. In a prospective, randomized study of intradermal hyaluronidase to reduce dermal augmentation from HA, in 2005, Vartanian et al. recommended initial injections of 5 to 10 U to minimize the risk of allergic reaction and because of worry that high concentrations could dissolve native HA in the face, resulting in cosmetic deformity.[10] Current doses in practice vary, but range from 0.05 to 0.1 mL (7.5 to 28 U) per injection. Slow injections are placed directly into the HA depot. Simple HA nodules generally respond within 24 to 48 hours. Nodules of unknown cause and cases of inflammation may require a greater length of time for complete resolution, though most patients experience some degree of improvement within a few days. Follow-up at 2 weeks is recommended to assess the result. Hyaluronidase can spread and worsen severe inflammation and suspected abscesses; in these cases, concomitant systemic antibiotic therapy should be initiated.

## Side effects and precautions

Adverse effects to hyaluronidase are rare. Local injection site reactions are the most commonly reported reactions. Allergic reactions, such as urticaria or edema, have been reported in less than 0.1% of patients and mostly occur after retrobulbar or intravenous injection during ophthalmic surgery, although Andre and Fléchet reported a case of angioedema after ovine hyaluronidase into the upper lip, in which swelling began in the lips and progressed all over the upper face within 15 minutes.[11] According to Balassiano and Bravo after a retrospective study of 50 patients after use of hyaluronidase for immediate HA injection,[12] 46% had some kind of reaction, such as erythema, edema, and burning, but nothing major, after hylauronidase injection (the author). Vitrase showed the lowest percentage of edema and erythema in injection site.

Preliminary skin testing is officially recommended prior to using all preparations, particularly those derived from animal sources. An injection of 0.02 mL (3 U) of a 150 U/mL solution is placed intradermally; a wheal appearing within 5 minutes and persisting for 20 to 30 minutes with localized itching indicates a positive reaction. However, allergic reaction may not be completely excluded by skin test.

Contraindications include hypersensitivity to any of the components, particularly in a patient with a history of allergic response to bovine collagen. Caution should be used in patients with a history of allergic reaction to bee stings because hyaluronidase is one of the many biologically active components in bee venom. As mentioned previously, in the presence of infection, hyaluronidase can spread infection and should only be used in conjunction with systemic antibiotics.

## Other enzymatic reversers

In February 2010 the FDA approval of collagenase Clostridium histolyticum (Xiaflex) for the treatment of patients with Dupuytren contracture (a genetic disorder of pathologic collagen production) has led to some debate about the enzyme's ability to reverse the effect of collagen-based fillers. However, collagenase is associated with serious potential side effects, including tendon

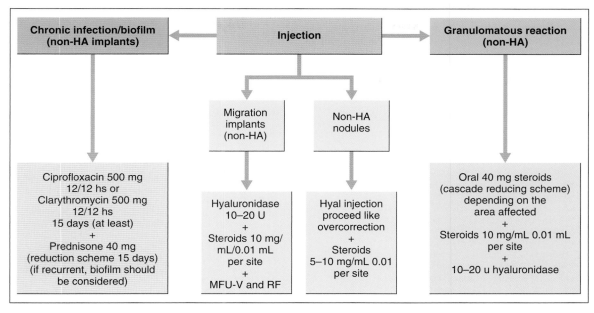

**Figure 31.8** Late-onset adverse events partially reversible.

rupture and ligament damage, complex regional pain syndrome, sensory abnormality, injection site hemorrhage, and severe allergic reactions after subsequent treatment sessions, and has not been studied for collagen reversal in the face.

## Partially reversible adverse events and reversers (Fig. 31.8)

Normally the partially reversible events are the late-onset ones and the more common are nodules (noninflammatory and nonpainful) after misplacement or accumulation of products, such as CaHA and PLLA (especially on chin area). Superficial injection of particulate fillers, such as CaHA, can produce skin discoloration at the injection site; this occurrence might be partially corrected with the use of a $CO_2$ laser to thicken the dermis and disguise the appearance.

Red, painful nodules appearing from 2 weeks up to 1 year after treatment could indicate infection due to biofilm and require immediate treatment with systemic antibiotics, incision and drainage, and hyaluronidase (that would help to destroy fibrotic tissue around the implant). Combination gels, such as PMMA or polyalkylimide, are most susceptible to complications from biofilms.

More severe infections require intravenous antibiotics followed by a course of oral antibiotics and judicial use of intralesional corticosteroids to assist in eliminating persistent inflammatory nodules. Because steroids can worsen inflammation and activate a biofilm, they should be injected only with concomitant use of antibiotics and should be used only in late-onset infections after erythema,

tenderness, and edema have subsided. If the nodule does not respond to antibiotics or corticosteroids, intralesional 5-fluorouracil (5-FU) mixed with triamcinolone has been shown to improve some granulomatous reactions. Surgery is generally considered the last option after failure of more conservative approaches and should only be performed by experienced physicians. Fifty-two percent of patients in the IFS study experienced adverse effects, such as scarring and asymmetry from surgical reversal. Cassuto et al. describe the use of two different types of laser-assisted treatments in 20 patients to heat and penetrate skin and mucosa, allowing melting and evacuation of organic and synthetic components of granulomatous filler reactions with lower morbidity and better cosmetic results than surgical excision.[13] Emerging technology, such as microfocused ultrasound energy devices, may theoretically have an application to these "adverse events" especially for resistant nodules or product migration that could have a benefit in breaking the fibrotic tissue around nodules.

## Conclusion

The rise in popularity of soft tissue augmentation for restoration of volume in the face mandates a greater understanding of treatment options and protocols for the management of related adverse effects. All injectable implants may present with complications, some of which can be treated by noninvasive approaches. Biodegradable fillers are less likely to cause more severe reactions; complications generally appear within 6 months and may be managed conservatively. **The availability of hyaluronidase** to "erase" unwanted effects makes the use of HA filling agents the product of choice for most practitioners.

Adverse events after placement of permanent fillers can appear years after initial treatment and often require invasive reversal techniques with the potential complication of tissue scaring and atrophy. Optimal management of these complications can be difficult and requires a thorough knowledge of available interventions and their likely outcomes.

## References

1. *ASAPS 2015—Statistics of non surgical procedures in 2015.* <http://www.surgery.org/sites/default/files/2015-quick-facts.pdf>.
2. Cohen J, Biesman BS, Dayan SH, et al. Treatment of hyaluronic acid filler-induced impending necrosis with hyaluronidase: consensus recommendations. *Aesthet Surg J.* 2015;35:1–6.
3. Soparkar CN, Patrinely JR, Tschen J. Erasing restylane. *Ophthal Plast Reconstr Surg.* 2004;20:317–318.
4. Lambros V. The use of hyaluronidase to reverse the effects of hyaluronic acid filler. *Plast Reconstr Surg.* 2004;114:277.
5. Brody HJ. Use of hyaluronidase in the treatment of granulomatous hyaluronic acid reactions or unwanted hyaluronic acid misplacement. *Dermatol Surg.* 2005;31(8 pt 1):893–897.
6. Hirsch RJ, Narurkar V, Carruthers J. Management of injected hyaluronic acid induced Tyndall effects. *Lasers Surg Med.* 2006;38:202–204.
7. Hirsch RJ, Cohen JL, Carruthers JD. Successful management of an unusual presentation of impending necrosis following a hyaluronic acid injection embolus and a proposed algorithm for management with hyaluronidase. *Dermatol Surg.* 2007;33:357–360.
8. Menon H, Thomas M, D'silva J. Low dose of hyaluronidase to treat over correction by HA filler—a case report. *J Plast Reconstr Aesthet Surg.* 2010;63:e416–e417.
9. Cavallini M, Antonioli B, Gazzola R, et al. Hyaluronidases for treating complications by hyaluronic acid dermal fillers evaluation of the effects on cell cultures and human skin. *Eur J Plast Surg.* 2013;36:477–484.
10. Vartanian AJ, Frankel AS, Rubin MG. Injected hyaluronidase reduces Restylane-mediated cutaneous augmentation. *Arch Facial Plast Surg.* 2005;7:231–237.
11. Andre P, Fléchet ML. Angioedema after ovine hyaluronidase injection for treating hyaluronic acid overcorrection. *J Cosmet Dermatol.* 2008;7:136–138.
12. Balassiano L, Bravo B. Hyaluronidase: a necessity for any dermatologist applying injectable hyaluronic acid. *Surg Cosmet Dermatol.* 2014;6(4):338–443.
13. Cassuto D, Marangoni O, De Santis G, Christensen L. Advanced laser techniques for filler-induced complications. *Dermatol Surg.* 2009;35(suppl 2):S1689–S1695.
14. Beleznay K, Carruthers JD, Carruthers A, Mummert ME, Humphrey S. Delayed-onset nodules secondary to a smooth cohesive 20 mg/mL hyaluronic acid filler: cause and management. *Dermatol Surg.* 2015;41:1–11.

## Further reading

Carruthers JD, Fagien S, Rohrich RJ, Weinkle S, Carruthers A. Blindness caused by cosmetic filler injection. *Plast Reconstr Surg.* 2014;134(6):1197–1201.

Conejo-Mir JS, Sanz Guirado S, Angel Muñoz M. Adverse granulomatous reaction to Artecoll treated by intralesional 5-fluorouracil and triamcinolone injections. *Dermatol Surg.* 2006;32:1079–1081.

Goldan O, Georgiou I, Grabov-Nardini G, et al. Early and late complications after a nonabsorbable hydrogel polymer injection: a series of 14 patients and novel management. *Dermatol Surg.* 2007;33(suppl 2):S199–S206.

Hurst LC, Badalamente MA, Hentz VR, et al. Injectable collagenase clostridium histolyticum for Dupuytren's contracture. *N Engl J Med.* 2009;361:968–979.

Marković-Housley Z, Miglierini G, Soldatova L, Rizkallah PJ, Müller U, Schirmer T. Crystal structure of hyaluronidase, a major allergen of bee venom. *Structure.* 2000;8:1025–1035.

Narins RS, Coleman WP 3rd, Glogau RG. Recommendations and treatment options for nodules and other filler complications. *Dermatol Surg.* 2009;35(suppl 2):1667–1671.

Starr CR, Engleberg NC. Role of hyaluronidase in subcutaneous spread and growth of group A streptococcus. *Infect Immun.* 2006;74:40–48.

Sundaram H, Fagien S. Cohesive polydensified matrix hyaluronic acid for fine lines. *Plast Reconstr Surg.* 2015;136;5(S):149–163.

Voigts R, DeVore DP, Grazer JM. Dispersion of calcium hydroxylapatite accumulations in the skin: animal studies and clinical practices. *Dermatol Surg.* 2010;36:798–803.

Watt AJ, Curtin CM, Hentz VR. Collagenase injection as nonsurgical treatment of Dupuytren's disease: 8-year follow-up. *J Hand Surg.* 2010;35:534–539.

Woodward J, Khan T, Martin J. Facial filler complications. *Facial Plast Surg Clin North Am.* 2015;23:447–458.

Yang B, Guo X, Zang H, Liu J. Determination of modification degree in BDDE-modified hyaluronic acid hydrogel by SEC/MS. *Carbohydr Polym.* 2015;131:233–239.

Voigts R, Devore D, Glazer J. Dispersion of calcium hydroxylapatite accumulations in the skin: animal studies and clinical practice. *Derm Surg* 2010;36(S1):798–803.

# 32

# Combinations

## Omer Ibrahim, Adele Haimovic, Jeffrey S. Dover

### Summary and Key Features

- There are a multitude of factors that contribute to skin aging, including volume loss, dyspigmentation, fine wrinkles, and changes in skin texture.
- A multifaceted approach targeting the various aspects of aging is often required to effectively rejuvenate the skin and ensure patient satisfaction.
- Literature suggests that a combination of treatments with fillers, neurotoxins, and light- and energy-based devices is both safe and provides synergistic beneficial effects for the treatment of aging skin.
- Further investigation into the efficacy, mechanisms of action, and optimal techniques is essential to advancing the treatment of photoaged skin.

## Introduction

Soft tissue fillers, such as hyaluronic acid (HA), are but a single tool in the physician's arsenal in the treatment of aging skin. To effectively treat the patient and yield desirable results, the physician as artist must globally visualize the entire subject and face as a whole. The physician must not only examine the types of lines and wrinkles, the fine or deep, static or dynamic, but he or she must look past the mere lines and wrinkles to assess volume deficits created with the passage of time, as well as studying skin texture changes, telangiectasias, pigmentation, and skin laxity in his or her assessment of the patient. In this chapter we discuss the efficacy and safety of combining fillers with different treatment modalities in the management of this multifaceted process of skin aging.

## Combining soft tissue fillers with neurotoxins

The use of injectable medications has revolutionized the treatment of facial rhytides. Neurotoxins, such as onabotulinumtoxin A (onaBot), abobotulinumtoxin A (aboBot), and incobotulinumtoxin A (incoBot), have become mainstays in the treatment of dynamic wrinkles, not only of the upper face but also in the perioral skin and the neck and jawline. To many patients, neuromodulators

are the starter or "gateway" treatments on their road to facial rejuvenation. Starting with neuromodulators alone is a good starting point, but knowledge of the efficacy and safety of combining neurotoxins with soft tissue fillers is essential to more advanced techniques and better results. As early as 2003, Carruthers and Carruthers demonstrated the superiority of combining HA filler and onaBot in the treatment of severe glabellar rhytides (Fig. 32.1).[1] Thirty-eight female subjects were randomized to either treatment with HA alone or with HA and onaBot. The combination group showed a better response both at rest and maximum frown, and this response was maintained for an average of 14 weeks longer than the HA group. No differences in adverse effects were noted. In a randomized split-face study by Dubina et al., patients' glabellar/forehead wrinkles were treated with aboBot alone on one side and aboBot and HA filler on the other side. Blinded ratings demonstrated longer-lasting effects and greater static and dynamic wrinkle reduction in the combination group without differences in side effects. Subjects also favored combination treatments over toxin alone.[2] These studies suggest that HA fillers and neurotoxins act synergistically in alleviating skin wrinkles. The effect of the toxin results in muscle relaxation and therefore slower breakdown of the HA. The effect of the HA filler results in a softer, more natural return to baseline after the toxin wears off.[2]

The combination of HA fillers and neurotoxins has been applied to other areas of the face (Fig. 32.2). In one study by Beer et al., aboBot was placed into the glabella and crow's feet and HA filler into the temples and glabella.[3] Investigators noted significant improvements in glabellar rhytids, periorbital areas, crow's feet, and temporal hollowing. Furthermore, 64% of patients who received toxin alone in the past preferred combination treatments. Carruthers et al. assessed the combination of HA and toxin in the lower face and perioral region.[4,5] Ninety female subjects were randomized to receive either HA filler alone, onaBot alone, or HA and onaBot in combination. Subjects in all three groups demonstrated statistically significant investigator-rated improvements in lower face appearance. The combination group had greater improvement from baseline than either modality alone. Adverse events were mild, transient, and typical of the procedures performed. Unique untoward side effects from combining treatments were not noted. Similar studies have shown comparable high rates of patient satisfaction and

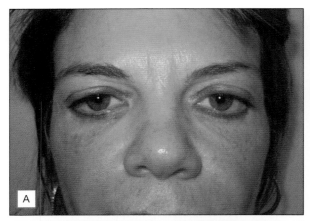

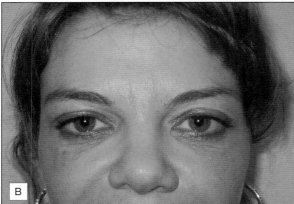

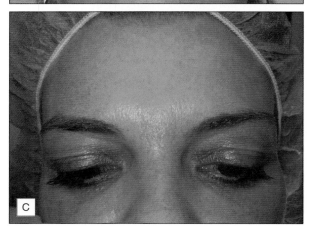

**Figure 32.1** Significant improvement of glabellar wrinkles with a combination of hyaluronic acid and botulinum toxin. **A, B** Before and after BTX. **C,** After BTX plus HA. *BTX,* Botulinum toxin; *HA,* hyaluronic acid. *Adapted from Romagnoli M, Belmontesi M. Hyaluronic acid-based fillers: theory and practice. Clin Dermatol. 2008;26(2):123–159.*

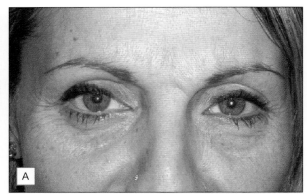

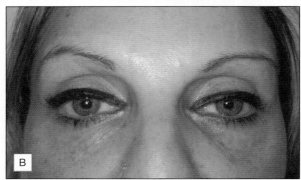

**Figure 32.2 A, B** Hyaluronic acid filler in the glabella and tear troughs combined with botulinum toxin to the glabella to produce marked rejuvenation. *Adapted from Romagnoli M, Belmontesi M. Hyaluronic acid-based fillers: theory and practice.* Clin Dermatol. *2008;26(2):123–159.*

efficacy when fillers were combined with neurotoxins in up to 13 facial zones.[6] In addition to treating aging skin, some investigators have used HA and neurotoxin to reshape aspects of the face in lieu of more traditional invasive cosmetic surgery. One such example is the combination of HA and toxin to redefine the contour of the nose (Fig. 32.3).[7]

The combination of filler and neurotoxin appears to be safe and effective. However, the physician must be aware that the majority of reports and studies on this subject have used HA fillers, and reports on other types of fillers are scarce. A firm grasp of facial anatomy including the vasculature is imperative to achieve desirable results and minimize adverse effects.

## Combining soft tissue fillers with light- and energy-based devices

Lasers and light-based treatments have gained popularity as noninvasive techniques to improve the appearance of aging skin, including color and texture. The high degree of improvement, low rates of adverse events, and minimal downtime associated with laser- and light-based therapies

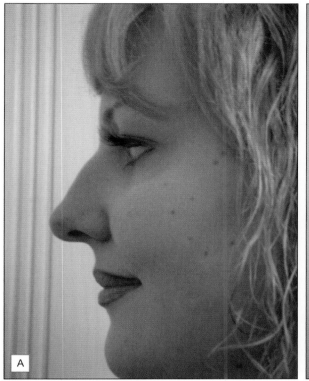 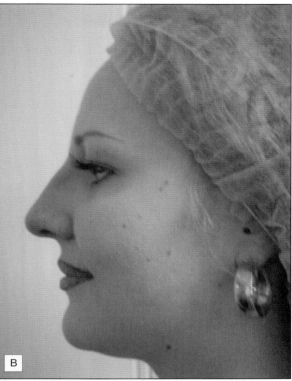

**Figure 32.3 A, B** Hyaluronic acid filler treatment to reshape the nasal bridge. *Adapted from Romagnoli M, Belmontesi M. Hyaluronic acid-based fillers: theory and practice. Clin Dermatol. 2008;26(2):123–159.*

have made them favorable options. Because these technologies target different aspects of the aging process than soft tissue fillers, investigators have studied whether concomitant use of these therapies with soft tissue augmentation can be performed safely and effectively to treat the various facets of photoaging. Many studies have suggested that combining fillers with devices, such as ablative and nonablative lasers, intense pulsed light (IPL), radiofrequency (RF), and ultrasound, is safe and efficacious in treating photoaged skin.

RF devices are used to tighten and contour skin; however, their ability to restore volume loss is limited. Several studies have examined the utility of combining RF therapy with fillers.[8] England et al. demonstrated that RF treatment 2 weeks after injections with fillers does not influence the rate of side effects or adversely affect filler duration.[9] A follow-up study concluded that RF treatment over fillers increased the inflammatory, foreign body, and fibrotic responses seen on histology.[10] However, these findings contrast with subsequent histologic reports by Alam et al. No histopathologic changes were appreciated in patients treated with either HA filler or calcium hydroxyapatite followed by treatment with a monopolar RF device.[11] Studies have not only demonstrated that combining RF devices with fillers appears to be safe, but

more recent work has suggested that combining RF therapy with HA fillers on the same day may work synergistically and provide long-lasting effects for the improvement of age-related volume loss.[12]

IPL is a nonablative device that targets melanin and hemoglobin, treating vascular and pigmented lesions seen in sun-damaged skin. Fabi and Goldman examined 90 patients treated with IPL immediately before or as early as 6 days after poly-L-lactic acid (PLLA) injection;[13] 86.7% of subjects reported at least mild photorejuvenating effects from the combination of treatments. There were no significant complications, including nodule formation after IPL treatment. They concluded that combination of PLLA injection and IPL for facial photorejuvenation is effective and does not result in increased adverse events than with each treatment modality alone.

In addition to RF devices and IPL, focused ultrasound is used to improve skin laxity. Friedmann et al. reviewed their experience with combination therapy with IPL, PLLA, and microfocused ultrasound (MFU).[14] They reported that all three photorejuvenation modalities can be safely performed in a single treatment session. They recommend that PLLA injections should be performed last to avoid blood contamination of the MFU or IPL equipment.

Lasers, such as the 1320-nm neodymium-doped yttrium aluminum garnet (Nd : YAG) laser and the 1450-nm diode laser, are thought to stimulate new collagen formation in the dermis. Goldman et al. performed a randomized trial to evaluate the effect of therapy with monopolar RF, IPL, 1320-nm Nd : YAG laser (14 to 16 J/cm$^2$, cooling 15 ms before, 10 ms during, 15 ms after; or 16 to 17 J/cm$^2$, 10 ms before, 5 ms during, and 10 ms after), or 1450-nm diode laser (6-mm spot, 12 to 14 J/cm$^2$ energy density) on HA injection.[15] They concluded that HA filler can be combined with either modality without altering efficacy or safety. Ribé and Ribé examined whether injections with HA followed immediately by fractional 1440-nm Nd : YAG laser for neck skin rejuvenation would have clinical and histologic effects.[16] They reported improvement in skin tightness, texture, and fine lines after combination therapy. Based on biopsy specimens they concluded that the fractional nonablative laser produced favorable epidermal and superficial changes, whereas the HA led to favorable changes deeper in the dermis.

Farkas et al. examined the histologic specimens from porcine models that were treated with HA fillers followed by different lasers 2 weeks later.[17] Based on histologic examination the fillers were not affected by IPL, nonablative lasers, or very superficial ablative treatments. However, the deep ablative therapies (such as deep carbon dioxide or erbium : YAG lasers) demonstrated interactions with the HA filler, such as migration of fillers into the ablated microchannels. These authors suggest that if deep resurfacing is planned, laser treatments should be performed before filler injections or on different days to optimize outcomes and limit side effects.

## Combining soft tissue fillers

The realm of soft tissue fillers is ever-growing and evolving. More and more products with varying constituents, concentrations of HA, degrees of cross-linking, flow characteristics, and tissue-lifting abilities surface on the market every year, expanding the physician's repertoire of injectables. With the advent of a more global or comprehensive approach to facial aging, the use of combinations of different types of fillers to address different aspects of aging has become commonplace (Fig. 32.4). Fillers can be approximately divided into those that add volume,

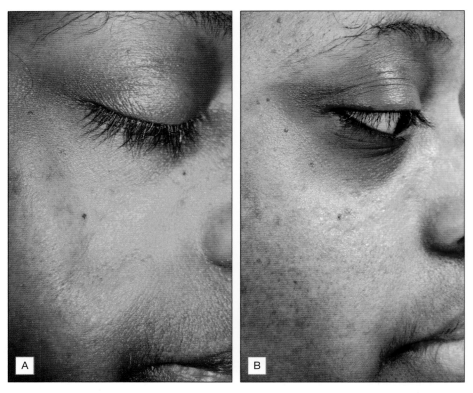

**Figure 32.4 A,** Significant midfacial atrophy secondary to lupus profundus. **B,** Significant improvement in facial atrophy after treatment with a combination of hyaluronic acid and poly-L-lactic acid fillers. *Adapted from Eastham AB, Liang CA, Femia AN, Lee TC, Vleugels RA, Merola JF. Lupus erythematosus panniculitis-induced facial atrophy: effective treatment with poly-L-lactic acid and hyaluronic acid dermal fillers. J Am Acad Dermatol. 2013;69(5):e260–e262.*

those that fill lines, those that provide lift, and those that are able to buttress.[18] These different fillers can be combined in the same location, on top of the other, or in different locations to achieve desirable effects. Of note, there is broad overlap of these products, and in some cases single versatile filler can be used for different indications, with or without dilution or blending with xylocaine. Blending filler with lidocaine or xylocaine, with or without epinephrine, decreases the viscosity and extrusion force of the filler and increases patient comfort without compromising the filler's integrity. Therefore thicker fillers more suited for deeper placement within tissue can be softened with blending to allow for easier flow and filling of fine lines, such as in the medial cheek, or feathering along the edge of a filled area, increasing the filler's versatility and applicability to different areas of the face.[19,20]

Among many changes that develop over time, the disappearance of the malar fat pad with resultant drooping of the midface is one of the more prominent.[21,22] Thicker HA products with higher degree of cross-linking or calcium hydroxyapatite injected deep into the malar area can help to lift the skin back closer to its original youthful state. However, not addressing the perioral lines with softer products retains an aged look. Therefore softer, lighter, less or differently cross-linked HA products can be injected into perioral lines, marionette lines, and superficial lip lines to concurrently rejuvenate the perioral area.[18] Thicker, more durable products or injectables that induce collagen formation can also be used to fill voids in the temples, cheeks, and jawline.[23] After the cheeks, malar areas, and perioral area are rejuvenated, the glabella, tear troughs, and lips can be restored with even lighter HA fillers, especially in people with thinner skin.[18]

In addition to combining fillers geographically on the face, they can be combined temporally. Products with shorter lifespans can be placed at the patient's first visit, to test the patient's response and satisfaction with the filler. After a patient is content, longer-lasting fillers can be injected at subsequent visits to achieve the same effects for longer duration.[18]

## Conclusion

Injectable soft tissue fillers have revolutionized the management of aging skin. Although they can tackle some aspects of volume deficit, skin laxity, and static wrinkles, they fall short of addressing the multitude of factors that contribute to the aged face, especially changes in color and texture. This has necessitated the coupling of soft tissue fillers with a multitude of modalities to radically rejuvenate the skin. Through literature ranging from randomized controlled trials to expert opinion, it has become apparent that combining fillers with one another, as well as with neurotoxins and light- and energy-based devices, is effective and safe in treating the aging patient and yielding superior results.

## References

1. Carruthers J, Carruthers A. A prospective, randomized, parallel group study analyzing the effect of BTX-A (Botox) and non-animal sourced hyaluronic acid (NASHA, Restylane) in combination compared with NASHA (Restylane) alone in severe glabellar rhytides in adult female subjects: treatment of severe glabellar rhytides with a hyaluronic acid derivative compared with the derivative and BTX-A. *Dermatol Surg.* 2003;29(8):802–809.

2. Dubina M, Tung R, Bolotin D, et al. Treatment of forehead/glabellar rhytide complex with combination botulinum toxin a and hyaluronic acid versus botulinum toxin A injection alone: a split-face, rater-blinded, randomized control trial. *J Cosmet Dermatol.* 2013;12(4):261–266.

3. Beer KR, Julius H, Dunn M, Wilson F. Remodeling of periorbital, temporal, glabellar, and crow's feet areas with hyaluronic acid and botulinum toxin. *J Cosmet Dermatol.* 2014;13(2):143–150.

4. Carruthers A, Carruthers J, Monheit GD, Davis PG, Tardie G. Multicenter, randomized, parallel-group study of the safety and effectiveness of onabotulinumtoxinA and hyaluronic acid dermal fillers (24-mg/mL smooth, cohesive gel) alone and in combination for lower facial rejuvenation. *Dermatol Surg.* 2010;36(suppl 4):2121–2134.

5. Carruthers J, Carruthers A, Monheit GD, Davis PG. Multicenter, randomized, parallel-group study of onabotulinumtoxinA and hyaluronic acid dermal fillers (24-mg/mL smooth, cohesive gel) alone and in combination for lower facial rejuvenation: satisfaction and patient-reported outcomes. *Dermatol Surg.* 2010;36(suppl 4):2135–2145.

6. Molina B, David M, Jain R, et al. Patient satisfaction and efficacy of full-facial rejuvenation using a combination of botulinum toxin type A and hyaluronic acid filler. *Dermatol Surg.* 2015;41(suppl 1):S325–S332.

7. Redaelli A. Medical rhinoplasty with hyaluronic acid and botulinum toxin A: a very simple and quite effective technique. *J Cosmet Dermatol.* 2008;7(3):210–220.

8. Cuerda-Galindo E, Palomar-Gallego MA, Linares-Garciavaldecasas R. Are combined same-day treatments the future for photorejuvenation? Review of the literature on combined treatments with lasers, intense pulsed light, radiofrequency, botulinum toxin, and fillers for rejuvenation. *J Cosmet Laser Ther.* 2015;17(1):49–54.

9. England LJ, Tan MH, Shumaker PR, et al. Effects of monopolar radiofrequency treatment over soft-tissue fillers in an animal model. *Lasers Surg Med.* 2005;37(5):356–365.

10. Shumaker PR, England LJ, Dover JS, et al. Effect of monopolar radiofrequency treatment over soft-tissue fillers in an animal model: part 2. *Lasers Surg Med.* 2006;38(3):211–217.

11. Alam M, Levy R, Pajvani U, et al. Safety of radiofrequency treatment over human skin previously injected with medium-term injectable soft-tissue augmentation materials: a controlled pilot trial. *Lasers Surg Med.* 2006;38(3):205–210.

12. Ko EJ, Kim H, Park WS, Kim BJ. Correction of midface volume deficiency using hyaluronic acid filler and intradermal radiofrequency. *J Cosmet Laser Ther.* 2015;17(1):46–48.

13. Fabi SG, Goldman MP. The safety and efficacy of combining poly-L-lactic acid with intense pulsed light in facial rejuvenation: a retrospective study of 90 patients. *Dermatol Surg.* 2012;38(7 Pt 2):1208–1216.

14. Friedmann DP, Fabi SG, Goldman MP. Combination of intense pulsed light, Sculptra, and Ultherapy for treatment of the aging face. *J Cosmet Dermatol.* 2014;13(2):109–118.

15. Goldman MP, Alster TS, Weiss R. A randomized trial to determine the influence of laser therapy, monopolar radiofrequency treatment, and intense pulsed light therapy

administered immediately after hyaluronic acid gel implantation. *Dermatol Surg.* 2007;33(5):535–542.

16. Ribé A, Ribé N. Neck skin rejuvenation: histological and clinical changes after combined therapy with a fractional non-ablative laser and stabilized hyaluronic acid-based gel of non-animal origin. *J Cosmet Laser Ther.* 2011;13(4):154–161.

17. Farkas JP, Richardson JA, Brown S, Hoopman JE, Kenkel JM. Effects of common laser treatments on hyaluronic acid fillers in a porcine model. *Aesthet Surg J.* 2008;28(5):503–511.

18. Beer K. Dermal fillers and combinations of fillers for facial rejuvenation. *Dermatol Clin.* 2009;27(4):427–432.

19. Fagien S. Variable reconstitution of injectable hyaluronic acid with local anesthetic for expanded applications in facial aesthetic enhancement. *Dermatol Surg.* 2010;36:815–821.

20. Fagien S, Cassuto D. Reconstituted injectable hyaluronic acid: expanded applications in facial aesthetics and additional thoughts on the mechanism of action in cosmetic medicine. *Plast Reconstr Surg.* 2012;130(1):208–217.

21. Rohrich RJ, Pessa JE. The fat compartments of the face: anatomy and clinical implications for cosmetic surgery. *Plast Reconstr Surg.* 2007;119(7):2219–2227; discussion 2228–2231.

22. Shaw Jr RB, Kahn DM. Aging of the midface bony elements: a three-dimensional computed tomographic study. *Plast Reconstr Surg.* 2007;119(2):675–681; discussion 682–683.

23. Sadick NS, Manhas-Bhutani S, Krueger N. A novel approach to structural facial volume replacement. *Aesthetic Plast Surg.* 2013;37(2):266–276.

# 33

# Legal aspects of soft tissue filler treatments

## Mathew M. Avram

## Summary and Key Features

- As with all medical interventions, soft tissue filler treatments involve several areas of law, including the law of negligence and informed consent.
- It is important to note that these two doctrines are distinct.
- Thus one legal doctrine cannot be used to protect a defendant from an action based under the other theory.
- State law governs most issues regarding soft tissue filler treatments, including delegation of soft tissue filler treatments to nonphysicians.
- Under the doctrine of respondeat superior, a physician is liable legally for any injuries caused by a nonphysician injector, so long as the nonphysician is performing within the scope of his or her duty.

## Introduction

Soft tissue filler treatments have revolutionized the practice of aesthetic medicine. They provide an essential component for safe and effective treatment of rhytides, lipoatrophy, tissue laxity, scars, and other conditions. Millions of treatments are performed each year. Indeed, among American Society for Dermatologic Surgery (ASDS) members alone, there were 1,366,848 soft tissue filler treatments performed in the United States in 2015. This does not include non-ASDS dermatologist treatments—not to mention all other nondermatologist injectors. For the most part, side effects are predictable, mild, and transient. As their popularity has increased, reports of adverse side effects naturally have also increased. As in all other fields of medicine, there are potential medicolegal aspects of complications and patient injury. This chapter will examine some of the basic legal principles that govern soft tissue filler treatments. This is by no means a comprehensive or exhaustive review. That is well beyond the scope of this chapter. Nor is it meant to provide legal advice. Rather, it is designed to give the reader an introduction to some of the potential legal issues involved with soft tissue filler injections.

## Informed consent

All patients have the right to an informed consent prior to treatment. This right exists regardless of the nature of treatment. Medical and cosmetic treatments require informed patient consent as do invasive and noninvasive treatments. The same is true for oral and topical medications. In each instance the patient has a right to an informed consent. This right is grounded in a strong judicial belief in patient autonomy that is a bedrock of US common law regarding health care treatments. As former US Supreme Court Justice Cardozo explained:

*"Every human being of adult years and sound mind has a right to determine what shall be done with his own body."*

Indeed, the failure to obtain an informed consent prior to treatment constitutes a battery, and the physician is liable for damages. At the same time a patient has a duty to disclose accurate information to their physician. If patient misleads physician, this can be defense to an informed consent action.

There are several requirements for an adequate informed consent. They are all geared towards informing the patient of the nature and purpose of the medical treatment. It requires a description of the diagnosis, along with the medical steps preceding the diagnosis. In terms of a soft tissue filler treatment, the discussion should address the purpose of treatment. Some examples include the improvement of fine lines and wrinkles, volumization of areas of lipoatrophy, and improvement of scars.

The risks of treatment must be disclosed because this is often a central concern of a patient undergoing a treatment. Thus a discussion regarding side effects should precede any treatment. The disclosure should provide sufficient information to enable the patient to choose knowledgeably among medical alternatives. In this way the patient is placed in control of the course of their medical treatment. This is not only important for legal reasons but more importantly for good patient care and understanding the procedure. Among the risks include pain, bruising, swelling, infection, poor cosmesis, overcorrection, undercorrection, allergic reaction, pigment changes, ulceration, scar, and loss of vision (see Chapters 30 and 31 on Complications) (Table 33.1). It is helpful to place these side effects into context as well. Pain,

**Table 33.1** Common medical terms translated to lay person terms

| Purpura | Bruising |
|---|---|
| Eythema | Redness |
| Ptosis | Drooping |
| Necrosis | Ulcer |
| Hyperpigmentation | Skin darkening |
| Hypopigmentation | Skin lightening |
| Edema | Swelling |
| Bullae | Blister |

bruising, and swelling are typically transient. Explaining these common side effects will educate the patient and prevent surprise or disappointment when these common adverse sequelae occur. From a more prosaic standpoint, a good explanation of expected side effects will decrease the volume of phone calls post procedure.

Infection can include herpes simplex outbreak, cellulitis, and biofilms. Due to the subjective nature of treatment, it is important to explain that the cosmetic outcome of a procedure may not match the expectations of the patient. The patient may find the treatment inadequate or excessive. Again, a thorough discussion prior to treatment is the best means to avoid patient surprise at a cosmetic outcome that does not match his or her expectations.

Furthermore, it is important to describe alternatives to treatment. For soft tissue fillers, there are a myriad of them. One important alternative is no treatment at all. Because the vast majority of these treatments are cosmetic in nature, there is no requirement that a physician inject a patient to improve his or her health. It is truly the patients' decision as to whether they wish to undergo an elective cosmetic treatment. On the other hand, there is no legal requirement for a physician to perform a cosmetic procedure on a patient.

Other alternatives depend on the indication for the procedure. Static rhytides can be improved with laser-, light-, and energy-based treatments. The same can be said for skin laxity. In many cases, surgical lifting procedures are the definitive therapy. By far the most common treatment alternative is other soft tissue fillers. These of course include hyaluronic acid, poly-L-lactic acid, calcium hydroxylapatite, and permanent fillers.

For any given side effect, it is important to examine its probability and severity. Serious side effects, even if rare, should be disclosed. For example, although quite rare, the risk for blindness as a result of soft tissue filler treatment has been documented in the literature. It happens more commonly in certain anatomic areas. Nonetheless, despite its rarity, given the serious nature of this particular side effect, it is best to alert patients as to its possibility.

When counseling a patient, it is important to address any peculiar susceptibilities of the patient that may increase the risk for an adverse side effect. A simple example is a patient on anticoagulation therapy. Such patients are far more likely to experience postprocedure bruising and/ or hematoma than patients who are not on such therapy. In addition, the duty to discuss specific risk factors for a patient expands as the patient asks more specific questions about the procedure and its risks. As with many of these legal concepts, good legal practice will also serve the goal of good patient care. Alerting a patient as to the increased risk for significant bruising will prevent surprise and disappointment at postprocedure side effects.

Importantly, physical injury is not required for a battery action. Rather, patients need only to show that they were not informed of the nature of medical touching. Thus the burden of proof for a plaintiff in a battery action can be easier than that in a negligence action. It does not require an expert witness, nor is there any need to establish a standard of care. Rather, one needs only to show a nonconsensual medical touching. Expanding an area of planned treatment can also constitute a battery if the patient did not give consent. For example, if a patient consents to treatment of nasolabial folds with soft tissue filler, extending the treatment to the temples without prior consent could be a battery. This would be particularly true for a patient who is anesthetized during treatment. Such a patient would have no means of knowing that a new area was being treated.

Patient comprehension is a key component of consent. A written consent is ineffective if the patient does not understand material information about the procedure. A patient cannot give an informed consent without understanding the material issues involved with a treatment's risks and benefits. For this reason it is important to avoid complicated scientific discussions and medical jargon during an initial consultation or when seeking consent prior to a procedure. For the same reason, written consents should be written using clear, simple layperson terms and avoiding polysyllabic, technical medical jargon.

Table 33.1 contains a list of common medical terms used in soft tissue filler and other aesthetic treatments translated into more simplified lay person terms (Table 33.1).

It is best to use bold-faced, enlarged print for these risks to highlight them for a patient signing a consent form. Anything that raises the awareness of a patient as to the risks of a procedure will confer greater legitimacy to an informed consent. Simplified consent forms achieve this far more effectively than complicated, small-type, lengthy verbiage. For similar reasons, courts view overbroad written consents with disfavor. Courts prefer more specificity to show an informed consent. Thus blanket authorizations are not a good idea legally.

The best means to memorialize patient comprehension and consent for any given procedure is a written consent. A signed, written document is the best evidence to protect against an action sounding in battery. It is best to obtain written consents prior to each soft tissue filler treatment, even if it has been performed previously. First, it is additional evidence of a patient who understands the risks and benefits of the procedure. In addition, as the patient's health or cosmetic concerns change, each signed written consent is timely evidence that the discussion of risks and benefits was performed.

For reasons of practicality, many oral and topical treatments are commonly performed without a written consent. In these circumstances it is best practice to include a discussion of risks and benefits in the patient's chart. Electronic medical records help this effort, but it is important to tailor "cut and paste" paragraph templates to conform to the patient being treated. Otherwise, such documentation of oral consent will appear bogus.

There are a few exceptions to the requirement for informed consent. In the practice of injectables these exceptions are very rare. In a true emergency, the doctor has the right to act without patient consent (i.e., unconscious patient). A patient having an acute medical emergency related to or unrelated to the treatment fits within this exception. In contrast, if a competent patient refuses, treatment cannot proceed.

A patient must have the mental capacity to make a medical decision. Courts presume patient comprehension. Thus the plaintiff has the burden of proof to show that the patient lacked mental competency to give an informed consent for a procedure. Although this is not a typical concern for soft tissue filler treatments, minors lack legal capacity. Parents must consent to medical or cosmetic procedures, including soft tissue fillers.

The patient has a duty to provide truthful and accurate information to the physician. If a patient misleads a physician with false information, this can be defense to an informed consent action (i.e., false denial of a prior hypersensitivity reaction to a soft tissue filler procedure).

To prevail in an action based on lack of informed consent, a plaintiff must first establish that the course of treatment carried an undisclosed risk. Next, the plaintiff must show that the physician's nondisclosure of that risk breached the applicable standard of care. Furthermore, it must be shown that the undisclosed risk caused the patient's injury. Finally, it must be established that with proper disclosure, the patient would have made a different treatment choice.

## Negligence and malpractice

The basic four elements of a suit for negligence are a breach of a duty that causes harm to the patient. Negligence, also known as malpractice, is a completely distinct legal concept from that of battery (i.e., failure to obtain informed consent). It is important to understand that a patient can successfully sue for battery but unsuccessfully for malpractice. On the contrary, a patient may have a cause of action under malpractice but not under failure

to obtain consent. A written consent is merely evidence of an informed discussion about the risks and benefits of a medical procedure. It does not act as a shield against malpractice claims.

The physician is held to a "reasonable duty" standard. This duty is the quality of care at a level consonant with medical knowledge and judgment that a physician is reasonably expected to possess. It is a duty based upon the adept use of such medical facilities, services, and equipment that are available to the physician. The reasonable duty standard varies based upon the facts and circumstances of each case. The most common ways for establishing the reasonable duty standard arise from expert testimony, the medical literature, standard practice, and clinical guidelines.

The trial judge determines whether an expert witness is qualified. The expert must have sufficient training to assess the physician's performance. There is no requirement that the expert witness be board-certified. Furthermore, the expert need not be in the same specialty as the defendant physician. The expert needs to establish a standard of care. In addition, the expert must establish that the defendant physician failed to meet that standard to a "reasonable degree of medical and scientific certainty."

There are also other means of establishing negligence. Effective cross-examination of the defendant's expert witness that acknowledges negligence can suffice. US Food and Drug Administration and Physicians' Desk Reference warnings can be used to establish a standard of care and that it has been breached. Learned treatises can do the same. Finally, a defendant's explicit admission of negligence can be used to establish malpractice. It is important to note that this should not be confused with a physician's expression of sympathy to a patient who has experienced an adverse side effect, injury, or poor outcome. Indeed, expressions of empathy may even decrease the chances of litigation.

## Defenses to a malpractice action

There are multiple defenses to a negligence action. The first is known as the "respectable minority exception." It holds that there can be more than one appropriate way to perform competent medical care. A physician is free to pursue more than one type of treatment regimen so long as a "considerate number of reputable and respected physicians" do the same. For example, volumization can be achieved with hyaluronic fillers, as well as poly-L-lactic acid fillers, because there are a number of physicians who use either filler for this purpose.

Contributory fault is another potential defense in certain circumstances in which a patient's mistakes or lifestyle choices contribute to injuries. Damages to plaintiff are mitigated by failure to exercise ordinary care (i.e., smoking and sunbathing after traditional resurfacing procedure against doctor's advice). Conversely, the physician also owes a duty to prevent patients from harming themselves (i.e., it is inadvisable to give sedatives to a patient who may be driving home back from office). In this case the physician needs to confirm that the patient will have a ride home and will not be driving.

Statute of limitations can provide an important means to help litigation to be brought in a timely manner. It is often set at 2 to 3 years after injury or malpractice, but the timing of when the statue begins is a crucial determining factor. The timing begins from when the defendant breaches his duty or when the plaintiff suffers injury. However, even these determinations require further subdividing. Indeed, the timing can begin when the patient plaintiff becomes aware or reasonably should be aware of the injury. This issue is particularly important in patients with permanent fillers. In some cases complications are not seen for years following the date of treatment. In these cases the statue of limitations may begin several years after the date of treatment.

## How to avoid litigation

Good communication and rapport are the most important means to avoid a lawsuit. Patients with a good relationship with their physician are far less likely to sue. Although it may seem obvious how to create that relationship, physicians and patients may fail to connect. There are a few simple ways to enhance the relationship. It is important to communicate clearly, eschewing the use of medical language in favor of straightforward terms. It is important to avoid rushing a consultation and to answer all questions. There is a legal requirement for a comprehensible discussion of the risks and benefits of any medical procedure. Taking the time to discuss a procedure before it is performed helps to set proper expectations and avoid postprocedure disappointment or surprise at side effects. It is also good medical practice.

It is crucial to assess the patient at consultation, particularly their expectations. It is important to make certain that their expectations are realistic. Patients who misunderstand a procedure are far more likely to be upset following a procedure. That insight can be gained by the physician or staff. It is important to trust your own and your staff's intuition about a patient. For elective cosmetic treatments, there is no legal obligation to perform a cosmetic treatment on a patient. Indeed, refusing treatment may be the best decision you make regarding caring for that particular patient. Taking the time to discuss a procedure before it is performed helps to set proper expectations and avoid postprocedure disappointment or surprise at side effects.

## Complications

Even in skilled hands, if you treat a sufficient number of patients, you will encounter challenging side effects. This is true in every area of medicine, and soft tissue filler treatments are no exception to the rule. If the patient calls

with an adverse event or feels their cosmetic appearance is poor, it is important to assess the patient. Often, side effects are temporary and mild, and reassurance is all that is needed. If possible, examine the patient the same day. Occasionally a patient will underestimate the severity of his or her side effect. Thus an office visit is the best opportunity to make a precise diagnosis and intervention. If you are uncertain as to what is happening, consult a colleague. Many physicians feel a sense of shame or embarrassment reaching out to a colleague regarding a complication or a poor result. This feeling needs to be suppressed. Indeed, calling a colleague demonstrates your dedication to the care of the patient. Furthermore, no expert physician practices without requiring the help of a colleague from time to time. With that being said, it is important not to perform a procedure that might produce a side effect that you cannot recognize and treat (i.e., herpetic infection following a soft tissue filler treatment).

Good documentation can be very helpful for dealing with dissatisfied patients. Photography can be especially helpful to document the pretreatment appearance of a patient claiming a side effect unrelated to treatment (i.e., preexisting rhytides). It is also helpful to document unrelated skin findings in a patient's chart in the unlikely event a patient attributes those findings to a soft tissue filler treatment, such as facial lipoatrophy outside the area of treatment or telangiectasias among other findings. On the other hand, poor photography or poor documentation can be problematic. A poor pretreatment photo may make demonstrating benefit far more difficult. Furthermore, "cut and paste" documentation that does not accurately describe the patient will be a sign of poor documentation and will undermine the accuracy of a physician's notes.

Liability for side effects will correlate with the degree of their duration. In general, permanent side effects will produce more liability than temporary ones. For example, bruising, swelling, and redness are expected temporary side effects that should not produce any liability. Handholding and time are the best course of treatment. The same holds for correctable side effects or those that endure for a longer period of time, such as Tyndall effect, poor cosmetic appearance, nodules, and allergic or hypersensitivity reactions. They typically can be corrected. Hyaluronidase can be quite helpful. Thus legal consequences are highly unlikely to attach. However, more permanent side effects are far more likely to result in litigation, such as scar and loss of vision. These side effects are permanent and also more serious. Thus damages attach.

The most feared complication of soft tissue filler injections is vascular occlusion. This is an emergent issue that requires immediate attention. The key to treatment is early diagnosis. It occurs with direct injection into a vessel producing occlusion at the local injection site or more distally. Blanching is often seen at the time of injection. With time, pain and a retiform purpura also become apparent (Fig. 33.1). Eventually skin breakdown and ulceration occur. It can present with erythema and pustules and thus can be misdiagnosed as bacterial or viral infection. Early

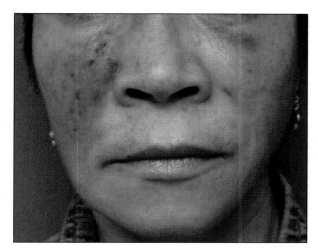

**Figure 33.1** Classic retiform purpura in a patient with vascular occlusion. *Courtesy of Jean and Alastair Carruthers.*

detection and treatment are crucial. Because the signs and symptoms may not be readily apparent, it is imperative that staff and physicians immediately recognize its clinical presentation. Even more dramatic is loss of vision. This symptom occurs at the time of occlusion and requires recognition and treatment within 90 minutes. Immediate loss of vision will make diagnosis quite obvious.

The first symptoms of vascular occlusion of nonocular vessels may not be recognized until a patient is home. In this case, whoever answers the phone at a physician's office will need to be aware of the signs and diagnosis and triage appropriately. Because of the seriousness of this complication, it is best that you do not perform soft tissue filler treatments if you *and your staff* cannot recognize an evolving necrosis (i.e., blanching; retiform purpura; pain). Your staff needs to know the signs of an impending necrosis, and they need to be able to ask the pertinent questions over the phone. Furthermore, do not perform soft tissue filler treatments if you do not have unexpired hyaluronidase, Acetyl salicylic acid (ASA), and nitropaste readily available in your office. Consent forms should be signed prior to each visit. The consent forms must contain the following serious risks: blindness, ulcer, and scar. If using hyaluronidase, it is best to document a discussion of relevant potential side effects.

## Physician extenders

Increasingly, physicians are delegating cosmetic procedures to nonphysicians. This trend is especially true for certain laser procedures and chemical peels. Some have chosen to also delegate injection of neurotoxins and soft tissue filler treatments. It is important to note that the law holds a supervising physician legally responsible for such practice under the legal doctrine of *respondeat superior*. Indeed, a physician is held liable for a physician extender's negligence provided that the provider is an employee receiving a salary and benefits and performing within the scope of his or her duty. This is true regardless of whether the physician saw the patient or not at that visit.

It is important to note that the law in the United States governing issues of who can legally perform soft tissue filler treatments is a state issue. It is determined by each state individually, and there is no national law addressing this issue. The required supervision of nonphysician procedures also varies state to state. Some jurisdictions require on-site supervision by physicians, whereas others do not. It is incumbent on the physician to become familiar with the applicable law in his or her state.

## Conclusion

There are several legal issues involved with soft tissue filler treatments. Among them include the need for informed consent and a duty to provide competent medical care to patients. However, these two doctrines, the doctrines of informed consent and malpractice, are distinct. Neither shields a physician defendant from an action under the other legal theory. Furthermore, it is incumbent on the physician to know the applicable state law before delegation of soft tissue filler treatments to nonphysicians. Furthermore, the physician is liable legally for any injuries that occur by a nonphysician injector so long as the nonphysician is performing within the scope of their duty.

## Further reading

Furrow BR, Greaney TL, Johnson SH, Jost TS, Schwartz RL. *Health Law*. ed 2. St Paul, MN: West Academic Publishing; 2000.

Hall MA, Ellman IM, Orentlicher D. *Health Care Law and Ethics in a Nut Shell*. ed 3. St Paul, MN: West Academic Publishing; 2011.

# 34

# Pretreatment and posttreatment photography

## Kevin C. Smith

### Summary and Key Features

- Photography is an essential part of the care of the aesthetic patient.
- To be credible in the eyes of patients and of maximum utility for follow-up, photos should be of consistent quality, with reproducible lighting, standard poses, camera angles, and color rendition.
- Pretreatment photos contribute to patient satisfaction and retention by helping patients to appreciate the benefits of treatment when they return for follow-up.
- Pretreatment photos are of great value in the efficient and satisfactory management and resolution of disappointments, misunderstandings, and complications.
- The efficient, consistent use of photography during the pretreatment consultation and at follow-up visits as the years go on saves time and makes money.
- The only photos I have ever regretted are the ones I did not get!

Credible, consistent photos of patients have been of great value to my patients, to my development as a physician specializing in the aesthetic care of patients, and to the development of my practice.

*Credible* photos accurately and reproducibly represent the true state of the patient. This requires a *consistent* and *systematic* approach to photography, which in the end is also most efficient and effective. Photography of patients always involves a trade-off between technical perfection and practical efficiency. In making this trade-off, I have taken comfort from Voltaire's observation (*La Bégueule* 1772)[1]: "*Le mieux est l'ennemi du bien.*" (The perfect is the enemy of the good.) When applied to routine daily photography of patients, this means that excessive concern for "perfect" lighting, the "perfect" camera, the "perfect" angle, etc. will seriously interfere with obtaining large numbers of routine high-value-but-not-"perfect" photos.

The only photos I have regretted have been the photos I did not get. Credible, consistent photos help to enhance and consolidate patient satisfaction with my treatment and care. In other situations, credible, consistent photos have helped to resolve misunderstandings, disappointments, or complications of treatment.

Consistent, symmetrical overhead lighting is vital for credible pretreatment and posttreatment photography of both the filler patient and the patient being treated with botulinum neurotoxin type-A (BoNT-A) (Fig. 34.1), and in a position in which the lines and contours of the face will be properly lit. If necessary, an electrician can install a couple of light-emitting diode (LED) panels on a single light switch to provide symmetrical illumination.

It is important NOT to use a camera-mounted flash when photographing patients before or after fillers or BoNT-A because the flash will fill in and obscure facial lines, creases, and contours (compare Fig. 34.2C vs. D, Table 34.1). Flash photography is excellent for the assessment of skin color and telangiectasia and so is essential in that aspect of the management of the aesthetic patient.

*Credible* and *consistent* color reproduction is vital for effective use of photos during follow-up. I have found it very practical to use a camera that has TWO "custom" settings—allowing me to have one custom setting for flash photography (skin color and telangiectasia) and a second custom setting for filler and BoNT-A patients. These custom settings control every aspect of camera operation (macro, flash, image stabilizer and focusing, color balance), so that I can simply and efficiently switch between the custom settings C1 and C2, depending on whether I want a flash or nonflash photo. There are only a few pocket-sized cameras on the market that have *two* custom settings. I have found Canon G-series[2] cameras to be very satisfactory. They can be carried comfortably in the hip pocket of my scrub shirt or lab coat all day long and have excellent lens and sensors and long battery life.

To ensure consistent color rendition, the settings I use are detailed in Table 34.2. You will probably end up using different settings, depending on lighting conditions in your office and the type of printer or display you are using. You will note that a relatively high ASA of 400 is used so that the shutter speed will be at least 1/125 second during handheld, nonflash shots, thus minimizing the effect of motion. Locking the controls down with transparent Duct tape reduces the risk of accidental changes to settings (Fig. 34.3).

There can be substantial variation between the color of an image as it is displayed on the camera, and the color

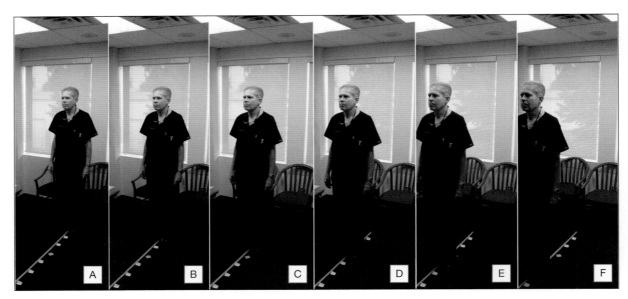

**Figure 34.1** Method to find standard position for subject to stand while being photographed. Markers are placed at 20-cm intervals along a line midway between two fluorescent overhead lights. The subject is photographed at each position, then the photos are printed and compared. It was determined that position C in this series produced the best balance of light and shadow. This procedure can then be repeated in additional rooms, and the final markers adjusted so that very similar photos will result when photos were taken in any of the rooms. A pair of LED panels can be mounted on the ceiling in cases where the orientation of fluorescent lights does not produce suitable symmetrical lighting.

**Table 34.1** Flash versus no flash

| Characteristic of photo | Camera-mounted flash | No-flash, symmetrical overhead lighting |
|---|---|---|
| Color rendition | Best | Good |
| Fine detail | Best | Good |
| Contour | Poor—filled in by flash | Good when properly lit |
| Lines and creases | Poor—filled in by flash | Good when properly lit |

of that image when displayed on a screen or printed by a color laser or inkjet printer. I have found it vital to set a custom color balance in each of C1 and C2 so that the color rendition of the *displayed* images will have maximum credibility and consistency. Custom color balancing is performed by taking a series of shots (**Fig. 34.4**) under standard lighting, varying only the color balance settings (green/magenta and blue/amber), printing out the results, picking the most accurate color rendition, then iterating if necessary until the best possible solution is found. The process is repeated to determine the best color balance for use with the built-in flash on the camera. Then, the custom color balance for C1 or C2 (if you are working with a Canon G-series camera, the author is using a G15)

is set. You will probably not need to change that setting until you switch to another camera or another color laser or inkjet printer, perhaps in a few years. You should carefully record a list of ALL of the settings on your camera, so that the settings can be restored if necessary (e.g., if you send the camera away to be serviced or repaired). You will probably also want to experiment with your color printer to optimize the printer settings, which should then be recorded and saved as a preset in your printer menu.

Until recently color inkjet printers were much more expensive to use, and the disposable ink cartridges were an ecologic concern. The author has switched to the Epson 4550 color inkjet printer, which has very large refillable ink tanks rather than cartridges. Color rendition and image detail, even on plain paper, is superior to any laser printer the author is aware of, and cost per page is very reasonable.

It is important to set the printing preferences in your software to print the serial number of the photo and the time and date of the photo under each image. This will make it easy for you to retrieve the digital original from your computer for reprinting or publication.

When dealing with patient photos, the issue of consent should be considered. In my practice (Ontario, Canada, 2016) verbal consent for photography is sufficient. Written consent may be necessary in some circumstances prior to publication, presentation, or dissemination of a patient's photo. A full discussion of consent as it relates to patient photos is beyond the scope of this chapter. The reader should keep abreast of the laws and customs in their jurisdiction.

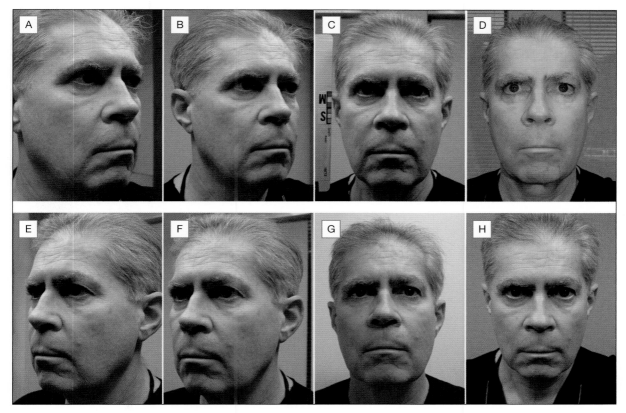

**Figure 34.2** Facial views commonly obtained before treatment with fillers. Camera approximately 40 cm from subject and held at the level of the subject's nose, except in H. **A, E** Tip of nose aligned with edge of cheek. **B, F** Tip of nose aligned with infraorbital foramen. **C,** Anterior. This image also illustrates inclusion of the chart tab showing patient's name and chart number, so that the individual in the series will be positively identified. The chart tab also provides objective black and white references to assist with color balancing for publication; and elements in the chart tab also provide an objective size reference, in case that is needed. **D,** Photo taken using built-in flash on camera. Note that flash fills in and obscures facial line, creases and contours, and skin texture, compared with nonflash image shot under symmetrical overhead lighting. **G,** Photo taken with the subject seated in the exam room, rather than standing (C) behind the photo marker, centered between two overhead fluorescent lights. When compared with (C), we see that *the appearance of the subject is altered and softened by asymmetrical and diffuse lighting,* so that comparison of standard photos (A–F) with the patient at follow-up can be misleading for the patient and the clinician unless the patient is standing *in the same position as was used for photography* when the comparison with pretreatment photos is made. **H,** Superior view, taken with the lens at the level of the top of the head, aiming down at an angle of approximately 30 degrees. This illustrates prejowl sulcus and sometimes also is useful to demonstrate midcheek volume loss related to aging or to disease.

It is vital to protect the photos being stored in your computer systems from unauthorized access or dissemination. To this end, it is best to use a desktop computer rather than an easily stolen laptop to process the photos. The computer must be password-protected, and the image files should be encrypted. Backup drives should also be encrypted. Photos can also be backed up to a secure off-site storage facility (e.g., Crashplan, Backblaze, Carbonite, or Spideroak). You should check your backup systems to make sure that they are performing as expected, perhaps every month (put this chore in your calendar!). Ideally, a dedicated computer should be used for storage and printing, and that computer should not be connected to the internet unless there is a good reason (e.g., to install a software update or during daily backup to off-site storage). The computer can be connected to a color printer by a USB cable, to avoid using the office network, which can be compromised. A trusted third party (e.g., your lawyer) should have a copy of the necessary passwords, for use in case you are dead or disabled.

Usual procedure for photography:

1. I briefly explain that before treatment I will take some photos to help the patient see how they are responding to treatment when they return for follow-up.

2. I ask the patient to stand centered behind the photo marker on the carpet (Fig. 34.5, inset) with his or her back to the window. By positioning the patient

**Table 34.2** Camera settings

| Example of custom settings for Canon G15 | C1: Flash | C2: No flash |
|---|---|---|
| *Exposure adjustment | 0 | 0 |
| *ASA | 400 | 400 |
| Exposure | Center weighted | Center weighted |
| Macro | on | on |
| Dynamic range correction | 0 | 0 |
| Light source & custom color balance (blue/amber and magenta/green) | Flash<br>B2, M2 | Fluorescent<br>B3, 0 |
| My colors | off | off |
| Bracketing | off | off |
| Single shot | on | on |
| Flash power adjustment | 0 | n/a |
| Flash | on | off |
| Neutral density filter | off | off |
| Aspect ratio | 4:3 | 4:3 |
| JPEG/RAW | JPEG | JPEG |
| Maximum resolution | on | on |

*Exposure adjustment and ASA dials are taped down, to reduce the chance that they will accidentally be changed.

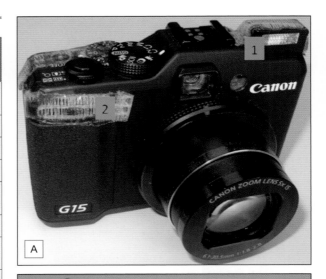

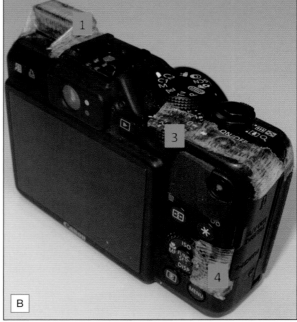

**Figure 34.3** Transparent Duct tape is used to lock down control dials on the camera, to reduce the chance that settings will be inadvertently changed, degrading image quality. Duct tape is much more durable that Scotch tape. 1. Flash; 2. Front control dial; 3. Exposure compensation dial; 4. Rear control dial.

with his or her back to the window, I eliminate window light as a variable.

3. The camera is switched to the appropriate preset mode (on my Canon G15: C1 is used for flash photos, C2 for nonflash photos).

4. The camera is held at the level of the patient's nose, at a distance of approximately 40 cm from the face.

5. For at least one photo in each series, the patient's chart tab is held close to the face, so that the patient's name and chart number are included in the photo (see Fig. 34.3C). This ensures positive identification when the photos are printed. The chart tab also provides objective black and white references, which can be helpful in rare cases in which a photo is being color-balanced for publication or litigation; and the chart tab also provides an objective size reference if it is necessary in the future to determine the size of a mole or other feature in the photo.

6. Anterior and oblique photos of the patient's relaxed face are obtained (see Fig. 34.3), as necessary, to illustrate the features that will be treated. If fillers are to be used on the nose, lateral photos are also taken. When the prejowl sulcus is to be treated, it can be helpful to take a photo with the camera held at the level of the top of the head, at a

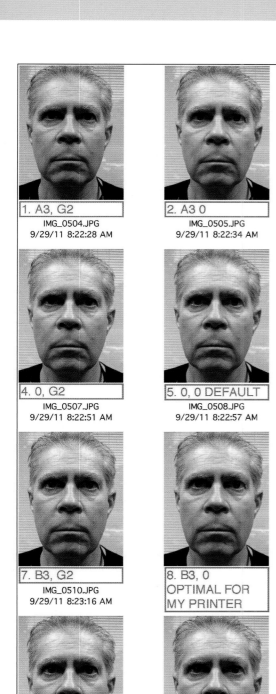
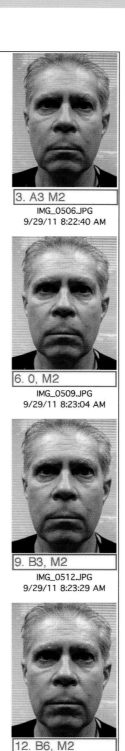

| 1. A3, G2 | 2. A3 0 | 3. A3 M2 |
| IMG_0504.JPG | IMG_0505.JPG | IMG_0506.JPG |
| 9/29/11 8:22:28 AM | 9/29/11 8:22:34 AM | 9/29/11 8:22:40 AM |

| 4. 0, G2 | 5. 0, 0 DEFAULT | 6. 0, M2 |
| IMG_0507.JPG | IMG_0508.JPG | IMG_0509.JPG |
| 9/29/11 8:22:51 AM | 9/29/11 8:22:57 AM | 9/29/11 8:23:04 AM |

| 7. B3, G2 | 8. B3, 0 OPTIMAL FOR MY PRINTER | 9. B3, M2 |
| IMG_0510.JPG | | IMG_0512.JPG |
| 9/29/11 8:23:16 AM | | 9/29/11 8:23:29 AM |

| 10. B6, G2 | 11. B6, 0 | 12. B6, M2 |
| IMG_0513.JPG | IMG_0514.JPG | IMG_0515.JPG |
| 9/29/11 8:23:38 AM | 9/29/11 8:23:43 AM | 9/29/11 8:23:50 AM |

**Figure 34.4** Method to find best color balance settings for standard flash or nonflash photos. This array of images illustrates a range of custom color balance settings. To determine the correct setting for accurate output on a given printer, simply shoot an array of standard photos, carefully recording the camera settings, then after printing the images pick the most accurate print(s), and take another array of photos with parameters tightly grouped around those used for the best photos from the first series. After a couple of iterations, you will zero in on the ideal parameters for your lighting and your printer (see Table 34.1: Camera settings).

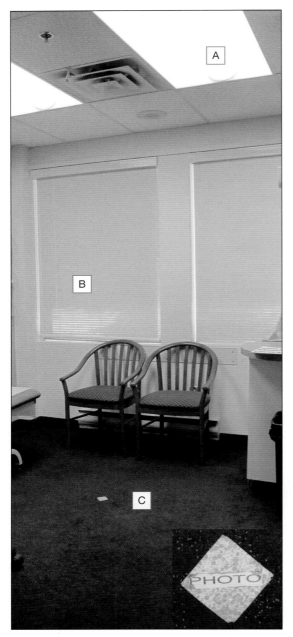

**Figure 34.5** Exam room layout for photography. **A,** Overhead fluorescent lights. If symmetrical overhead lights are not available, a pair of light-emitting diode panels can be installed to provide illumination during nonflash photography. **B,** Roller blinds in front of Venetian blinds on windows, providing a neutral backdrop and privacy if the patient disrobes; it also reduces glare and heat load on bright days. **C,** Marker on floor which patient stands behind with their back to the window when being photographed before and after filler and BoNT-A treatment. Marker is equidistant between overhead lights and is at the point determined as shown in Figure 34.1, which gives the best balance of light and shadow. Marker is a 5-cm square of SOLAS Marine tape, with a label saying "PHOTO" (inset). (Without the label, many patients try to peel the tape off the carpet and put it in the garbage for me.) Patients also stand behind this marker during flash photography, before and after laser and intense pulsed-light treatment for telangiectasia and dyschromia.

distance of approximately 40 cm, pointing down at approximately a 30-degree angle at the face (see **Fig. 34.3H**).

7. If treatment of the lips with fillers is anticipated, it is quick, cheap, and easy to obtain the pretreatment series shown in **Fig. 34.6**. Without these baseline images, follow-up visits can occasionally be stressful and difficult to resolve.

8. If treatment with BoNT-A is anticipated, photos of the face showing activity of the facial muscles are taken (e.g., before treatment of the forehead the sequence would be: "relax, brows up, scowl, crinkle your nose" [to illustrate "bunny lines"]. For crow's feet oblique photos are taken: "relax, close your eyes tightly [orbicularis occuli], relax your face, now give me a big TOOTHY smile [zygomaticus major and minor, with and without orbicularis occuli]). Similarly, relaxed and full contraction photos are taken of other muscle groups to be treated (Box 34.1).

Makeup is not generally removed before nonflash photos that will be used for follow-up of filler or BoNT-A treatment. Photos without makeup would be "perfect" but as a practical matter add little value and patients often do not wish to remove their makeup.

Removal of makeup is *essential* before flash photos that will be used to illustrate erythema, telangiectasia, and/or dyschromia.

Procedure for viewing photos at follow-up:

Patients who are allowed to view their pretreatment photos have been found to estimate their degree of improvement as being greater and have higher satisfaction than patients who are not allowed to view their pretreatment photos.[3] It is often helpful to give the patient a large, square hand mirror (**Fig. 34.7**) and to hold the pretreatment photo beside the patient's face, so that the patient can look in the mirror and simultaneously see his or her face and also see the pretreatment image. This helps many patients to assess their response to treatment and to discuss additional treatment. For the most accurate comparison, the patient is sometimes invited to stand at the same point in the room under symmetrical lighting where the pretreatment photos were shot, so that posttreatment lighting will be very similar to that which was used when the photos were taken.

## Patient instructions for emailing photos

There are some circumstances where it is helpful for patients to email photos to the treating physician. To ensure the highest-quality images, I have prepared a standard set of instructions for patients to follow:

1. Please set your cellphone or camera to the highest possible resolution (number of pixels).

2. Shoot from AT LEAST ARM'S LENGTH (2 FEET AWAY). If the camera is closer than that the photo

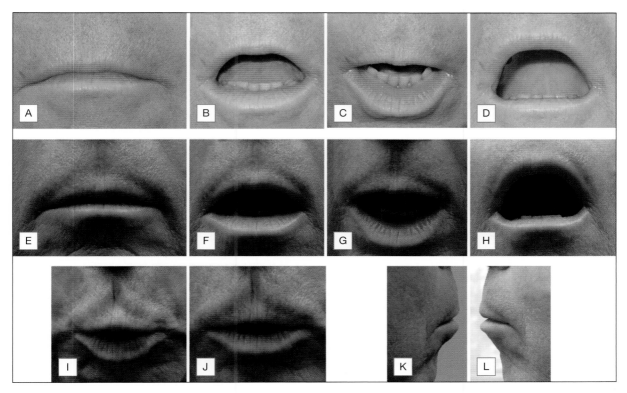

**Figure 34.6** Photos before treatment of the lips with fillers and/or BoNT-A. Anterior (A–H) and lateral (K and L) views of the lips, with (A–D) and with flash (E–H, K and L), with the lips together and relaxed (A, E), and with the lips parted and level with the camera (B, F), from above (C, G) and from below (D, H) provide the information necessary to maximize patient satisfaction and to resolve common complaints and concerns. Where vertical lines above the lips are a potential target for treatment or for future discussion with the patient, relaxed (E), full contraction (I) and partial contraction (J) images are very valuable, both during the consultation and at follow-up.

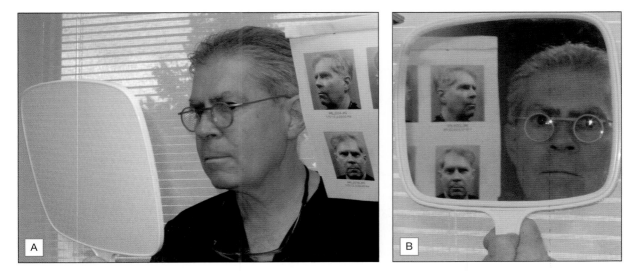

**Figure 34.7** Method for the display of pretreatment photos to patients during follow-up visits. In (A) the subject is examining himself in a large square hand mirror, and pretreatment photos held beside his face so that he can see *both* his face *and* his pretreatment image in the mirror *simultaneously*, as shown in (B). This technique is very helpful at follow-up, usually to consolidate the patient's satisfaction with treatment and occasionally to plan future treatment or to help the patient resolve misunderstandings, disappointments, or complications.

---

**Box 34.1**
**Standard poses**

Except as otherwise noted, all images are obtained with the patient standing behind the "photo" marker on floor with light falling symmetrically from above on the patient's face, lens at same height as nose, camera approximately 40 cm from the patient's nose, patient's head level, and patient looking straight ahead.* denotes baseline images obtained routinely on almost all patients:

**Anterior view**

*Relaxed—to illustrate relaxed state, and to visualize static lines and creases, and areas of volume depletion or excess, alignment and contours of the nose and lips

*Brows up—frontalis

*Frown—glabellar complex

Crinkle nose—bunny lines: nasalis and levator labii superioris alaeque nasii

Perioral wrinkles—orbicularis oris

Clench chin—mentalis

Turn corners of mouth down—depressor angui oris and platysma

Clench neck muscles—platysmal bands

**Anterior-superior view (similar to Towne view in radiology)**

Patient standing in standard position, looking straight ahead, relaxed.

Photo taken from above at a 30-degree angle pointing downward, patient relaxed, to illustrate in particular prejowl sulcus, and upper-medial cheek volume loss related to the malar fat pad. As a practical matter, like other photos this is taken from a distance of approximately 40 cm from the patient's nose, and for this photo the camera is held so that the lens is at the level of the top of the patient's head, instead of at nose level.

**Right and left oblique view**

Lens at height of nose, tip of nose aligned with edge of cheek, patient's head level:

*Relaxed—static lines and creases, areas of excess and deficient volume, contours of the nose and lips, contours of nose

*Close eyes tightly—orbicularis occuli

*Open eyes, big toothy grin—zygomaticus major and minor, and orbicularis occuli

Crinkle nose—bunny lines: nasalis and levator labii superioris alaeque nasii

Perioral wrinkles—orbicularis oris

Clench chin—mentalis

Turn corners of mouth down—depressor angui oris and platysma

Clench neck muscles—platysmal bands

**Oblique view**

Lens at height of nose, tip of nose aligned with location of infraorbital foramen in midcheek, patient's head level.

Visualize ogee curve, and malar cheek, contours of the nose and lips, postjowl sulcus, and infra malar volume status, static lines, and creases.

**Lateral view**

Lens at height of nose, centered on the cheek midway between the tip of the nose and the antitragus of the ear, patient looking straight ahead: to visualize areas of volume depletion or excess, contours of the nose and lips, static lines, and creases.

**Handheld oblique lighting (e.g., using a Streamlight Stylus Pro pocket LED light)**

To better visualize scars from acne or injuries. Handheld oblique lighting is useful both for photography and sometimes during injection of scars with fillers.

---

is more likely to be out of focus and/or wrongly exposed.

3. Please write the time, date, and your initials on a white piece of paper and hold that next to the area being photographed. The white paper will help me to color balance the image, if necessary, when it arrives.

4. Please do not attempt to color balance or otherwise adjust the image before sending it.

5. Please send photos taken with and without flash because certain elements like color and texture can be easier to interpret if BOTH types of photos are available.

6. Please also email me answers to the following questions:
   a. When did this problem start?
   b. How bad is it today compared with what it is like at its worst?
   c. What do you think is causing this problem?
   d. What have you been doing to try to make this better (prescription and over-the-counter medicines, and home remedies).
   e. Have you ever had a problem like this in the past?
   f. Do you have any other skin problems?

This approach helped the author and his patients (e.g., in one case facilitating within minutes the early detection and treatment of a case of vascular occlusion with impending necrosis on the midforehead after filler injection).

**Pearl 1**

Choose a camera you can comfortably carry in your pocket all day because if the camera is not IN YOUR POCKET you will fail to take many of the photos that are necessary for the proper care of the aesthetic patient.

## Pearl 2

Use transparent Duct tape to lock down the controls on your camera, so that they do not get accidentally reset to unwanted values and so degrade image quality.

## Pearl 3

Hold the chart tab, with the patient's name and chart number, close to the area being photographed in at least some photos in each session, so that there will be no confusion as to the identity of the patient.

## Pearl 4

Print out the photos at the end of every day, and initial all of them before they are filed, so that you can monitor the quality of your photography. Prints are much more practical at follow-up visits than images on a screen.

## Pearl 5

Set your preferences so that the time, date, and serial number are automatically printed under every photo. This will help your staff when they are trying to identify the occasional photo that did not include the chart tab and will help you to retrieve the original digital image from your computer in cases, for example, in which you want to reprint the image.

## Pearl 6

When doing demonstration treatments at meetings, if your camera is not available be sure to use your cellphone camera to obtain baseline and posttreatment photos of individuals you treat or consult on, and also photograph their consent forms and treatment records. A chart should be made on each of these individuals when you return to your office and should be kept with the records of other patients.

## References

1. Voltaire: La Bégueule (The Prude, A Moral Tale). 1772 <http://fr.wikisource.org/wiki/La_B%C3%A9gueule>. Accessed 02.10.11.
2. <http://www.steves-digicams.com/camera-reviews/canon/powershot-g12/canon-powershot-g12-review.html>. Accessed 02.10.11.
3. Hawkins SS, DeSantis C, Matzke M, Weinkauf R. Consumer evaluation of before and after photographs increases perception of anti-aging benefits. Poster Abstracts. *J Am Acad Dermatol*. 2004;50(suppl 3):27.

# Index

Page numbers followed by "*f*" indicate figures, "*t*" indicate tables, and "*b*" indicate boxes.